DISEASES OF SHEEP

Diseases of Sheep

Editor:

Sarika Garg

Delve Publishing

www.delvepublishing.com

Diseases of Sheep

Editor: **Sarika Garg**

708 3rd Avenue, 6th Floor
New York, NY 10017
United States of America
www.delvepublishing.com

ISBN: 978-1-68095-863-8
Library of Congress Control Number: 2016951616

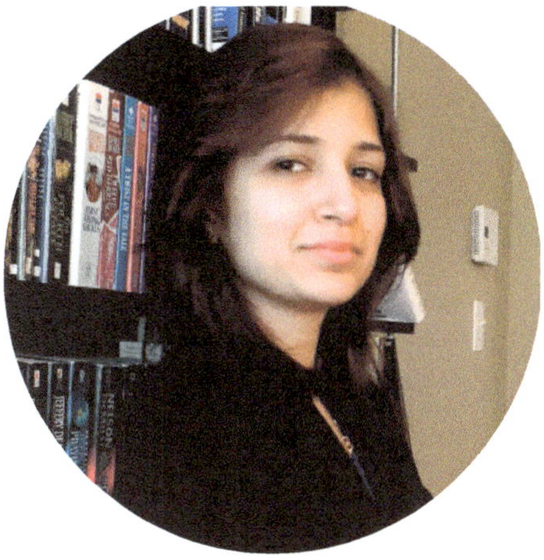

About the Editor

Sarika Garg

Ph.D. Montreal, Canada

Sarika Garg procured her doctoral degree at the Max Planck Unit For Structural Molecular Biology, University of Hamburg, Germany in 2011. This was followed by Postdoctoral Scientist position at University of Saskatchewan, Canada. Later, she moved to CRCHUM, University of Montreal for her second Postdoc. She has diverse research interests and has contributed immensely in many research fields viz. Enzyme Technology, Environmental Science, and Neuroscience. She has numerous research papers and review articles to her credit. She has coauthored two books 'Enzymes & Enzyme Technology'; and 'Biochemical Tests: Principles and Protocols'. She has also contributed several chapters in various books including a chapter on Regulation of Gene Expression in Encyclopedia of Molecular Cell Biology and Molecular Medicine. She is a recipient of 2012 SHRF Postdoctoral Fellowship Award and 2012 Laura E. Chapman Research Award. She is currently working as a Career Counselor in her very own venture 'higherstudiescounseling.com', Montreal, Canada and as a freelancer science writer.

Contents

List of Contributors

Ludovic Martinelle
Research Unit of Epidemiology and Risk Analysis Applied to Veterinary Sciences (UREAR-ULg), Fundamental and Applied Research for Animals & Health (FARAH), Faculty of Veterinary Medicine, University of Liège, Liège, Belgium

Antoine Poskin
Research Unit of Epidemiology and Risk Analysis Applied to Veterinary Sciences (UREAR-ULg), Fundamental and Applied Research for Animals & Health (FARAH), Faculty of Veterinary Medicine, University of Liège, Liège, Belgium
Operational Directorate Viral Diseases, Veterinary and Agrochemical Research Centre (CODA-CERVA), Brussels, Belgium

Fabiana Dal Pozzo
Research Unit of Epidemiology and Risk Analysis Applied to Veterinary Sciences (UREAR-ULg), Fundamental and Applied Research for Animals & Health (FARAH), Faculty of Veterinary Medicine, University of Liège, Liège, Belgium

Nick De Regge
Operational Directorate Viral Diseases, Veterinary and Agrochemical Research Centre (CODA-CERVA), Brussels, Belgium

Brigitte Cay
Operational Directorate Viral Diseases, Veterinary and Agrochemical Research Centre (CODA-CERVA), Brussels, Belgium

Claude Saegerman
Research Unit of Epidemiology and Risk Analysis Applied to Veterinary Sciences (UREAR-ULg), Fundamental and Applied Research for Animals & Health (FARAH), Faculty of Veterinary Medicine, University of Liège, Liège, Belgium

Daniel Oladimeji Oluwayelu
Department of Veterinary Microbiology and Parasitology, University of Ibadan, Ibadan 20005, Nigeria

Comfort Oluladun Aiki-Raji
Department of Veterinary Microbiology and Parasitology, University of Ibadan, Ibadan 20005, Nigeria

Emmanuel Chibuzor Umeh
Department of Veterinary Microbiology and Parasitology, University of Ibadan, Ibadan 20005, Nigeria

Samat Odunayo Mustapha
Department of Veterinary Microbiology and Parasitology, University of Ibadan, Ibadan 20005, Nigeria

Adebowale Idris Adebiyi
Department of Veterinary Microbiology and Parasitology, University of Ibadan, Ibadan 20005, Nigeria

Aliasghar Tehrani
Department of Pathology, Faculty of Veterinary Medicine, University of Urmia, Urmia, Iran

Javad Javanbakht
Department of Pathology, Faculty of Veterinary Medicine, University of Tehran, Tehran, Iran

Meysam Jani
Graduate Faculty of Veterinary Medicine, University of Tehran, Tehran, Iran

Farhang Sasani
Department of Pathology, Faculty of Veterinary Medicine, University of Tehran, Tehran, Iran

Amirali Solati
Department of Veterinary Medicine, Islamic Azad University, Saveh branch, Saveh, Iran

Mojtaba Rajabian
Graduate Faculty of Veterinary Medicine, University of Tehran, Tehran, Iran

Farshid Khadivar
Graduate Faculty of Veterinary Medicine, University of Tehran, Tehran, Iran

Hamid Akbari
Department of Clinical Science, Faculty of Veterinary Medicine, University of Urmia, Urmia, Iran

Mohammadreza Mohammadian
Graduate Faculty of Veterinary Medicine, University of Tehran, Tehran, Iran

Li Mao
Institute of Veterinary Medicine, Jiangsu Academy of Agricultural Sciences; Key Laboratory of Veterinary Biological Engineering and Technology, Ministry of Agriculture; National Center for Engineering Research of Veterinary Bio-products, Nanjing 210014, China
Jiangsu Co-innovation Center for Prevention and Control of Important Animal Infectious Diseases and Zoonoses, Yangzhou 225009, China

Xia Liu
Institute of Veterinary Medicine, Jiangsu Academy of Agricultural Sciences; Key Laboratory of Veterinary Biological Engineering and Technology, Ministry of Agriculture; National Center for Engineering Research of Veterinary Bio-products, Nanjing 210014, China
Jiangsu Co-innovation Center for Prevention and Control of Important Animal Infectious Diseases and Zoonoses, Yangzhou 225009, China

Wenliang Li
Institute of Veterinary Medicine, Jiangsu Academy of Agricultural Sciences; Key Laboratory of Veterinary Biological Engineering and Technology, Ministry of Agriculture; National Center for Engineering Research of Veterinary Bio-products, Nanjing 210014, China
Jiangsu Co-innovation Center for Prevention and Control of Important Animal Infectious Diseases and Zoonoses, Yangzhou 225009, China

Leilei Yang
Institute of Veterinary Medicine, Jiangsu Academy of Agricultural Sciences; Key Laboratory of Veterinary Biological Engineering and Technology, Ministry of Agriculture; National Center for Engineering Research of Veterinary Bio-products, Nanjing 210014, China
Jiangsu Co-innovation Center for Prevention and Control of Important Animal Infectious Diseases and Zoonoses, Yangzhou 225009, China

Wenwen Zhang
Institute of Veterinary Medicine, Jiangsu Academy of Agricultural Sciences; Key Laboratory of Veterinary Biological Engineering and Technology, Ministry of Agriculture; National Center for Engineering Research of Veterinary Bio-products, Nanjing 210014, China
Jiangsu Co-innovation Center for Prevention and Control of Important Animal Infectious Diseases and Zoonoses, Yangzhou 225009, China

Jieyuan Jiang
Institute of Veterinary Medicine, Jiangsu Academy of Agricultural Sciences; Key Laboratory of Veterinary Biological Engineering and Technology, Ministry of Agriculture; National Center for Engineering Research of Veterinary Bio-products, Nanjing 210014, China
Jiangsu Co-innovation Center for Prevention and Control of Important Animal Infectious Diseases and Zoonoses, Yangzhou 225009, China

Xia Liu
College of Animal Science and Technology, Anhui Agricultural University, Hefei, Anhui, China
Institute of Veterinary Medicine, Jiangsu Academy of Agricultural Sciences, Key Laboratory of Veterinary Biological Engineering and Technology, Ministry of Agriculture, National Center for Engineering Research of Veterinary Bio-products, Nanjing, Jiangsu, China

Li Mao
Institute of Veterinary Medicine, Jiangsu Academy of Agricultural Sciences, Key Laboratory of Veterinary Biological Engineering and Technology, Ministry of Agriculture, National Center for Engineering Research of Veterinary Bio-products, Nanjing, Jiangsu, China

Wenliang Li
Institute of Veterinary Medicine, Jiangsu Academy of Agricultural Sciences, Key Laboratory of Veterinary Biological Engineering and Technology, Ministry of Agriculture, National Center for Engineering Research of Veterinary Bio-products, Nanjing, Jiangsu, China

Leilei Yang
Institute of Veterinary Medicine, Jiangsu Academy of Agricultural Sciences, Key Laboratory of Veterinary Biological Engineering and Technology, Ministry of Agriculture, National Center for Engineering Research of Veterinary Bio-products, Nanjing, Jiangsu, China

Wenwen Zhang
Institute of Veterinary Medicine, Jiangsu Academy of Agricultural Sciences, Key Laboratory of Veterinary Biological Engineering and Technology, Ministry of Agriculture, National Center for Engineering Research of Veterinary Bio-products, Nanjing, Jiangsu, China

Jianzhong Wei
College of Animal Science and Technology, Anhui Agricultural University, Hefei, Anhui, China

Jieyuan Jiang
Institute of Veterinary Medicine, Jiangsu Academy of Agricultural Sciences, Key Laboratory of Veterinary Biological Engineering and Technology, Ministry of Agriculture, National Center for Engineering Research of Veterinary Bio-products, Nanjing, Jiangsu, China

Mohammad Khezri
Department of Veterinary Medicine, Agricultural and Natural Resources Research Center of Kurdistan, Sanandaj, Iran

Seyed Mahmud Azimi
Department of Foot-and-Mouth Disease Vaccine, Razi Vaccine and Serum Research Institute, Karaj, Iran

Yasmin Bano
Department of Microbiology, All India Institute of Medical Sciences, Tatibandh, GE Road, Raipur, Chhattisgarh, India

Sajad Ahmad Lone
National Institute for Research in Tribal Health (ICMR), Nagpur Road, Jabalpur, Madhya Pradesh, India

Deborah Greber
Clinic for Ruminants, Vetsuisse Faculty, University of Bern, Bremgartenstrasse 109a, Bern 3001, Switzerland
Institute of Genetics, Vetsuisse Faculty, University of Bern, Bremgartenstrasse 109a, Bern 3001, Switzerland

Marcus Doherr
Veterinary Public Health Institute, Vetsuisse Faculty, University of Bern, Schwarzenburgstrasse 155, Liebefeld 3097, Switzerland

Cord Drögemüller
Institute of Genetics, Vetsuisse Faculty, University of Bern, Bremgartenstrasse 109a, Bern 3001, Switzerland

Adrian Steiner
Clinic for Ruminants, Vetsuisse Faculty, University of Bern, Bremgartenstrasse 109a, Bern 3001, Switzerland

Michelle R. Mousel
Range Sheep Production Efficiency Research Unit, Agricultural Research Service, Department of Agriculture, Dubois, ID, United States of America

James O. Reynolds
Animal Disease Research Unit, Agricultural Research Service, Department of Agriculture, Pullman, WA, United States of America

Stephen N. White
Department of Veterinary Microbiology and Pathology, Washington State University, Pullman, WA, United States of America

Dora Romero-Salas
Laboratorio de Parasitología. UD PZTM. Facultad de Medicina Veterinaria y Zootecnia, Universidad Veracruzana, Veracruz, Mexico

Cosme Alvarado-Esquivel
Laboratorio de Investigación Biomédica. Facultad de Medicina y Nutrición, Juárez University of Durango State, Avenida Universidad S/N, 34000 Durango, Mexico

Anabel Cruz-Romero
Laboratorio de Parasitología. UD PZTM. Facultad de Medicina Veterinaria y Zootecnia, Universidad Veracruzana, Veracruz, Mexico

Mariel Aguilar-Domínguez
Laboratorio de Parasitología. UD PZTM. Facultad de Medicina Veterinaria y Zootecnia, Universidad Veracruzana, Veracruz, Mexico

Nelly Ibarra-Priego
Laboratorio de Parasitología. UD PZTM. Facultad de Medicina Veterinaria y Zootecnia, Universidad Veracruzana, Veracruz, Mexico

José O. Merino-Charrez
Facultad de Medicina Veterinaria y Zootecnia, Universidad Autónoma de Tamaulipas, Cd. Victoria, Tamaulipas, Mexico

Adalberto A. Pérez de León
USDA-ARS Knipling-Bushland U.S. Livestock Insects Research Laboratory, and Veterinary Pest Genomics Center, Kerrville, TX, USA

Jesús Hernández-Tinoco
Institute for Scientific Research "Dr. Roberto Rivera Damm", Juárez University of Durango State, Durango, Mexico

Sarvan Kumar
Department of Veterinary Pathology, Lala Lajpat Rai University of Veterinary & Animal Sciences, Hisar, Haryana, India

K. K. Jakhar
Department of Veterinary Pathology, Lala Lajpat Rai University of Veterinary & Animal Sciences, Hisar, Haryana, India

Satyavir Singh
Department of Veterinary Parasitology, Lala Lajpat Rai University of Veterinary & Animal Sciences, Hisar, Haryana, India

Sandeep Potliya
Department of Veterinary Surgery and Radiology, Lala Lajpat Rai University of Veterinary & Animal Sciences, Hisar, Haryana, India

Kailash Kumar
Department of Veterinary Gynaecology and Obstetrics, Lala Lajpat Rai University of Veterinary & Animal Sciences, Hisar, Haryana, India

Madan Pal
Department of Veterinary Surgery and Radiology, Lala Lajpat Rai University of Veterinary & Animal Sciences, Hisar, Haryana, India

Sarvan Kumar
Department of Veterinary Pathology, Lala Lajpat Rai University of Veterinary & Animal Sciences, Hisar, Haryana, India

K. K. Jakhar
Department of Veterinary Pathology, Lala Lajpat Rai University of Veterinary & Animal Sciences, Hisar, Haryana, India

Vikas Nehra
Department of Veterinary Pathology, Lala Lajpat Rai University of Veterinary & Animal Sciences, Hisar, Haryana, India

Madan Pal
Department of Veterinary Surgery and Radiology, Lala Lajpat Rai University of Veterinary & Animal Sciences, Hisar, Haryana, India

Priscila Barbante
Department of Veterinary Hygiene and Public Health, School of Veterinary Medicine and Animal Husbandry, São Paulo State University (UNESP – Univ Estadual Paulista), Botucatu, São Paulo State, Brazil

Fabio H Shimabukuro
Adolfo Lutz Institute, Sorocaba, São Paulo State, Brazil

Helio Langoni
Department of Veterinary Hygiene and Public Health, School of Veterinary Medicine and Animal Husbandry, São Paulo State University (UNESP – Univ Estadual Paulista), Botucatu, São Paulo State, Brazil

Virgínia B Richini-Pereira
Adolfo Lutz Institute – CLR II, Bauru, São Paulo State, Brazil

Simone B Lucheis
Paulista Agency of Agribusiness Technology (APTA/SAA), Av. Rodrigues Alves, 40-40, Bauru, SP CEP 17030-000, Brazil

Rahmeto Abebe
School of Veterinary Medicine, Hawassa University, Hawassa, Ethiopia

Mulugeta Melesse
Hadiya Zone Animal and Fisheries Resources Development Department, South Ethiopia, Hossana, Ethiopia

Solomon Mekuria
School of Veterinary Medicine, Hawassa University, Hawassa, Ethiopia

Tormod Mørk
Department of Animal Health, National Veterinary Institute, Dep, N-0033 Oslo, Norway

Steinar Waage
Department of Production Animal Clinical Sciences, Norwegian School of Veterinary Science, Dep, N-0033 Oslo, Norway

Tore Tollersrud
Department of Animal Health, National Veterinary Institute, Dep, N-0033 Oslo, Norway

Bjørg Kvitle
Department of Animal Health, National Veterinary Institute, Dep, N-0033 Oslo, Norway

Ståle Sviland
Department of Animal Health, National Veterinary Institute, Dep, N-0033 Oslo, Norway

Abid bin Tarif,
The Pirbright Institute, Ash Road, Pirbright, Woking, Surrey GU24 0NF, United Kingdom

Lidia Lasecka,
The Pirbright Institute, Ash Road, Pirbright, Woking, Surrey GU24 0NF, United Kingdom

Barbara Holzer
The Pirbright Institute, Ash Road, Pirbright, Woking, Surrey GU24 0NF, United Kingdom

Michael D Baron
The Pirbright Institute, Ash Road, Pirbright, Woking, Surrey GU24 0NF, United Kingdom

James Patrick Crilly
University of Cambridge, farm animal health and production (sheep) at the Royal (Dick) School of Veterinary Studies (R[D] SVS) in Edinburgh

Nina Rzechorzek
University of Cambridge, PhD on hypothermic preconditioning of cortical neurons residency in neurology at the R(D)SVS

Philip Scott
Farm animal medicine and surgery at the University of Edinburgh

Thomas E. Besser
Department of Veterinary Microbiology and Pathology, Washington State University, Pullman, Washington, United States of America
Washington Animal Disease Diagnostic Laboratory, Washington State University, Pullman Washington, United States of America,

E. Frances Cassirer
Idaho Department of Fish and Game, Lewiston, Idaho, United States of America

Kathleen A. Potter
Department of Veterinary Microbiology and Pathology, Washington State University, Pullman, Washington, United States of America
Washington Animal Disease Diagnostic Laboratory, Washington State University, Pullman Washington, United States of America,

Kevin Lahmers
Department of Veterinary Microbiology and Pathology, Washington State University, Pullman, Washington, United States of America

J. Lindsay Oaks
Department of Veterinary Microbiology and Pathology, Washington State University, Pullman, Washington, United States of America
Washington Animal Disease Diagnostic Laboratory, Washington State University, Pullman Washington, United States of America,

Sudarvili Shanthalingam
Department of Veterinary Microbiology and Pathology, Washington State University, Pullman, Washington, United States of America

Subramaniam Srikumaran
Department of Veterinary Microbiology and Pathology, Washington State University, Pullman, Washington, United States of America

William J. Foreyt
Department of Veterinary Microbiology and Pathology, Washington State University, Pullman, Washington, United States of America

Francisco Ruiz-Fons
NEIKER- Instituto Vasco de Investigación y Desarrollo Agrario, Department of Animal Health, Berreaga 1, 48160 Derio, Bizkaia, Spain

Ianire Astobiza
NEIKER- Instituto Vasco de Investigación y Desarrollo Agrario, Department of Animal Health, Berreaga 1, 48160 Derio, Bizkaia, Spain

Jesús F Barandika
NEIKER- Instituto Vasco de Investigación y Desarrollo Agrario, Department of Animal Health, Berreaga 1, 48160 Derio, Bizkaia, Spain

Ana Hurtado
NEIKER- Instituto Vasco de Investigación y Desarrollo Agrario, Department of Animal Health, Berreaga 1, 48160 Derio, Bizkaia, Spain

Raquel Atxaerandio
NEIKER- Instituto Vasco de Investigación y Desarrollo Agrario, Department of Animal Health, Berreaga 1, 48160 Derio, Bizkaia, Spain

Ramón A Juste
NEIKER- Instituto Vasco de Investigación y Desarrollo Agrario, Department of Animal Health, Berreaga 1, 48160 Derio, Bizkaia, Spain

Ana L García-Pérez
NEIKER- Instituto Vasco de Investigación y Desarrollo Agrario, Department of Animal Health, Berreaga 1, 48160 Derio, Bizkaia, Spain

Amaia Larruskain
Genomics and Health Group, Department of Genetics, Physical Anthropology and Animal Physiology, Faculty of Science and Technology, University of the Basque Country UPV/EHU, Bilbao 48080, Spain

Begoña M. Jugo
Genomics and Health Group, Department of Genetics, Physical Anthropology and Animal Physiology, Faculty of Science and Technology, University of the Basque Country UPV/EHU, Bilbao 48080, Spain

Xia Zhao
Department of Animal Science and Center for Integrated Animal Genomics, Iowa State University, Ames, Iowa, United States of America

Keren E. Dittmer
Institute of Veterinary, Animal and Biomedical Sciences, Massey University, Palmerston North, New Zealand

Hugh T. Blair
Institute of Veterinary, Animal and Biomedical Sciences, Massey University, Palmerston North, New Zealand

Keith G. Thompson
Institute of Veterinary, Animal and Biomedical Sciences, Massey University, Palmerston North, New Zealand

Max F. Rothschild
Department of Animal Science and Center for Integrated Animal Genomics, Iowa State University, Ames, Iowa, United States of America

Dorian J. Garrick
Department of Animal Science and Center for Integrated Animal Genomics, Iowa State University, Ames, Iowa, United States of America
Institute of Veterinary, Animal and Biomedical Sciences, Massey University, Palmerston North, New Zealand

Stefano Reale
Molecular Biology Department, Istituto Zooprofilattico Sperimentale della Sicilia "A. Mirri", Palermo, Italy

Mario Cosenza
Molecular Biology Department, Istituto Zooprofilattico Sperimentale della Sicilia "A. Mirri", Palermo, Italy

Luca Sìneo
Laboratory of Anthropology, STEBICEF Department, University of Palermo, Palermo, Italy

Letizia Arcoleo
Laboratory of Anthropology, STEBICEF Department, University of Palermo, Palermo, Italy

Gabriele Zaffora
Molecular Biology Department, Istituto Zooprofilattico Sperimentale della Sicilia "A. Mirri", Palermo, Italy

Daniele Macrì
Molecular Biology Department, Istituto Zooprofilattico Sperimentale della Sicilia "A. Mirri", Palermo, Italy

Fabrizio Vitale
Molecular Biology Department, Istituto Zooprofilattico Sperimentale della Sicilia "A. Mirri", Palermo, Italy

Esayas Gelaye
Animal Production and Health Laboratory, Joint FAO/IAEA Division of Nuclear Techniques in Food and Agriculture, Department of Nuclear Sciences and Applications, International Atomic Energy Agency, Wagramer Strasse 5, Vienna, Austria
Institute of Applied Genetics and Cell Biology, University of Natural Resources and Life Sciences, Muthgasse 18, A-1190 Vienna, Austria
Research and Diagnostic Laboratories, National Veterinary Institute, Debre Zeit, Ethiopia

Jenna Elizabeth Achenbach
Animal Production and Health Laboratory, Joint FAO/IAEA Division of Nuclear Techniques in Food and Agriculture, Department of Nuclear Sciences and Applications, International Atomic Energy Agency, Wagramer Strasse 5, Vienna, Austria

Shiferaw Jenberie
Research and Diagnostic Laboratories, National Veterinary Institute, Debre Zeit, Ethiopia

Gelagay Ayelet
Research and Diagnostic Laboratories, National Veterinary Institute, Debre Zeit, Ethiopia

Alebachew Belay
Research and Diagnostic Laboratories, National Veterinary Institute, Debre Zeit, Ethiopia

Martha Yami
Research and Diagnostic Laboratories, National Veterinary Institute, Debre Zeit, Ethiopia

Angelika Loitsch
Institute for Veterinary Disease Control, Austrian Agency for Health and Food Safety, Robert Koch-Gasse 17, A-2340 Mödling, Austria

Reingard Grabherr
[5]Institute of Applied Microbiology, University of Natural Resources and Life Sciences, Muthgasse 11, 1190 Vienna, Austria

Adama Diallo
Animal Production and Health Laboratory, Joint FAO/IAEA Division of Nuclear Techniques in Food and Agriculture, Department of Nuclear Sciences and Applications, International Atomic Energy Agency, Wagramer Strasse 5, Vienna, Austria

Charles Euloge Lamien
Animal Production and Health Laboratory, Joint FAO/IAEA Division of Nuclear Techniques in Food and Agriculture, Department of Nuclear Sciences and Applications, International Atomic Energy Agency, Wagramer Strasse 5, Vienna, Austria

Mohammad Naser Nazem
Department of Basic Sciences, Faculty of Veterinary Medicine, Shahid Bahonar University of Kerman, Kerman, Iran

Bahador Shojaei
Department of Basic Sciences, Faculty of Veterinary Medicine, Shahid Bahonar University of Kerman, Kerman, Iran

Akbar Asadi
Department of Basic Sciences, Faculty of Veterinary Medicine, Islamic Azad University, Shahre Babak Branch, Kerman, Iran

Mohammad Hasanzadeh
Department of Basic Sciences, Faculty of Veterinary Medicine, Shahid Bahonar University of Kerman, Kerman, Iran

Preface

In the past few years, diseases in sheep have grabbed the headlines several times. The repercussions of a disease range from a sheep slaughter to an impediment in livestock yield. Some diseases are zoonotic diseases that can be passed from sheep to humans. Considering the major consequences of the diseases in sheep, several biologists are working towards providing an early warning system for sheep producers. Many diseases can be prevented through the proper control strategy or vet consultancy, if applied in a timely manner. However, to evaluate the symptoms of a disease, it is critical to be well versed with it. Therefore, in this book, efforts have been done to assemble a wide range of published research studies under this central theme.

The first Chapter reports the colonization of the placenta without congenital malformations in sheep infected with Schmallenberg virus (SBV). The second Chapter describes the presence of antibodies against Akabane virus (AKAV) in ruminants in Nigeria. AKAV is a pathogen responsible for abortions and congenital malformations in ruminants. Chapter 3 accounts the popularity of Haemonchus contortus, a blood sucking parasite causing anemia, in slaughtered sheep in Iran. The characterization of one Chinese sheep Border disease virus (BDV) and the complete coding sequence of BDV strain JSLS12-01 are described in Chapters 4 and 5, respectively. Chapter 6 features the seroprevalence rates of Bluetongue disease in sheep in many areas of Iran. Brucellosis, world's major zoonosis, leads to abortion, infertility, and low milk yield. This disease has been reviewed in Chapter 7. Congenital disorders in sheep are discussed in the following two Chapters. Cryptosporidiosis is a zoonotic disease affecting human populations and domestic animal. Its prevalence in small ruminants in Mexico is discussed in Chapter 10. The gastrointestinal tract disorders in sheep are presented in the following two Chapters. Leptospirosis infection in sheep flocks in Southeast Brazil is described in Chapter 13. The prevalence of Lungworm infection in small ruminants in Southern Ethiopia is reported in Chapter 14. The bacteria and the characteristics of Mastitis in sheep are illustrated in Chapter 15. Nairobi sheep disease virus and the major cytokine responses in infected sheep are discussed in Chapter 16. Paresis and paralysis in sheep are described in Chapter 17. The transmission of bronchopneumonia infection from one infected animal to all sheep is talked about in Chapter 18. The epidemiological pattern of Q fever in domestic ruminants in described in Chapter 19. Retroviral infections and inherited Rickets in sheep are explained in Chapters 20 and 21, respectively. The evaluation of the haplotypes distribution in ancient sheep and the modern population is accounted in the following Chapter. The characterization of the orf virus and the spider lamb syndrome in sheep are discussed in Chapters 23 and 24, respectively.

I hope that this book will be beneficial for students, researchers, teachers, and sheep producers.

Editor
Sarika Garg, Ph.D.
Montreal, Canada

CHAPTER 1

EXPERIMENTAL INFECTION OF SHEEP AT 45 AND 60 DAYS OF GESTATION WITH SCHMALLENBERG VIRUS READILY LED TO PLACENTAL COLONIZATION WITHOUT CAUSING CONGENITAL MALFORMATIONS

Ludovic Martinelle[1], Antoine Poskin[1, 2], Fabiana Dal Pozzo[1], Nick De Regge[2], Brigitte Cay[2], Claude Saegerman[1]

[1]Research Unit of Epidemiology and Risk Analysis Applied to Veterinary Sciences (UREAR-ULg), Fundamental and Applied Research for Animals & Health (FARAH), Faculty of Veterinary Medicine, University of Liège, Liège, Belgium

[2]Operational Directorate Viral Diseases, Veterinary and Agrochemical Research Centre (CODA-CERVA), Brussels, Belgium

ABSTRACT

Background

Main impact of Schmallenberg virus (SBV) on livestock consists in reproductive disorders, with teratogenic effects, abortions and stillbirths. SBV pathogenesis and viral placental crossing remain currently poorly understood. Therefore, we implemented an experimental infection of ewes, inoculated with SBV at 45 or 60 days of gestation (dg).

Methodology

"Mourerous" breed ewes were randomly separated in three groups: eight and nine ewes were subcutaneously inoculated with 1 ml of SBV infectious serum at 45 and 60 dg, respectively (G45 and G60). Six other ewes were inoculated subcutaneously with sterile phosphate buffer saline as control group. All SBV inoculated ewes showed RNAemia consistent with previously published studies, they seroconverted and no clinical sign was reported. Lambs were born at term via caesarian-section, and right after birth they were blood sampled and clinically examined. Then both lambs and ewes were euthanized and necropsied.

Principal Findings/Significance

No lambs showed any malformation suggestive of SBV infection and none of them had RNAemia or anti-SBV antibodies prior to colostrum uptake. Positive SBV RNA detection in organs was rare in both G45 and G60 lambs (2/11 and 1/10, respectively). Nevertheless most of the lambs in G45 (9/11) and G60 (9/10) had at least one extraembryonic structure SBV positive by RTqPCR. The number of positive extraembryonic structures was significantly higher in G60 lambs. Time of

Citation: Martinelle L, Poskin A, Dal Pozzo F, De Regge N, Cay B, Saegerman C (2015) Experimental Infection of Sheep at 45 and 60 Days of Gestation with Schmallenberg Virus Readily Led to Placental Colonization without Causing Congenital Malformations. PLoS ONE 10(9): e0139375. doi:10.1371/journal.pone.0139375.

inoculation (45 or 60 dg) had no impact on the placental colonization success rate but affected the frequency of detecting the virus in the offspring extraembryonic structures by the time of lambing. SBV readily colonized the placenta when ewes were infected at 45 or 60 dg but infection of the fetuses was limited and did not lead to congenital malformations.

INTRODUCTION

In summer 2011, a new unspecific clinical syndrome was first described in adult cattle in Germany causing febrile disease, milk drop and diarrhoea [1], later attributed to a novel*Orthobunyavirus* (family *Bunyaviridae*) named Schmallenberg virus (SBV). Palearctic telmophagous midges of the genus *Culicoides* [2–4] were identified as the vector of SBV. However the most striking consequence of SBV spreading throughout Europe was the epizootic of malformations in ruminant offspring, leading to abortions, peripartum mortality and stillbirths. Indeed, SBV was linked to an arthrogryposis / hydranencephaly syndrome in ruminant newborns following *in utero* infection [5].

According to literature about Akabane virus (AKAV), a closely related *Orthobunyavirus*, the moment of the gestation when the mother gets infected influences the outcome of an *in utero*infection. In sheep, Parsonson et al. suggested that AKAV might only be able to reach the fetus if placenta is developed and vascularized enough [6], whereas Hashiguchi et al. considered congenital malformations highly unlikely to occur if infection took place after 50 days post insemination [7]. So far, susceptible gestation periods leading to congenital malformations need to be clarified in the different SBV host species.

In several European countries, SBV had a greater impact on sheep flock than in cattle herds [8, 9]. As a matter of fact, dairy cattle give birth basically all year round while lambing are mostly seasonal, with mating of the sheep concentrated in July-August or October-November, depending on the breed [10]. Indeed, sheep breeding seasons are widely overlapping with some of the highest vector activity periods in Europe [11]. Moreover, increased odds of malformations were reported in sheep flock with an early mating season in 2011 [12]. Thus considering the breeding season as a risk factor in correlation with the vector activity, the management of the breeding season could be a key element to avoid congenital malformations and to get ewes infected before or after the critical period of susceptibility for the fetus. Based on the pathogenesis of Akabane virus and epidemiological studies of the SBV outbreaks, it is assumed that teratogenic infection takes place in the first trimester. Stockhofe et al. performed SBV experimental infection of sheep at 38 and 45 days of pregnancy [13], however the infected ewes were slaughtered one week after inoculation. The aim of the current study was to investigate the occurrence of malformation at term in ewes infected later in the course of gestation. Thus we implemented an experimental study performed on groups of pregnant ewes subcutaneously infected with infectious SBV serum at day 45 and 60 of gestation. Therefore we could get a better insight on SBV pathogenesis in pregnant ewes and rate of transplacental transmission and colonization following two different gestation times of inoculation.

MATERIALS AND METHODS

Ethical Statements

The experiments, maintenance and care of ewes complied with the guidelines of the European Convention for the Protection of Vertebrate Animals used for Experimental and other Scientific Purposes (CETS n° 123). The protocol used in this study was approved by the Ethical Committee of the IPH-VAR (Scientific Institute of Public Health—Veterinary and Agrochemical Research Center (VAR), number of project: 121017–01) on the 11th February 2013. All surgery was performed using xylazin (Paxman®, Virbac, France) and local anesthesia (procaine hydrochloride 4%, VMD, Belgium), and all efforts were made to minimize suffering.

Animals

A total of 23 "Mourerous" ewes of about 1 year-old and originating from a SBV free area in France were used in this experiment (original sheep flock from the *Alpes-Maritimes* department (ISO code FR-06), animals selected after a last serological screening carried out on the 08/11/2012). The Mourerous is a middle-size rustic breed from south of France. All the animals were serologically and virologically negative for SBV as determined by ELISA, SNT and RTqPCR (see below) before and after arrival at the experimental animal centre of CODA-CERVA where they were kept in Biosafety Level 3 facilities. The ewes also tested negative for bluetongue virus (BTV) and Maedi-Visna virus. The animals were only implemented in the experiments after a thorough clinical examination to ensure their asymptomatic state and good clinical condition in range with the physiological parameters [14].

Inoculum

The infectious serum used for inoculation of the sheep was obtained from Friedrich Loeffler Institute (Riems, Germany) and was already successfully tested in calves and sheep [1, 15,16]. Briefly, the infectious serum originated from a heifer sampled two and three days after inoculation with infectious whole blood from a SBV-positive cow. The inoculum contained about 2 x 10^3 50% tissue culture infective dose/ml ($TCID_{50}$/ml) [15] and 7.3 x 10^6 RNA copies/ml of SBV S-Segment as determined by a RTqPCR detecting the SBV-S segment (see below).

Insemination and Diagnosis of Gestation

The animals were synchronised using Veramix sponges (60 mg Medroxyprogesterone Acetate, Zoetis®, Louvain-La-Neuve, Belgium). The sponges were removed 12 days after insertion and the ewes received 500 IU Pregnant Mare Serum Gonadotrophin through intramuscular route. Intracervical artificial insemination (AI) has been realized 52 hours after sponge removal, with a double dose of semen.

A total of four rams, from 1 to 6 years old, were used to get semen doses: 3 *Ile-de-France* and one crossbred Texel X Ile-de-France. These rams originated from a Maedi-Visna negative flock, and despite being SBV seropositive, their semen has been tested negative twice, one week apart, for SBV RNA (RTqPCR). A sample of each of the semen doses used for the actual AI has been also tested negative for SBV RNA *a posteriori*.

Gestation diagnostic has been performed by detection of pregnancy associated glycoprotein (PAG) by radio immune-assay (RIA) at 27 days post AI as previously described [17] and then by ultrasonography at 40/55 and 95/110 dg for the groups inoculated at 45 and 60 dg, respectively.

Experimental Design

During the whole duration of the experiment insect light/glue traps were displayed and regularly removed and replaced, allowing identification of the caught insects to ensure the absence of*Culicoides*.

The ewes were inoculated subcutaneously (SC) in the left axilla with 1 ml of infectious serum. Eight ewes were inoculated at 45 dg (G45, ewe1 to ewe8) and nine ewes at 60 dg (G60, ewe9 to ewe17). Two control groups of three animals each were inoculated SC with sterile phosphate buffer saline respectively at 45 and 60 dg (control G45 and control G60, ewes18 to 20 and ewes21 to 23).

During the first two weeks of the experiment, clinical, virological and serological monitoring was realized on a daily basis, then once a week until the end of the experiment.

At the expected lambing period for each respective group, ewes were closely monitored and when first signs of labor could be identified, the ewe was anesthetized with xylazin (Paxman®, Virbac, France) intravenously (IV) and local anesthesia (procaine hydrochloride 4%, VMD, Belgium), and lambing was perform by Caesarian section. Once the Caesarian section was realized, the ewe was euthanatized with IV injection of 5 ml of T61® (MSD Animal Health BVBA, Belgium) and subsequently necropsied.

Lambs were identified following their mother (ewe1 gives birth to lamb1; plus a, b or c in case of multiple gestation). When the lambs were born alive they were revived to allow the evaluation of any neurological trouble. Ability of standing up and suckling reflex were evaluated and a morphologic examination, with special emphasis on skull and limbs, was also performed. Blood samples were taken and lambs were then euthanatized with 1 ml T61® IV and necropsied. Tissue samples were taken from extraembryonic structures (intercotyledonary membrane, placentome, umbilical cord, amniotic fluid, meconium), and organs including CNS (brain, cerebellum, brainstem, spinal cord), lymphoid organs (prescapular, mesenteric, submandibular, mediastinic lymphnodes, thymus and spleen), other inner organs and tissues (gonads, adrenal gland, liver and lung) and musculoskeletal structures (femoral cartilage,*Musculus Semitendinosus*) for viral RNA detection. Placentomes were collected, longitudinally cut and separated in two halves for subsequent SBV RNA detection. The Intercotyledonary membrane was sampled in the area surrounding the collected placentomes. Samples (2 cm long) of the umbilical cord were collected 4–5 cm distal to the newborns.

SBV Detection by RTqPCR

The extraction of RNA from organs, feces, blood and serum and the detection of SBV-S segment by a one-step RTqPCR were performed as previously described [18].

The Cq values were converted into S-segment copy numbers using a RNA standard curve that was tested in each PCR run [19]. Briefly, RNA was extracted from SBV infectious serum with the RNeasyMini kit (Qiagen) following manufaturer's instructions and reverse transcribed with M-MLV Reverse Transcriptase (Life Technologies). A PCR amplification using primers targeting a 839bp fragment of the S gene of SBV (forward: 5'-CTAGCACGTTGGATTGCTGA-3'; reverse:5'-TGTCCTTGAGGACCCTATGC-3'; Integrated DNA Technologies) was performed using the FastStart PCR Master kit (Roche). The fragment was cloned in the 2.1-TOPO cloning vector (Life Technologies) and transformed into competent *Escherichia Coli* TOP10 cells and multiplied. The plasmids were isolated and then linearized with BamHI, followed by *in vitro*transcription with the TranscriptAid T7 High Yield kit (Thermo Scientific) following manufacturer's instructions. Remaining DNA plasmids were eliminated by 2 successive Turbo DNA free treatments (Life Technologies) following manufacturer's instructions and the RNA was purified using the RNeasyMini kit (Qiagen). The copy number was calculated based on the predicted molecular weight of the RNA transcripts. Aliquots of the RNA transcripts were stored at −80°.

The RNA standard curve consisted of a ten-fold serial dilution of the RNA transcripts in TE buffer. The dilution series ranging from 3.9×10^7 to 3.9 copies/μL were run together with samples of blood or organ and the standard curve was constructed by plotting the Cq values against the log of the input RNA copy number. A linear regression was fitted to the scattered points and was used to calculate the number of copies in the samples ran during the same RTqPCR.

Serology

The presence of neutralizing anti-SBV antibodies was assessed by seroneutralization (SNT), following the method described by De Regge et al. [20] and using an SBV isolate obtained from brain tissue of a lamb aborted in Belgium in 2011 which was passaged four times in Vero cells. Two positive and one negative control were added systematically to each assay. The titer was determined as the reciprocal of the highest serum dilution in which the entire monolayer was still intact. Sera were considered positive if the titer was ≥4 (specificity of 100% [20]).

Statistical Analysis

Differences in RNAemia of the different groups through time were assessed by two-way ANOVA with repeated measures. Difference between mean maximum copy numbers by group was evaluated with Welch test for unequal variance. Differences in positive detection of viral RNA in lambs, organs and reproductive performances (viability at birth, prolificacy) were evaluated by Chi^2 test or Fisher's exact test for count data depending on the sample size.

P values ≤ 0.05 were considered significant. Statistical analyses were performed using the R software/environment

(R-3.0.1, R Foundation for Statistical Computing, http://www.r-project.org/).

RESULTS

Clinical Impact and Lambing

No clinical impact following inoculation was measured in ewes. The temperatures stayed within the physiological range upon euthanasia. All the animals conserved a good appetite and remained in good general condition.

Table 1 reports sex ratio, prolificacy rate and the percentage of living lambs at birth. No significant different was reported in the viability of the offspring between infected groups and between infected and control groups (Chi² test = 0.7, $P = 0.4$ and Chi² test = 0.3, $P = 0.6$, respectively; df = 1). Prolificity rate was also not significantly different between infected groups and between infected and control groups (Chi² test = 0.1, $P = 0.74$ and Chi² test = 0.008, $P = 0.93$, respectively; df = 1). None of the lambs had malformation evocative of SBV infection (arthrogryposis-hydranencephaly syndrome, stiff neck, scoliosis, brachygnathism). Only one lamb was born three days before the expected date and was in good health. All other lambs were born at term, no malformation was observed and they were able to stand up and showed a good suction reflex.

Table 1: Reproductive performances

Group	Number of lambs	Sex ratio	Weight at birth (Kg)^a	Prolificacy rate (%)	% of healthy living lambs
G45	11	0.8	4^a(0.7); 3.1^b(1.1); 2^c(0.3)	137.5	63.6
G60	10	1.5	4^a(0.5); 3.3^b(0.5)	111.1	80.0
Control G45	4	1.0	5^a(1)	133.3	50.0
Control G60	3	2.0	4.5^a(0.5); 3^b(1.8)	100.0	67.0
Total	28	1.2	3.7(1.2)	121.7	67.9

Sex ratio is the ratio of male lambs to female lambs. Prolificacy is defined as the number of progenies born per parturition.
^{a}: Single lambs
^{b}: Twins
^{c}: Triplets
Standard deviation follows in curved brackets.

SBV RNA Detection

SBV Detection in the Blood and Organs of the Ewes.

No viral RNA was detected in the blood of the ewes from the control groups. SBV genome was first detectable at 2 dpi in both G45 and G60 groups and could be detected for maximum 5 days (Fig 1). The mean SBV genome copy numbers detected in the blood of sheep with RNAemia were not significantly different between G45 and G60 groups through time (two-way ANOVA for repeated measures; group effect: $P = 0.4$; group-time interaction: $P = 0.44$). The mean of the maximal SBV RNA copy number was not significantly different between G45 and G60 (Welch test for unequal variance; $P = 0.83$).

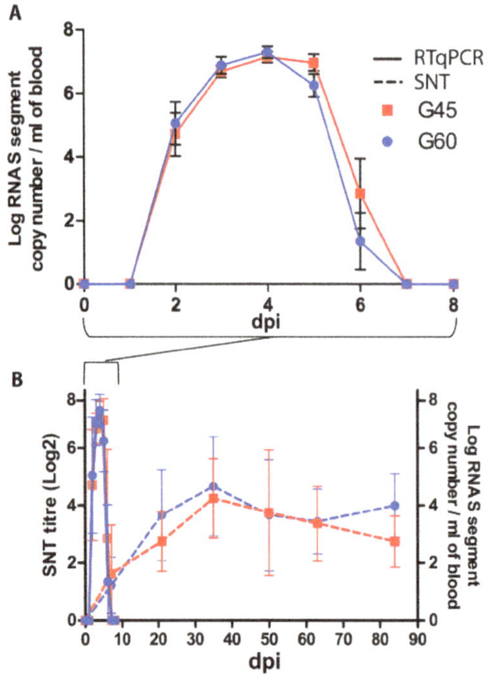

Figure 1: SBV viral RNA detection and neutralizing antibodies detection in the serum of the pregnant ewes.

Detection of SBV genome in serum for G45 and G60 ewes (A). Results of SNT for G45 and G60 ewes and SBV genome detection downscaled to 90 days (B). Full line represents SBV genome detection and dashed line represents SNT.

http://dx.doi.org/10.1371/journal.pone.0139375.g001

SBV genome could be detected in the ovaries of ewe9, in the ovaries and the spleen of ewe11 and only in the spleen ewe16, all belonging to G60. No SBV nucleic acid could be detected in any of the G45 ewes or control groups' organ samples.

SBV Detection in the Blood and Organs of the Lambs.

No SBV RNA could be detected in the blood of any of the lambs, from any of either the infected or control groups.

SBV RNA was shown in the brainstem and spinal cord of lamb10 and in the femoral joint cartilage, prescapular lymph node and muscle *M. semitendinosus* of lamb11 (both G60); in G45 viral genome could only be demonstrated in the lung of lamb4b (Fig 2).

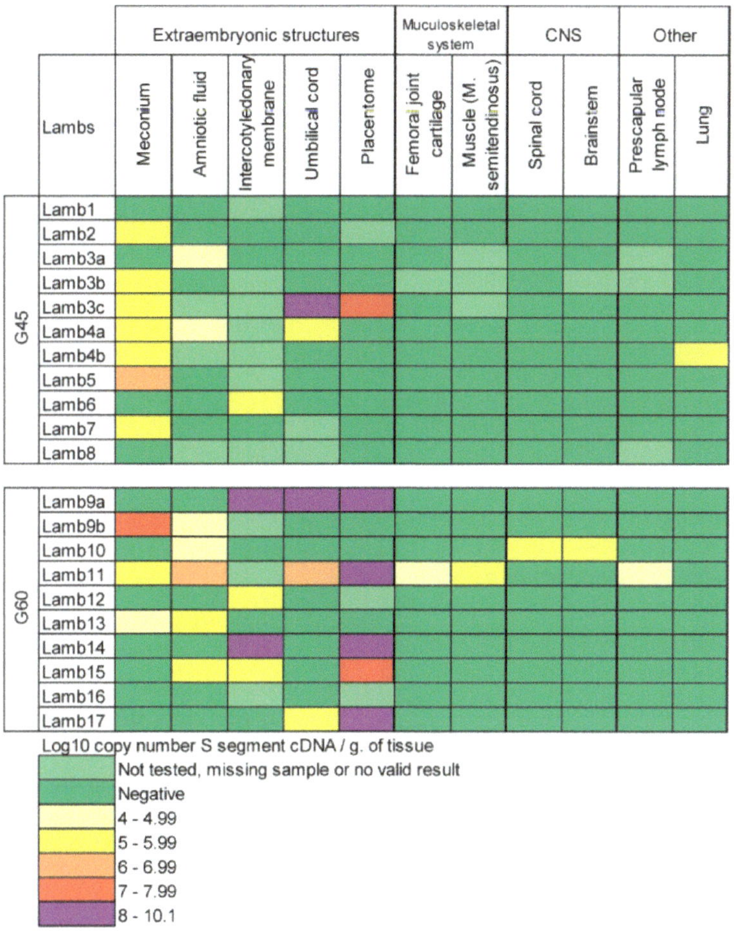

Figure 2: Mondrian matrix of SBV viral RNA detection in organs at necropsy.

Rectangles color-coded according to SBV detection level. CNS: Central nervous system.

http://dx.doi.org/10.1371/journal.pone.0139375.g002

SBV Detection in Extraembryonic Structures

Intercotyledonary membrane was the most frequently SBV positive extraembryonic structure in both G45 and G60, (50% of tested samples; 5/10) followed by amniotic fluid (38,9%; 7/18), umbilical cord (38.5%; 5/18) and placentomes (33.3%; 6/18) (Fig 2). Percentage of positive detection was higher in G60 (47.2%; 17/36) versus G45 (19.4%; 6/31) for each of the latter structures, and overall difference was significant (Chi² test = 5.74, df = 1, $P = 0.017$). For individual extraembryonic structure, detection was only significantly more frequent in G60 (55.6%; 5/9) versus G45 (10%; 1/10) for placentome (Chi² test = 4.55, df = 1; $P = 0.033$). Meconium of G45 lambs was found more often positive than G60 ones (7/11 versus 3/10), but that difference was not significant (Chi² test = 3.38, df = 1, $P = 0.12$).

The rate of placenta colonization, as defined as the number of lambs with at least one positive extraembryonic structure divided by the total number of lamb, was however not significantly different between G60 (90%; 9/10) and G45 (82%; 9/11), respectively (Fisher's exact test for count data = 1.94; $P = 1$).

Serology

All the inoculated ewes seroconverted within three weeks, with first positive detection at 7 dpi for several ewes of both G45 and G60. Then all the inoculated ewes remained seropositive until the end of the experiment (Fig 1B).

No newborn lamb had anti-SBV neutralizing Abs before colostrum uptake.

DISCUSSION

Viral placental crossing is defined as the passage of the virus from the mother through the placenta to fetal tissues. Thus, placental colonization does not necessarily imply passage of the pathogen to the fetus itself [21]. In this study SBV placental colonization could be demonstrated after experimental infection in most of pregnant ewes at 45 and 60 days of gestation. Extraembryonic structures were found frequently positive, as previously described after natural infection [18, 20].

However no teratogenic effect could be reproduced. Congenital malformations caused by SBV remain a rare phenomenon in the field; teratogenesis associated with SBV infection has been observed only in 1 malformed calf out of 72 ones born from infected dams in natural conditions [22]. In addition, Veldhuis et al. (2014) estimated in cattle the malformation rate at about 0.5% of infected fetuses [23]. Therefore with respect to the number of newborn lambs considered in the current study, the lack of malformations is not especially surprising, despite lambs being thought to display more often malformations caused by SBV than calves [9, 24–25].

In both G45 and G60, the percentage of successful placental colonization was high (9/11–82% and 9/10–90%, respectively) and consistent with previous experimental data reporting a 100% placental colonization with or without placental crossing in ewes infected with SBV at 38 or 42 dg [13]. However, in our study significantly more positive samples, from both extraembryonic structures and lamb organs, were found in newborn lambs originating from ewes that were infected at 60 dg compared to those infected at 45 dg. It is likely that infection in most of G45 fetuses was about to be resolved with SBV eliminated from many organs whereas G60 fetuses could not clear the virus as much, the infection being more recent in the latter. Indeed the G60 group had a shorter period to eliminate the virus (85–87 days for G60 instead of 100–102 for G45). Another explanation could derive from the hypothesis emitted by Parsonson et al. regarding AKAV, a close related *Orthobunyaviruses*. These authors hypothesized the efficiency of the placental crossing being related to the development and vascularization of the placentomes, possibly explaining the highest detection rate in G60 when compared to G45 [6]. The higher development of placentomes at 60 dg might provide more target cells to infect and therefore lead to prolonged positive detection in the infected tissues. According to Parsonson et al., fetal trophoblastic cells constitute privileged target cells for AKAV, and SBV was reported to readily replicate in ovine trophoblast cells both *in vitro* [26] and *in vivo* [8], possibly being important target cells for SBV as well. Lawn et al. [27] reported that in sheep placenta examined at 42 days of gestation, placentomes are rather undifferentiated with only a few displaying rudimentary villi and crypts. Therefore placentomes at 45 days of gestation might be insufficiently developed to support intensive viral replication, yet allowing placental colonization. By contrast, placentomes at 60 days of gestation could better sustain SBV replication, as reported for AKAV [6]. A strong correlation between malformations and precolostral anti-AKAV antibodies has been reported [28], and growing evidences suggest that this pattern is shared by SBV, with 79 to 91% of naturally infected malformed lambs reported to be seropositive before colostrum uptake [29, 30]. Therefore in the current study, with no lamb showing SBV-associated abnormalities it is not surprising that all the precolostral sera were negative.

To produce Abs, the fetus has to be immunocompetent and the virus has to reach the systemic blood circulation of the fetus. In sheep *in utero* acquisition of humoral immune competence can be roughly estimated to span from 66 to about 100 dg [31]. For AKAV production of neutralizing antibodies is considered to start at 65–75 dg in sheep [32]. However Parsonson et al. reported ewes infected between 30 and 36 dg giving birth to malformed lambs with precolostral neutralizing antibodies against AKAV [33]. In the latter study a significant individual variation in humoral response of fetuses to AKAV was reported and no stage of gestation could be associated to seroconversion in 100% of the infected animals.

Therefore, despite a frequent successful placental colonization of SBV, infection of the fetus itself might be far less common, since SBV RNA could only be detected in some organs of lamb4b (G45), lamb10 (G60) and lamb11 (G60). Together the rare productive infection of the fetus and the individual variation could explain the absence of precolostral Abs against SBV in this study.

Although SBV RNA was detected at least once in almost all the extraembryonic structures of the lambs born from infected ewes, SBV positive detection in central nervous system (CNS) was very scarce with only one brainstem and one spinal cord sample found positive from lamb10 (G60 lamb). In ruminant newborns showing congenital defects suggestive of SBV infection, CNS is very often positive by RTqPCR [18, 20]. Here, despite SBV detected in several organs but CNS (with the exception of lamb10 with SBV RNA in spinal cord and brainstem), no malformations were reported, supporting a CNS invasion and SBV genome detected at birth possibly being associated to congenital malformations.

From the infected pregnant ewe to the CNS of the fetus the virus has to cross two major histological obstacles, namely placenta and blood-brain barriers (BBB).

It has been suggested that the development of the BBB was the reason that adult animals only show asymptomatic or very mild SBV infection [26]. In sheep BBB to sucrose (small and metabolically inert molecule) starts to develop around 50–60 dg, undergo a large decrease of permeability at about 70 dg and keep developing until 123 dg [34]. Nevertheless no malformed lambs were found in G45 and G60 although G45 ewes were infected before the assumed establishment of the BBB. Orthobunyaviruses are considerably larger (about 100 nm in diameter [35]) when compared to sucrose (0.44–0.53 nm); hence viral particles crossing might be hindered already at an earlier stage of gestation. A delayed transmission from the mother to the fetus is unlikely since Stockhofe et al. reported a 100% placental crossing 7 days after the infection of pregnant ewes with SBV [13]. The critical period of gestation leading to malformation in lambs might be narrower, possibly closer to the lower estimate for AKAV, from 28 to 36 dg [8], or to the one reported by Sedda et al. for SBV, between 37 and 42 dg [36]. Herder et al. [37] described SBV antigens in ruminants CNS mostly detected in temporal and parietal lobes, mesencephalon and hippocampus. Besides, cerebellar hypoplasia was frequently reported. Several critical neurologic events related to these structures occur during the first third of gestation in sheep: post-proliferative zone appears in the cerebellum between 21 and 31 dg; hippocampus CA1/CA3 neurogenesis spans from 22 dg to 59 dg, and neurogenesis of the cortical layer VI peaks around 40 dg [38]. Moreover in the spinal cord motor neurons are differentiated and develop mostly between 31–35 dg, corresponding to the time the embryos become motile [39]. Thus most of these decisive steps were over or about to be finished by 45 dg. As a consequence SBV infecting fetuses after 45 dg might be able to cross the BBB but might fail to invade CNS because of the scarcity of developing target cells.

It was assumed that SBV induced malformations are secondary to CNS lesions since SBV shows a clear tropism for nervous tissues [29, 33]. Infection by pestiviruses like border disease virus and bovine viral diarrhea virus are characterized by CNS dysplasia and hypomyelinogenesis in a similar way than following AKAV infection [40]. However since arthrogryposis induced by pestiviruses is neither as frequent nor as severe than in cases caused by AKAV infection, authors hypothesized that the increased frequency of musculoskeletal troubles following *in utero* AKAV infection might be related not only to CNS damages but also to primary infection of fetal muscles [41, 42]. Indeed, primary infection of muscle cells was confirmed in ruminant fetuses infected by AKAV [6, 43]. The presence of SBV in muscle tissues is less frequently evaluated, and if so, quite often by IHC or *in situ*hybridization, with frequent negative results [30, 26, 44]. In the current study one muscle sample from a G60 lamb was found positive by RTqPCR, without signs of gross pathology. The lack of SBV positive detection in the serum of any of the lambs excludes a blood origin by the time of the test. In line with this result, Balseiro et al. reported a higher detection level of SBV RNA in muscles than in the brain or spinal cord of malformed calves [45]. These data suggest that primary infection of fetal muscles might act as an auxiliary mechanism to CNS infection in the pathogenesis of the hydranencephaly/arthrogryposis syndrome caused by SBV, as well as speculated for AKAV.

Yet not statistically significant, an intriguing finding was the SBV RNA higher detection rate in meconium from G45 lambs (7/11) than from G60 ones (3/10). Meconium was reported to be a matrix either rarely or frequently found positive by RTqPCR, depending on the considered study [18, 22]. It is noteworthy to underline that at the same time, amniotic fluid was found more often positive in G60 lambs (5/10) than in G45 lambs (2/11) but not statistically significant as well. As meconium is an end-product of the amniotic fluid being swallowed by the fetus during gestation time, it is likely that SBV detection in the meconium could reflect the former transient presence of the virus in the amniotic fluid. Fecal shedding was reported following SBV experimental infection in heifers [46] and ewes [47]. Hence positive SBV RNA detection in meconium might be the *in utero* version of the previously reported positive detection in the feces of adult animals.

CONCLUSION

The current study demonstrated a very high placental colonization rate when infection occurred at 45 or 60 days of gestation in an experimental context. As an extension of field data where congenital malformations were highly associated with SBV RNA detection in CNS, the absence of gross pathology evocative of SBV infection was reported along with RTqPCR negative results in CNS. In most of the cases, SBV did not reach CNS or could not produce an infection lasting long enough to be detected at birth. In addition, the lack of reported malformations supports the need of an established SBV infection in the CNS of the fetus to become teratogenic. Quite surprisingly, as the placental barrier along with the increasing immunocompetence were assumed to decrease the likelihood of a positive RNA detection at birth, the closer the infection from the term, the higher was the frequency of organs still positive. SBV could infect the placenta of most of the infected ewes. By contrast, viral genome could only be detected in organs of three new-born lambs, of which only one showed positive detection in CNS. No anti-SBV Abs could be detected before colostrum uptake. These results suggest SBV can readily colonize the placenta, but subsequent infection of the fetus is either rare or short lasting. Consequently CNS infection is even less common and so are malformations, at least following infection of the ewes at 45 or 60 days of gestation. *In situ*hybridization and immunohistochemistry might provide more detailed characterization of the cells involved in placental and fetal colonization. Additional experimental infections of pregnant ewes at earlier times in gestation would allow a further clarification of the limits of the specific stages of gestation leading to congenital defects.

ACKNOWLEDGMENTS

We warmly thank all the staff of CODA-CERVA Machelen for taking care of the animals, especially Laurent Mostin and Willem Van Campe. We would like to thank Nathalie Kirschvink and the team of the *Centre du Mouton*, University of Namur, Belgium, for precious advices and collaboration in AI and diagnostic of gestation. We also thank Martin Beer and Bernd Hoffmann from the FLI for providing the inoculum. Many thanks to ID Vet, France, for graciously providing the anti-SBV nucleoprotein MAbs.

AUTHOR CONTRIBUTIONS

Conceived and designed the experiments: LM AP FDP NDR BC CS. Performed the experiments: LM AP. Analyzed the data: LM AP CS. Contributed reagents/materials/analysis tools: LM AP NDR BC CS. Wrote the paper: LM AP FDP NDR BC CS.

REFERENCES

1. Hoffmann B, Scheuch M, Hoper D, Jungblut R, Holsteg M, Schirrmeier H, et al. Novel orthobunyavirus in Cattle, Europe, 2011. Emerging infectious diseases. 2012;18(3):469–72. doi: 10.3201/eid1803.111905. pmid:22376991
2. De Regge N, Deblauwe I, De Deken R, Vantieghem P, Madder M, Geysen D, et al. Detection of Schmallenberg virus in different Culicoides spp. by real-time RT-PCR. Transboundary and emerging diseases. 2012;59(6):471–

5. doi: 10.1111/tbed.12000. pmid:23025501

3. De Regge N, Madder M, Deblauwe I, Losson B, Fassotte C, Demeulemeester J, et al. Schmallenberg virus circulation in culicoides in Belgium in 2012: field validation of a real time RT-PCR approach to assess virus replication and dissemination in midges. PloS one. 2014;9(1):e87005. doi: 10.1371/journal.pone.0087005. pmid:24466312
4. Veronesi E, Henstock M, Gubbins S, Batten C, Manley R, Barber J, et al. Implicating Culicoides biting midges as vectors of Schmallenberg virus using semi-quantitative RT-PCR. PloS one. 2013;8(3):e57747. doi: 10.1371/journal.pone.0057747. pmid:23520481
5. Herder V, Wohlsein P, Peters M, Hansmann F, Baumgartner W. Salient lesions in domestic ruminants infected with the emerging so-called Schmallenberg virus in Germany. Veterinary pathology. 2012;49(4):588–91. doi: 10.1177/0300985812447831. pmid:22610033
6. Parsonson IM, McPhee DA, Della-Porta AJ, McClure S, McCullagh P. Transmission of Akabane virus from the ewe to the early fetus (32 to 53 days). Journal of comparative pathology. 1988;99(2):215–27. pmid:3141487 doi: 10.1016/0021-9975(88)90073-4
7. Hashiguchi Y, Nanba K, Kumagai T. Congenital abnormalities in newborn lambs following Akabane virus infection in pregnant ewes. National Institute of Animal Health quarterly. 1979;19(1–2):1–11. pmid:537648
8. EU consortium. Schmallenberg virus Technical and scientific studies Final report. Wageningen: March 2014.
9. Dominguez M, Gache K, Touratier A, Perrin JB, Fediaevsky A, Collin E, et al. Spread and impact of the Schmallenberg virus epidemic in France in 2012–2013. BMC veterinary research. 2014;10(1):248. doi: 10.1186/s12917-014-0248-x
10. Abecia JA, Forcada F, Gonzalez-Bulnes A. Pharmaceutical control of reproduction in sheep and goats. The Veterinary clinics of North America. 2011;27(1):67–79. doi: 10.1016/j.cvfa.2010.10.001. pmid:21215891
11. Takken W, Verhulst N, Scholte EJ, Jacobs F, Jongema Y, van Lammeren R. The phenology and population dynamics of Culicoides spp. in different ecosystems in The Netherlands. Preventive veterinary medicine. 2008;87(1–2):41–54. doi: 10.1016/j.prevetmed.2008.06.015. pmid:18639947
12. Luttikholt S, Veldhuis A, van den Brom R, Moll L, Lievaart-Peterson K, Peperkamp K, et al. Risk factors for malformations and impact on reproductive performance and mortality rates of Schmallenberg virus in sheep flocks in the Netherlands. PloS one. 2014;9(6):e100135. doi: 10.1371/journal.pone.0100135. pmid:24937443
13. Stockhofe N, Hulst M, Hakze. R, Vellema P, Van der Poel W, editors. Transplacental infection of Schmallenberg Virus in the first trimester of gestation is highly efficient in sheep. Epizone 7th Annual Meeting; 2013 1–4 October; Bruxelles.
14. Jackson P, Cockcroft PD. Clinical Examination of Farm Animals. Oxford, United Kingdom: Blackwell Science Ltd.; 2002.
15. Wernike K, Eschbaumer M, Breithaupt A, Hoffmann B, Beer M. Schmallenberg virus challenge models in cattle: infectious serum or culture-grown virus? Veterinary research. 2012;43:84. doi: 10.1186/1297-9716-43-84. pmid:23231006
16. Wernike K, Hoffmann B, Breard E, Botner A, Ponsart C, Zientara S, et al. Schmallenberg virus experimental infection of sheep. Veterinary microbiology. 2013;166(3–4):461–6. doi: 10.1016/j.vetmic.2013.06.030. pmid:23972950
17. Barbato O, Sousa NM, Debenedetti A, Canali C, Todini L, Beckers JF. Validation of a new pregnancy-associated glycoprotein radioimmunoassay method for the detection of early pregnancy in ewes. Theriogenology. 2009;72(7):993–1000. doi: 10.1016/j.theriogenology.2009.06.020. pmid:19726076
18. Bilk S, Schulze C, Fischer M, Beer M, Hlinak A, Hoffmann B. Organ distribution of Schmallenberg virus RNA in malformed newborns. Veterinary microbiology. 2012;159(1–2):236–8. doi: 10.1016/j.vetmic.2012.03.035. pmid:22516190
19. Poskin A, Martinelle L, Mostin L, Van Campe W, Dal Pozzo F, Saegerman C, et al. Dose-dependent effect of experimental Schmallenberg virus infection in sheep. Vet J. 2014;201(3):419–22. doi: 10.1016/j.tvjl.2014.05.031. pmid:24954869
20. De Regge N, van den Berg T, Georges L, Cay B. Diagnosis of Schmallenberg virus infection in malformed lambs and calves and first indications for virus clearance in the fetus. Veterinary microbiology. 2013;162(2–4):595–600. doi: 10.1016/j.vetmic.2012.11.029. pmid:23265245
21. Robbins JR, Bakardjiev AI. Pathogens and the placental fortress. Curr Opin Microbiol. 2012;15(1):36–43. doi: 10.1016/j.mib.2011.11.006. pmid:22169833
22. Wernike K, Holsteg M, Schirrmeier H, Hoffmann B, Beer M. Natural infection of pregnant cows with Schmallenberg virus—a follow-up study. PloS one. 2014;9(5):e98223.Bilk doi: 10.1371/journal.pone.0098223. pmid:24853555
23. Veldhuis AM, Carp-van Dijken S, van Wuijckhuise L, Witteveen G, van Schaik G. Schmallenberg virus in Dutch dairy herds: potential risk factors for high within-herd seroprevalence and malformations in calves, and its impact on productivity. Veterinary microbiology. 2014;168(2–4):281–93. doi: 10.1016/j.vetmic.2013.11.021. pmid:24360813
24. Afonso A, Abrahantes JC, Conraths F, Veldhuis A, Elbers A, Roberts H, et al. The Schmallenberg virus epidemic in Europe-2011-2013. Preventive veterinary medicine. 2014;116(4):391–403. doi: 10.1016/j.prevetmed.2014.02.012. pmid:24656341
25. Gubbins S, Richardson J, Baylis M, Wilson AJ, Abrahantes JC. Modelling the continental-scale spread of Schmallenberg virus in Europe: approaches and challenges. Preventive veterinary medicine. 2014;116(4):404–11. doi: 10.1016/j.prevetmed.2014.02.004. pmid:24630403
26. Varela M, Schnettler E, Caporale M, Murgia C, Barry G, McFarlane M, et al. Schmallenberg virus pathogenesis,

tropism and interaction with the innate immune system of the host. PLoS pathogens. 2013;9(1):e1003133. doi: 10.1371/journal.ppat.1003133. pmid:23326235

27. Lawn AM, Chiquoine AD, Amoroso EC. The development of the placenta in the sheep and goat: an electron microscope study. J Anat. 1969;105(Pt 3):557–78. pmid:5387511

28. Kurogi H, Inaba Y, Goto Y, Miura Y, Takahashi H. Serologic evidence for etiologic role of Akabane virus in epizootic abortion-arthrogryposis-hydranencephaly in cattle in Japan, 1972–1974. Archives of virology. 1975;47(1):71–83. pmid:1170831 doi: 10.1007/bf01315594

29. van Maanen C, van der Heijden H, Wellenberg GJ, Witteveen G, Luttikholt S, Bouwstra R, et al. Schmallenberg virus antibodies in bovine and ovine fetuses. The Veterinary record. 2012;171(12):299. pmid:22922706 doi: 10.1136/vr.101061

30. Peperkamp NH, Luttikholt SJ, Dijkman R, Vos JH, Junker K, Greijdanus S, et al. Ovine and Bovine Congenital Abnormalities Associated With Intrauterine Infection With Schmallenberg Virus. Veterinary pathology. 2014. doi: 10.1177/0300985814560231

31. Silverstein AM, Uhr JW, Kraner KL, Lukes RJ. Fetal response to antigenic stimulus. II. Antibody production by the fetal lamb. The Journal of experimental medicine. 1963;117:799–812. pmid:13992961 doi: 10.1084/jem.117.5.799

32. Wernike K, Hoffmann B, Beer M. Schmallenberg virus. Developments in biologicals. 2013;135:175–82. doi: 10.1159/000312546. pmid:23689895

33. Parsonson IM, Della-Porta AJ, Snowdon WA. Congenital abnormalities in newborn lambs after infection of pregnant sheep with Akabane virus. Infection and immunity. 1977;15(1):254–62. pmid:832900

34. Evans CA, Reynolds JM, Reynolds ML, Saunders NR, Segal MB. The development of a blood-brain barrier mechanism in foetal sheep. The Journal of physiology. 1974;238(2):371–86. pmid:4601383 doi: 10.1113/jphysiol.1974.sp010530

35. Elliott RM. Bunyaviruses and climate change. Clinical microbiology and infection: the official publication of the European Society of Clinical Microbiology and Infectious Diseases. 2009;15(6):510–7. doi: 10.1111/j.1469-0691.2009.02849.x

36. Sedda L, Rogers DJ. The influence of the wind in the Schmallenberg virus outbreak in Europe. Scientific reports. 2013;3:3361. doi: 10.1038/srep03361. pmid:24285292

37. Herder V, Hansmann F, Wohlsein P, Peters M, Varela M, Palmarini M, et al. Immunophenotyping of inflammatory cells associated with Schmallenberg virus infection of the central nervous system of ruminants. PloS one. 2013;8(5):e62939. doi: 10.1371/journal.pone.0062939. pmid:23667545

38. Workman AD, Charvet CJ, Clancy B, Darlington RB, Finlay BL. Modeling transformations of neurodevelopmental sequences across mammalian species. The Journal of neuroscience: the official journal of the Society for Neuroscience. 2013;33(17):7368–83. doi: 10.1523/jneurosci.5746-12.2013

39. Scharpenberg LG, Windle WF. A Study of Spinal Cord Development in Silver-stained Sheep Embryos correlated with Early Somatic Movements. Journal of Anatomy. 1938;72(Pt 3):344–51. pmid:17104702

40. Clarke GL, Osburn BI. Transmissible congenital demyelinating encephalopathy of lambs. Veterinary pathology. 1978;15(1):68–82. pmid:625870 doi: 10.1177/030098587801500109

41. Edwards JF, Livingston CW, Chung SI, Collisson EC. Ovine arthrogryposis and central nervous system malformations associated with in utero Cache Valley virus infection: spontaneous disease. Veterinary pathology. 1989;26(1):33–9. pmid:2492399 doi: 10.1177/030098588902600106

42. Kurogi H, Inaba Y, Takahashi E, Sato K, Satoda K. Congenital abnormalities in newborn calves after inoculation of pregnant cows with Akabane virus. Infection and immunity. 1977;17(2):338–43. pmid:892909

43. Kurogi H, Inaba Y, Takahashi E, Sato K, Omori T, Miura Y, et al. Epizootic congenital arthrogryposis-hydranencephaly syndrome in cattle: isolation of Akabane virus from affected fetuses. Archives of virology. 1976;51(1–2):67–74. pmid:962588 doi: 10.1007/bf01317835

44. Seehusen F, Hahn K, Herder V, Weigand M, Habierski A, Gerhauser I, et al. Skeletal muscle hypoplasia represents the only significant lesion in peripheral organs of ruminants infected with Schmallenberg virus during gestation. Journal of comparative pathology. 2014;151(2–3):148–52. doi: 10.1016/j.jcpa.2014.04.006. pmid:24975894

45. Balseiro A, Royo LJ, Gomez Antona A, Garcia Marin JF. First Confirmation of Schmallenberg Virus in Cattle in Spain: Tissue Distribution and Pathology. Transboundary and emerging diseases. 2013. doi: 10.1111/tbed.12185

46. Wernike K, Eschbaumer M, Schirrmeier H, Blohm U, Breithaupt A, Hoffmann B, et al. Oral exposure, reinfection and cellular immunity to Schmallenberg virus in cattle. Veterinary microbiology. 2013;165(1–2):155–9. doi: 10.1016/j.vetmic.2013.01.040. pmid:23452751

47. Martinelle L, Poskin A, Dal Pozzo F, Mostin L, van Campe W, Cay AB, et al. Three Different Routes of Inoculation for Experimental Infection with Schmallenberg Virus in Sheep. Transboundary and emerging diseases. 2015; doi: 10.1111/tbed.12356 (in press).

CHAPTER 2

SEROLOGICAL INVESTIGATION OF AKABANE VIRUS INFECTION IN CATTLE AND SHEEP IN NIGERIA

Daniel Oladimeji Oluwayelu, Comfort Oluladun Aiki-Raji, Emmanuel Chibuzor Umeh, Samat Odunayo Mustapha, and Adebowale Idris Adebiyi

Department of Veterinary Microbiology and Parasitology, University of Ibadan, Ibadan 20005, Nigeria

ABSTRACT

Akabane virus (AKAV) is recognized as an important pathogen that causes abortions and congenital malformations in ruminants. However, it has not received adequate attention in Nigeria. Therefore, in investigating this disease, serum samples from 184 (abattoir and farm) head of cattle and 184 intensively reared sheep from two states in southwest Nigeria were screened for antibodies against AKAV using enzyme-linked immunosorbent assay. An overall seropositivity of 70.1% (129/184) was obtained with antibodies being detectable in 73.8% of abattoir (trade) cattle and 40.0% in farm cattle, while 4.3% (8/184) seropositivity was observed in sheep. All the age groups of cattle tested had seropositive animals, 0-1 year (1/7, 14.3%), 2-3 years (17/34, 50.0%), 4-5 years (92/121, 76.0%), and >5 years (19/22, 86.4%), while in sheep only the age groups of 2-3 and 4-5 years showed seropositivity of 4.1% (4/97) and 8.2% (4/49), respectively. The detection of antibody-positive animals among unvaccinated cattle and sheep provides evidence of AKAV infection in Nigeria. These findings call for continuous monitoring of the disease among ruminants in order to ascertain the actual burden and increase awareness of the disease. This will facilitate early detection and aid the development of appropriate control measures against the disease in Nigeria.

INTRODUCTION

The family Bunyaviridae is the largest virus family with over 350 member viruses that are classified into five genera, including the Orthobunyavirus genus which contains a large number of viruses that share common genetic features [1]. Based on serological relationships, viruses in this genus have been divided into serogroups with the Simbu serogroup being one of the largest. Several Simbu serogroup viruses isolated from domestic and wild animals as well as mosquito and Culicoides vectors have been found in Africa, Australia, Asia, and the Middle East [2–6]. This serogroup, which includes Akabane, Aino, and Shamonda viruses, plays a significant role as pathogens of ruminants with Akabane virus (AKAV) being the most recognized [7]. In particular, Akabane virus, a teratogenic, Culicoides-borne virus, replicates in many kinds of natural host species and in several experimental animals [8]. Based on serological evidence, cattle, horses, donkeys, sheep, goats, pigs, camels, and buffaloes appear to be infected in natural situations [9, 10]. AKAV has been identified as a cause of seasonal epizootics of reproductive disorders (abortions, premature births, and stillbirths) and congenital arthrogryposis, hydranencephaly, or microencephaly in cattle,

Citation: Daniel Oladimeji Oluwayelu, Comfort Oluladun Aiki-Raji, Emmanuel Chibuzor Umeh, Samat Odunayo Mustapha, and Adebowale Idris Adebiyi, "Serological Investigation of Akabane Virus Infection in Cattle and Sheep in Nigeria," Advances in Virology, vol. 2016, Article ID 2936082, 4 pages, 2016. doi:10.1155/2016/2936082.

sheep, and goats, sometimes resulting in significant economic losses [1, 6, 11].

Although virus isolation [2], histopathology, immunohistochemistry, serology, and genetic analysis [12] have been used for laboratory confirmation of AKAV infections, serology is the most practical and commonly used technique. Specific antibodies against AKAV have been detected using virus neutralization test (VNT) and enzyme-linked immunosorbent assay (ELISA) [13, 14]. In Africa, limited information based on virus isolation and/or serology revealed the presence of AKAV in Kenya [2, 10], Sudan [15, 16], South Africa [5, 17], Zimbabwe [18], and Tanzania [19] with limited information from Nigeria and perhaps West Africa. In Nigeria, although abortions and congenital malformations associated with AKAV such as arthrogryposis, kyphosis, and scoliosis have been reported in ruminants [20–22], the virus has not received adequate attention as a possible cause of these conditions. Therefore, as part of ongoing surveillance for Culicoides-borne arboviruses of livestock in Nigeria, we investigated the presence of specific antibodies against AKAV in cattle and sheep from Oyo and Ogun states, southwest Nigeria.

MATERIALS AND METHODS

Study Area

This study was based on a cross-sectional design and conducted between May and September 2015 in Ogun and Oyo states of southwest Nigeria. The study area extended from latitudes 7°00′ to 8°00′ north and longitudes 3°35′ to 4°00′ east. Sera were collected in Oyo state from 184 head of trade cattle at the central municipal abattoirs in Bodija and Ogbomoso and a privately owned farm at Ido where they were kept semi-intensively. Cattle slaughtered at the abattoirs are sourced mainly from the northern part of the country and neighbouring countries, where they were reared on free-range management system that exposes them to insect vectors. Also, 184 sera were collected from semi-intensively reared sheep from farms and backyard flocks in Akinyele, Egbeda, Ido, Ibadan North, and Ona-Ara in Oyo state as well as from Imeko and Odeda in Ogun state. The semi-intensively managed cattle and sheep were allowed to graze on pastures during the day and kept indoors at night. However, the animal houses were not insect-proof.

Sample Collection

Blood (about 5 mL) was collected at slaughter from abattoir cattle while farm cattle and sheep were bled via the jugular vein into sterile plain bottles without anticoagulant. The blood was allowed to clot at room temperature after which sera were decanted into sterile Eppendorf tubes and stored at −20°C until tested.

Detection of AKAV Antibodies by Competitive ELISA

All the collected sera were analyzed using a commercially available ID Screen® competition ELISA kit (IDvet, Montpellier, France) that detects anti-G1 antibodies directed against AKAV in ruminant serum and plasma. The test, which was reported by the manufacturer to lack cross-reactivity with other viruses in the Bunyaviridaefamily, such as Schmallenberg virus (SBV), Rift Valley fever virus (RVFV), and Aino virus, and to have a high (96.52%) correlation with the VNT, was performed according to the kit protocol. For each sample, results were expressed as sample/negative percentage (S/N%) using the optical densities (OD) from the ELISA reader: S/N% = = $OD_{sample}/OD_{negative\ control} \times 100$. Samples that presented S/N% lower than 30%, between 30% and 40%, and >40% were considered positive, doubtful, and negative, respectively.

Statistical Analysis

Results of serology were analyzed using the statistical package GraphPad Prism version 5.01 (San Diego, USA). Differences in AKAV antibody seroprevalence between cattle and sheep, abattoir and farm cattle, and male and female animals were evaluated using chi-square (χ^2) test. Furthermore, seroprevalence results based on breed, age group, and location were subjected to one-way ANOVA and subsequently to Tukey's posttest for performing multiple comparisons in order to assess statistically significant differences between all possible pairs of groups. The level of statistical significance was $p<0.05$.

RESULTS

Out of 184 sheep sera tested, 8 (4.4%), 22 (12.0%), and 154 (83.7%) were positive, doubtful, and negative, respectively, for AKAV anti-G1 antibodies while, of the 184 cattle sera tested, 129 (70.1%), 37 (20.1%), and 18 (9.8%) were positive, doubtful, and negative, respectively (Table 1). The prevalence of AKAV antibodies was significantly ($P<0.05$) higher in abattoir cattle compared to farm cattle (Table 2). For the abattoir cattle, AKAV antibody prevalence was significantly higher in Bodija central abattoir compared to the Ogbomosho abattoir. Overall, based on cattle breed, AKAV antibody prevalence was 66.4% (75/113), 77.8% (28/36), 75.0% (3/4), 83.3% (10/12), and 76.5% (13/17) for White Fulani, Sokoto Gudali, Kuri, Red Bororo, and crossbreeds, respectively. However, comparison of the AKAV seroprevalence rates in sheep based on age, sex, breed, and location of sample collection revealed no significant differences.

Table 1: Prevalence of AKAV antibodies in sheep and cattle in the study area

	Number sampled	Positive (%)	Doubtful (%)	Negative (%)
Sheep	184	8 (4.4)	22 (12.0)	154 (83.7)
Cattle	184	129 (70.1)*	37 (20.1)	18 (9.8)
Total	364	137 (37.6)	59 (16.2)	172 (47.3)

*$P = 0.0001$.

Table 2: Seroprevalence of AKAV in cattle in the study area

Variable	Group	Number sampled	Positive (%)
Sex	Female	131	92 (70.2)
	Male	53	37 (69.8)
Age (years)	0-1	7	1 (14.3)*
	2-3	34	17 (50.0)
	4-5	121	92 (76.0)
	>5	22	19 (86.4)*
Source	Abattoir	164	121 (73.8)*
	Farm	20	8 (40.0)

*$P = 0.0001$.

DISCUSSION

Akabane virus has been shown to be an important pathogen causing abortions and congenital malformations in ruminants [23]. Antibodies to this Culicoides-borne, Simbu serogroup virus have been found in ruminants from countries of Australia, Asia, Southeast Asia, the Middle East, and Africa [6, 10, 16, 24, 25]. However, since the initial isolation of Simbu group viruses from cattle and Culicoides biting midges in Nigeria [26, 27], there has been no report on the presence of AKAV in Nigeria. In the present study, which is part of ongoing surveillance for Culicoides-borne arboviruses in Nigeria [28, 29], AKAV antibody prevalence of 70.1% and 4.3%, respectively, was obtained for cattle and sheep in two states (Ogun and Oyo) of southwest Nigeria using a competition ELISA. According to the internal validation report of the kit manufacturer on the assay, known SBV-, RVFV-, and Aino virus-positive sera produced negative results with the AKAV ELISA kit, demonstrating the absence of cross-reactions with antisera against these viruses. To our knowledge, this is the first report of AKAV antibody-positive animals in Nigeria. As AKAV vaccines are currently not administered to livestock in the country, the detection of seropositive cattle and sheep in this study suggests natural exposure of these animals to AKAV. The higher seroprevalence obtained for cattle, which is similar to the findings of a recent study in Sudan [16], is an indication that they were more likely to be infected with AKAV than sheep. This possibility is buttressed by the knowledge that cattle are allowed to graze more extensively, thus making them more exposed to the Culicoides vectors of AKAV than sheep. Moreover, it has previously been reported [30] that some Culicoides species have distinct feeding preference for cattle over sheep even when kept in the same vicinity.

Furthermore, it was observed in this study that AKAV antibodies were more prevalent in trade cattle from abattoirs than in farm cattle. This higher seroprevalence may be due to the fact that, compared to farm cattle which are domiciled in one location, trade cattle for slaughter at these abattoirs are sourced from different parts of Nigeria and neighbouring countries where they are kept mostly on free-range. This makes the abattoirs convergence points for animals from diverse geographical locations where they could have had contact with infected Culicoides vectors. Since there is unregulated transborder movement of ruminants from neighbouring West African countries into Nigeria, it is possible that some of the seropositive cattle could have imported the disease into the country. Also, the detection of seropositive animals among trade cattle of different breeds suggests that the disease is not breed-restricted.

Previous reports of congenital malformations in cattle and sheep in Nigeria suggested that these defects have no clearly established cause [20–22, 31]. However, the increased prevalence of AKAV antibodies observed with increasing age of cattle and sheep in this study (Table 2) suggests AKAV as a possible cause of these conditions. Since it has been reported that inapparent Akabane infection in adults can lead to abortions, stillbirth, and congenital defects in newborns [10, 32], this finding suggests that AKAV may significantly increase abortion risk among adult cattle and sheep, thus constituting a potential health risk to the animals. Therefore, the findings of this study corroborate the fact that AKAV is endemic in sub-Saharan Africa and underscore the need for large-scale surveillance of the virus in Nigeria in order to establish its role as a possible cause of economic losses in ruminants through abortions, stillbirths, and congenital malformations and develop effective prevention and control strategies. Additionally, virus isolation and genetic characterization of isolates will be essential for understanding the molecular epidemiology and evolution of AKAV in Nigeria.

REFERENCES

1. N. J. MacLachlan and E. J. Dubovi, "Bunyaviridae," in Fenner's Veterinary Virology, pp. 371–383, Academic Press, London, UK, 4th edition, 2011.
2. D. Metselaar and Y. Robin, "Akabane virus isolated in Kenya," Veterinary Record, vol. 99, no. 5, p. 86, 1976. · View at Scopus
3. W. J. Hartley and R. A. Wanner, "Bovine congenital arthrogryposis in New South Wales," Australian Veterinary Journal, vol. 50, no. 5, pp. 185–188, 1974.
4. Y. Miura, Y. Inaba, T. Tsuda et al., "A survey of antibodies to arthropod-borne viruses in Indonesian cattle," Japanese Journal of Veterinary Science, vol. 44, no. 6, pp. 857–863, 1982.
5. H. Zeller and M. Bouloy, "Infections by viruses of the families Bunyaviridae and Filoviridae," Revue Scientifique et Technique, vol. 19, no. 1, pp. 79–91, 2000.
6. O. Markusfield and E. Mayer, "An arthrogryposis and hydranencephaly syndrome in calves in Israel, 1969-70: epidemiological and clinical aspects," Refuah Veterinarith, vol. 28, pp. 51–61, 1971.
7. T. D. St George and P. D. Kirkland, "Diseases caused by Akabane and related Simbu-group viruses," inInfectious Diseases of Livestock, J. A. W. Coetzer and R. C. Tustin, Eds., pp. 1029–1036, Oxford University Press, Oxford, UK, 2nd edition, 2004.
8. C.-C. Huang, T.-S. Huang, M.-C. Deng, M.-H. Jong, and S.-Y. Lin, "Natural infections of pigs with Akabane virus," Veterinary Microbiology, vol. 94, no. 1, pp. 1–11, 2003.
9. S. Al-Busaidy, C. Hamblin, and W. P. Taylor, "Neutralising antibodies to Akabane virus in free-living wild animals in Africa," Tropical Animal Health and Production, vol. 19, no. 4, pp. 197–202, 1987.
10. F. G. Davies and D. M. Jessett, "A study of the host range and distribution of antibody to Akabane virus (genus bunyavirus, family Bunyaviridae) in Kenya," Journal of Hygiene, vol. 95, no. 1, pp. 191–196, 1985.
11. H. Kurogi, Y. Inaba, Y. Goto et al., "Serologic evidence for etiologic role of Akabane virus in epizootic abortion-arthrogryposis-hydranencephaly in cattle in Japan, 1972–1974," Archives of Virology, vol. 47, no. 1, pp. 71–83, 1975.
12. J.-K. Oem, H.-J. Yoon, H.-R. Kim et al., "Genetic and pathogenic characterization of Akabane viruses isolated from cattle with encephalomyelitis in Korea," Veterinary Microbiology, vol. 158, no. 3-4, pp. 259–266, 2012.
13. Y. Miura, S. Hayashi, T. Ishihara, Y. Inaba, T. Omori, and M. Matumoto, "Neutralizing antibody against Akabane

virus in precolostral sera from calves with congenital arthrogryposis-hydranencephaly syndrome," Archiv für die Gesamte Virusforschung, vol. 46, no. 3-4, pp. 377–380, 1974.

14. T. Tsuda, K. Yoshida, T. Yanase, S. Ohashi, and M. Yamakawa, "Competitive enzyme-linked immunosorbent assay for the detection of the antibodies specific to Akabane virus," Journal of Veterinary Diagnostic Investigation, vol. 16, no. 6, pp. 571–576, 2004.
15. M. E. Mohamed, P. S. Mellor, and W. P. Taylor, "Akabane virus: serological survey of antibodies in livestock in the Sudan," Revue d›Elevage et de Médecine Vétérinaire des pays Tropicaux, vol. 49, no. 4, pp. 285–288, 1996.
16. A. M. Elhassan, M. E. A. Mansour, A. A. A. Shamon, and A. M. El Hussein, "A serological survey of Akabane virus infection in cattle in Sudan," ISRN Veterinary Science, vol. 2014, Article ID 123904, 4 pages, 2014.
17. A. Theodoridis, E. M. Nevill, H. J. Els, and S. T. Boshoff, "Viruses isolated from Culicoides midges in South Africa during unsuccessful attempts to isolate bovine ephemeral fever virus," Onderstepoort Journal of Veterinary Research, vol. 46, no. 4, pp. 191–198, 1979.
18. N. K. Blackburn, I. Searle, and B. J. Phelps, "Viruses isolated from Culicoides (Diptera: Ceratopogonidae) caught at the veterinary research farm, Mazowe, Zimbabwe," Journal of the Entomological Society of South Africa, vol. 48, no. 2, pp. 331–336, 1985.
19. C. Mathew, S. Klevar, A. R. W. Elbers et al., "Detection of serum neutralizing antibodies to Simbu sero-group viruses in cattle in Tanzania," BMC Veterinary Research, vol. 11, article 208, 2015.
20. I. U. Ate and L. Allam, "Multiple congenital skeletal malformations in a lamb associated with dystocia in a Yankasa ewe," Nigerian Veterinary Journal, vol. 23, no. 1, pp. 61–63, 2002.
21. M. M. Bukar, M. Waziri, and U. I. Ibrahim, "Dystocia due to arthrogryposis and associated with a mummified twin in a crossed (Yankassa/Uda) ewe: a case report," Tropical Veterinarian, vol. 24, no. 4, pp. 85–88, 2006.
22. N. D. Ibrahim, S. Adamu, S. M. Useh, et al., "Multiple congenital defects in a Bunaji bull," Nigerian Veterinary Journal, vol. 27, no. 3, pp. 80–86, 2006.
23. O. R. Coverdale, D. H. Cybinski, and T. D. St George, "Congenital abnormalities in calves associated with Akabane virus and Aino virus," Australian Veterinary Journal, vol. 54, no. 3, pp. 151–152, 1978.
24. W. J. Hartley, R. A. Wanner, A. J. Della-Porta, and W. A. Snowdon, "Serological evidence for the association of Akabane virus with epizootic bovine congenital arthrogryposis and hydranencephaly syndromes in New South Wales," Australian Veterinary Journal, vol. 51, no. 2, pp. 103–104, 1975.
25. S. M. Al-Busaidy, P. S. Mellor, and W. P. Taylor, "Prevalence of neutralising antibodies to Akabane virus in the Arabian Peninsula," Veterinary Microbiology, vol. 17, no. 2, pp. 141–149, 1988.
26. O. R. Causey, G. E. Kemp, C. E. Causey, and V. H. Lee, "Isolation of Simbu-group viruses in Ibadan, Nigeria 1964–69, including the new types Sango, Shamonda, Sabo and Shuni," Annals of Tropical Medicine and Parasitology, vol. 66, no. 3, pp. 357–362, 1972.
27. V. H. Lee, "Isolation of viruses from field populations of Culicoides (Diptera: Ceratopogonidae) in Nigeria," Journal of Medical Entomology, vol. 16, no. 1, pp. 76–79, 1979.
28. D. O. Oluwayelu, O. Olatoye, M. Akanbi, and B. Hoffmann, "Seroprevalence of bluetongue virus infection in Oyo state, Nigeria," Journal of Commonwealth Veterinary Association, vol. 27, no. 2, pp. 234–238, 2011.
29. D. O. Oluwayelu, C. O. Meseko, and A. I. Adebiyi, "Serological screening for Schmallenberg virus in exotic and indigenous cattle in Nigeria," Sokoto Journal of Veterinary Sciences, vol. 13, no. 3, pp. 14–18, 2015.
30. S. Bartsch, B. Bauer, A. Wiemann, P.-H. Clausen, and S. Steuber, "Feeding patterns of biting midges of the Culicoides obsoletus and Culicoides pulicaris groups on selected farms in Brandenburg, Germany,"Parasitology Research, vol. 105, no. 2, pp. 373–380, 2009.
31. A. A. Bello, I. A. Nwanena, I. Hamman, and C. T. Aba, "Foetal monster in a four-year old Yankassa ewe with dystocia: a case report," Tropical Veterinarian, vol. 24, no. 4, pp. 89–94, 2006.
32. P. D. Kirkland, R. D. Barry, P. A. Harper, and R. Z. Zelski, "The development of Akabane virus-induced congenital abnormalities in cattle," Veterinary Record, vol. 122, no. 24, pp. 582–586, 1988.

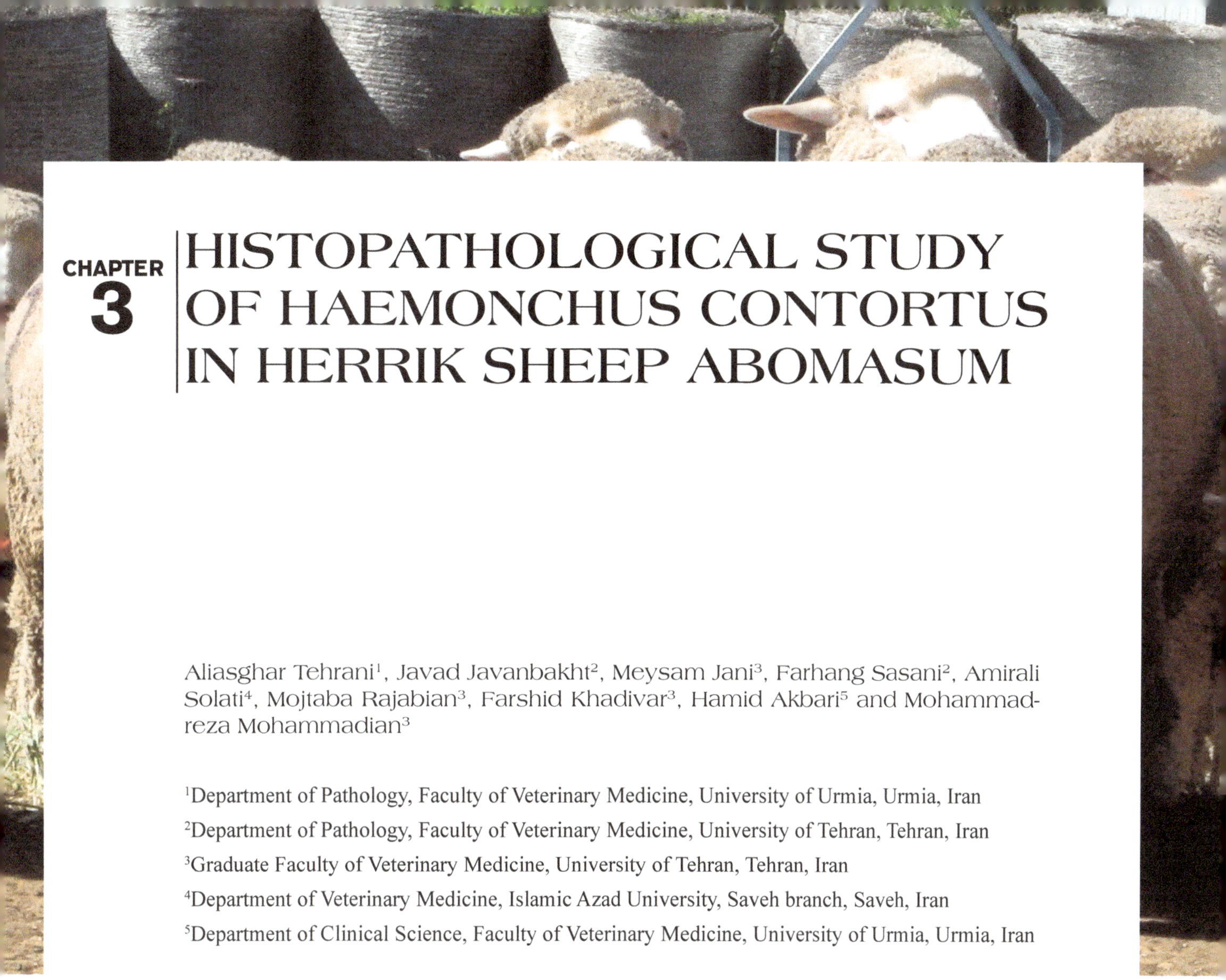

CHAPTER 3

HISTOPATHOLOGICAL STUDY OF HAEMONCHUS CONTORTUS IN HERRIK SHEEP ABOMASUM

Aliasghar Tehrani[1], Javad Javanbakht[2], Meysam Jani[3], Farhang Sasani[2], Amirali Solati[4], Mojtaba Rajabian[3], Farshid Khadivar[3], Hamid Akbari[5] and Mohammad-reza Mohammadian[3]

[1]Department of Pathology, Faculty of Veterinary Medicine, University of Urmia, Urmia, Iran

[2]Department of Pathology, Faculty of Veterinary Medicine, University of Tehran, Tehran, Iran

[3]Graduate Faculty of Veterinary Medicine, University of Tehran, Tehran, Iran

[4]Department of Veterinary Medicine, Islamic Azad University, Saveh branch, Saveh, Iran

[5]Department of Clinical Science, Faculty of Veterinary Medicine, University of Urmia, Urmia, Iran

ABSTRACT

Hemonchosis is a very common disease in small ruminants caused by Haemonchus contortus, a blood sucking parasite causing anaemia that may be fatal particularly to young animals. The present study was conducted to determine the prevalence of Haemonchus contortus in slaughtered sheep's at Urmia abattoir located in the North West of Iran. A total of 2421animals were slaughtered and examined from July 2010 to July 2011 in Urmia abattoir. In case of sheep, 225 out of 2421 were positive and prevalence of Haemonchus contortus infestation was 9.3%. Sex wise prevalence of Haemonchus contortus in sheep was 33.08% (76/229) in male and 66.22% (149/225) in female. The females indicated significantly (P<0.05) higher prevalence (66.22%) as compared to males (33.08%). The highest prevalence was recorded in the spring (April) and the lowest was in summer (July), respectively. On microscopic examination, infiltration of mononuclear cells and eosinophils in gastric glands, periglandular hyperemia and hemorrhage, mucous gland hyperplasia, connective tissue proliferation and necrosis was observed. Also, in mixed abomasal infection with Haemonchus and Ostertagia species, mucosal hyperplasia and increased mucous glands and sometimes cystic glands were seen. Statistical analysis using SPSS software, and chi-square test, demonstrated a non-significant difference between ages and abomasal pH values of infected and healthy sheep (p<0.05). But the difference between sexes, seasons and abomasal lesions was significant (p>0.05).

INTRODUCTION

Abomasum is one of the most important sites for living bursate nematodes belonging to Trichostrongylidae family in small ruminants, because it is the site location for 3 pathogen species of GI nematodes e.g., Haemonchus spp., Teladorsagia spp., Ostertagia spp.and Trichostrongylus spp., meanwhile it was shown that gastrointestinal nematodes could be harmful to the health mortalities, reduce weight gain and other production losses [1,2]. Small ruminants play an important role in maintaining family stability by providing meat, milk, skin and wool, earn cash income and play traditional social and religious roles. Health disorders in all classes of small ruminants represent the major problems and largely on the economics of sheep and goat production [3]. The gastrointestinal nematode, Haemonchus contortus (Barber's pole worm), is a major pathogen of ovine throughout the temperate and tropical regions of the world and is a significant cause of production losses. Debilitating infection with this parasite is most commonly

Citation: Tehrani A, Javanbakht J, Jani M, Sasani F, Solati A, et al. (2012) Histopathological Study of Haemonchus contortus in Herrik Sheep Abomasum. J Bacteriol Parasitol 3:144. doi:10.4172/2155-9597.1000144.

seen in young animals while resistance to infection develops, with exposure, in older ovine [4]. Female worms are 18-30 mm long and are easily recognized by the 'barbers pole' appearance of the white ovaries and uteri twisting for the length of the worm around a red blood-filled intestine and males are 10-20 mm long and uniformly reddish-brown [5]. This parasite is a gastrointestinal nematode of special importance in associated with to small ruminant production in warm climates [6] and is a blood feeding nematode which parasitises the abomasum and presents a serious constraint to ovine production in areas with predominantly summer rainfall [7]. The fourth larval (L4) and adult stages of this worm suck blood and in addition, move and leave wounds that hemorrhage from the abomasal wall of the host. A blood sucking H.contortus can suck about 0.05 ml blood per day in ovine [8]. H.contortus is of primary concern since it is a highly pathogenic blood-feeder helminth that causes anaemia and reduced productivity and can lead to death in infected animals [9] and the diagnosis of Haemonchosis is usually based upon clinical signs and fecal examinations. Eggs are found in feces when the damage has already been done. So ELISA enables detection of sub clinical infection [10]. Fayza Ahmed Omer et al. [11] showed that histopathological changes of the abomasum were of severe mucosal and submucosal haemorrhages. Epithelial cells indicated degeneration and other revealed hypertrophy. Gastric glands domonstrated some changes and contained, mononuclear cells dominated with eosinophils. Terefe et al. [12] observed that sheep infected with Oestrus ovis and H.contortus in a natural way eliminated smaller quantities of eggs in feces than those infected with only H.contortus. Previous infection with O. ovis in the nasal cavity also reduces the development and fertility of H.contortus in the abomasum. This reduction is associated with eosinophilia, an increase in abomasal eosinophils and globular leukocytes, as well as an inflammatory response in the abomasal mucosa [12,13]. Among the diseases that impose the survival and productivity of ovine and goats, gastrointestinal nematode infection ranks highest on a global index, with Barber's pole worm being of overwhelming importance [14]. The objective of this study was to histopathological study of Haemonchus contortus in Herrik sheep abomasums.

MATERIALS AND METHODS

Study Area

The district Urmia of agro-ecological zone was selected for the present study. Climatically, the study region is subtropical and receives an annual rainfall of about 150-350mm. The temperature is highest in June, before the onset of monsoon season. During summer, the daily maximum temperature exceeds 45°C and rarely declines below 22°C. Relative humidity is lowest during April-May and rises during the monsoon season. One year cycle is divided into four seasons viz. winter (December-February) spring (March-April) summer (May-September and autumn (October-November). summer also includes monsoon season (July-August).

Animals

During the period from July 2010 to July 2011, a total of 2421Herrik sheep ranging from 2 to 5 years of both sexes were subjected to a careful post-mortem examination during abattoir inspection in Urmia slaughter houses in West Azarbijan province (coordinates: 37°33N, 45°04E) Iran. The Herrik and Afshari sheep were selected to be examined as they are the most important and numerous native breed. The resulting samples were sent to the Laboratory of Parasitology and pathology, Faculty of Veterinary Medicine, Urmia University, Urmia, Iran, for parasitological and histopathological examination.

Parasitological Investigation

Abomasa of total 2421 sheeps slaughtered at Urmia abattoir were examined for the presence of adult worm of H.contortus. Sheep were comprising on male (n=859) and female (n=1562). Each abomasum was separated from the small intestine and the abomasums transferred to the parasitology laboratory, and examined within 3h of slaughter. The abomasum was slit open and their contects washed gently with water in separate buckets and collected. In addition, the abomasum was divided longitudinally in two equal parts (towards the greater curvature with a pair of scissors) and the whole mucosa of one part was scraped off and digested in a pepsin-HC1solution for 10 h at 37°C. The digest was concentrated over a 400-meshsieve (aperture diameter 51 pm) under a water-jet and the entire sieve contents examined [15,16].

Histopathological Examination

A 10-mm-long sample of the abomasa segment without any injury was removed, fixed, and prepared for histopathological examination. Tissue fragments were fixed in 10% neutral buffered formalin solution (for 72 hours), after stabilizing embedded in paraffin, sectioned at 5 μm thickness and then, stained with hematoxylin and eosin (H&E).

Statistical Analysis

Statistical analysis using spss software and Chi-square test was applied for the statistical analysis of the data [17].

RESULTS

Overall Prevalence of H.Contortus in Sheep

In this study, 225abomasa (9.3%) were infected with Haemonchus contortus. Sex wise prevalence of H.contortus in sheep was 33.08% (76/229) in male and 66.22% (149/225) in female. In the monthly survey, the highest rate of infection was in April (22.9%) and the lowest was in July (14.9%). The seasonal survey shows that the highest and lowest infection rates are in the spring (13.6%) and in summer (2.4%), respectively. In statistical analysis, there was a significant difference between seasons and the prevalence of the parasite ($P<0.05$). The study of parasites in the abomasa of 2421 sheep revealed that acute and chronic forms of haemonchosis are common in the region. And pre acute form of infection has no sign of presence or is utterly rare in above-mentioned region (Table 1, 2 and Figure 1).

Macroscopic and Microscopic Findings

Petechial hemorrhage in the abomasal mucosa (Probably due to the attachment of the parasite) (Figure 2), extensive mucosal hemorrhage, inflammation, mucous secretions around lesions and paleness of internal organs were seen (Figure 3). Also abomasal contents were fluidal and partially covered with free blood; the carcasses were paled and have generalized edema and fluid throughout of the body cavities secondary to hypoproteinemia. Moreover, following findings were witnessed: mononuclear cells infiltration (lymphocytes, monocytes and plasma cells), prominent eosinophilic infiltration in mucous glands and some even penetrated to the sub mucosa (Figure 4), perivascular hyperemia and lymphocytic infiltration, tissue thickening due to an increase in mucous glands and mucous secretion (Figures 5 and 6), connective tissue proliferation and necrosis (in chronic abomasal inflammation and wound healing) (Figure 7).

Table 1: Abomasum monthly contamination with Haemonchus contort

Seasons	Intact	Infested	Total number of inspections
July Count	160	0	160
Expected Count	145.1	14.9	160.0
Monthly Summary (%)	100.0%	.0%	100.0%
August Count	221	2	223
Expected Count	202.2	20.8	223.0
Monthly Summary (%)	99.1%	.9%	100.0%
September Count	231	13	224
Expected Count	221.2	22.8	224.0
Monthly Summary (%)	94.7%	5.3%	100.0%
October Count	186	27	213
Expected Count	193.1	19.9	213.0
Monthly Summary (%)	87.3%	12.7%	100.0%
November Count	138	18	156
Expected Count	141.4	14.6	156.0
Monthly Summary (%)	88.5%	11.5%	100.0%
December Count	158	23	181
Expected Count	164.1	16.9	181.0
Monthly Summary (%)	87.3%	12.7%	100.0%
January Count	171	11	182
Expected Count	165.0	17.0	182.0
Monthly Summary (%	94.0%	6.0%	100.0%
February Count	122	10	132
Expected Count	119.7	12.3	132.0
Monthly Summary (%)	92.4%	7.6%	100.0%
March Count	73	6	79
Expected Count	71.6	7.4	79.0
Monthly Summary (%)	92.4%	7.6%	100.0%
April Count	194	51	245
Expected Count	222.1	22.9	245.0
Monthly Summary (%)	79.2%	20.8%	100.0%
May Count	270	58	328
Expected Count	297.4	30.6	328.0
Monthly Summary (%)	82.3%	17.7%	100.0%
June Count	271	7	278
Expected Count	252.0	26.0	378.0
Monthly Summary (%)	97.5%	2.5%	100.0%
Total Count	2195	226	2421
Expected Count	2195.0	226.0	2421.0
Monthly Summary (%)	90.7%	9.3%	100.0%

Table 2: Abomasum seasonal contamination with Haemonchus contortus

Seasons	Intact (%)	Infected (%)	Total number of inspections (%)
Spring	735(86.4%)	116(13.6%)	851(100%)
Summer	612(97.6%)	15(2.4%)	627(100%)
Autumn	482(87.6%)	68(12.4%)	550(100%)
Winter	366(93.1%)	27(6.9%)	393(100%)
Total	2195(90.7%)	226(9.3%)	2421(100%)

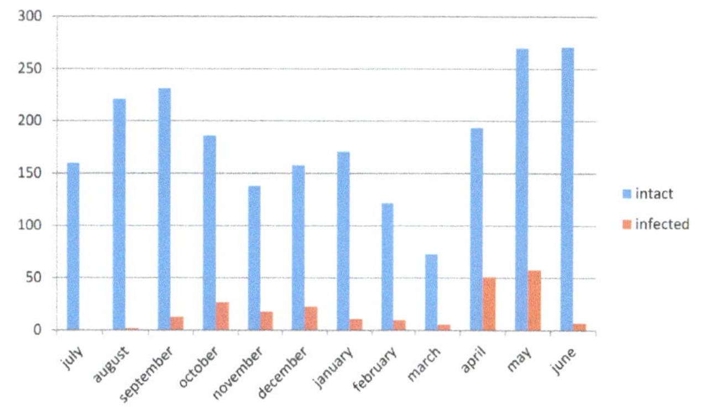

Figure 1: Abomasum monthly contamination with Haemonchus contortus.

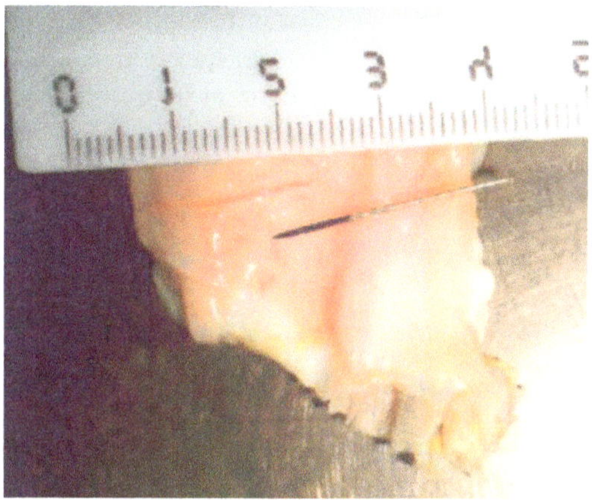

Figure 2: Petechial in the mucosa of the abomasum.

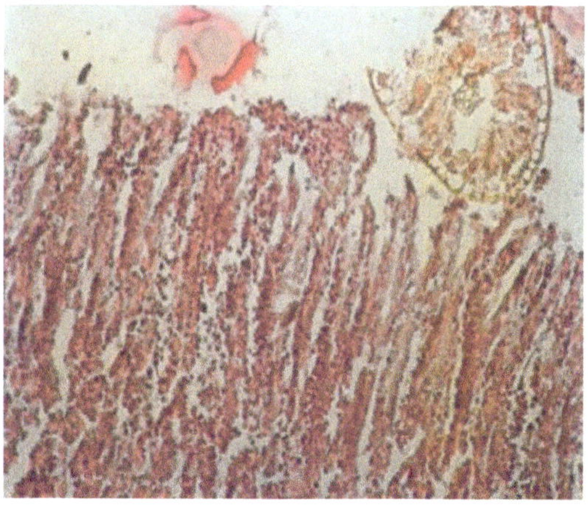

Figure 3: hemorrhage in between the glands and inflammatory cell infiltration.

Abomasal pH Values and Relationship between Sex, Ages, Season and Prevalence in Sheep

With regard to determination of infected abomasal pH values, slight increase in PH was seen (3.5 to 4.5), but there wasn't a close correlation between pH values of parasitized and healthy abomasa (P> 0.05). Also there wasn't a significant difference between ages of infected sheep (P> 0.05). But the difference between sexes, seasons and abomasal lesions was significant (p>0.05). Pertaining to seasons in which amount of rainfalls are considerable, temperature would result in dramatic increase of parasite frequency. Subsequently more sheep are afflicted. Needless to say, lesions would be widely seen in the abomasa either. So, there is a direct relevance between season and prevalence of lesions in the abomasa ($P < 0.05$). And this issue occurs during the spring in the North West region of Iran (West Azerbaijan).

DISCUSSION

Haemonchosis is a serious health problem which causes lower production due to high morbidity, mortality, and cost of treatment and control measures [18]. The results revealed that the infected animals (sheeps) harbour H.contortus infection throughout the year at all the studied sites with varied incidence. It could be inferred from the infection level that the permanent flocks in azerbaijan west Urmia areas had substantial worm burdens of H.contortus. The present study demonstrated that prevalence of infection was 9.3% and the average rate of infection is 49 % in Iran [19]. So this rate is much less than average of infection in Iran. This is probably due to cold winters and hot summers that destroy the parasite. According to studies by Eslami et al. [19] rate of infection in sheep is 49%, and 40.8% in goats, 0.8% in wild sheep, 22% in cattle, and 12% in camels. The seasonal survey demonstrated that the highest and lowest infection rates are in the spring (13.6%) and in summer (2.4%), successively. Recently O'Sullivan and Donald suggested that spring rise was due to a temporary depression of immunological capacity brought about by endocrine changes associated with lactation, which could result in a resumption of development of arrested larvae, an increased rate of establishment of newly ingested larvae and increased fecundity of female worms.

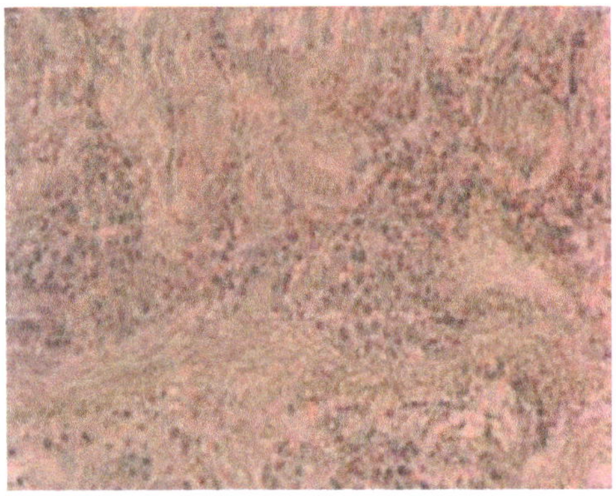

Figure 4: Infiltration of inflammatory cells in the mucosa of the abomasum.

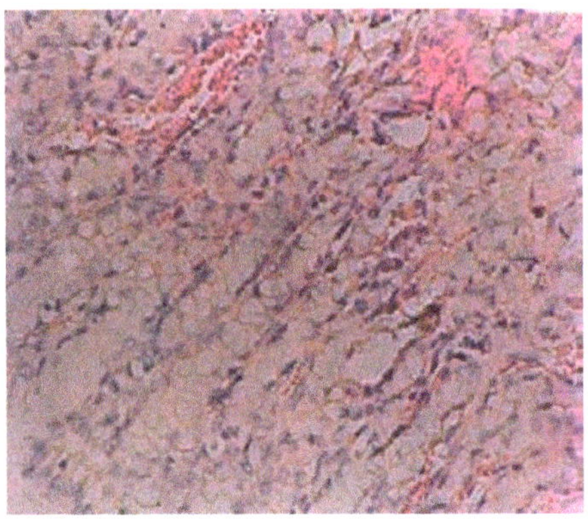

Figure 5: Increase in mucous glands and hemorrhage in between the glands.

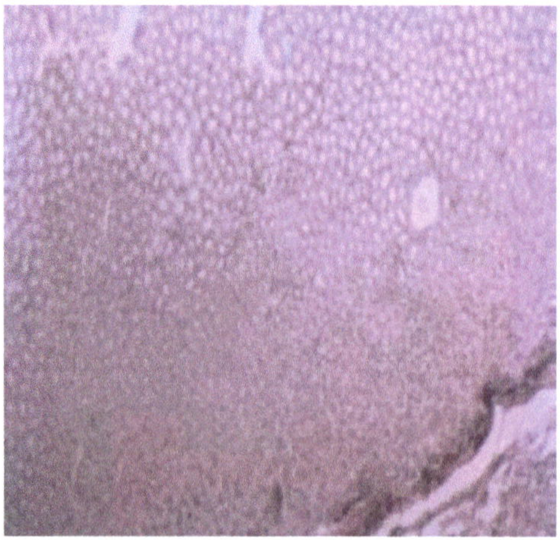

Figure 6: Hyperplasia and cystic glands in the abomasum.

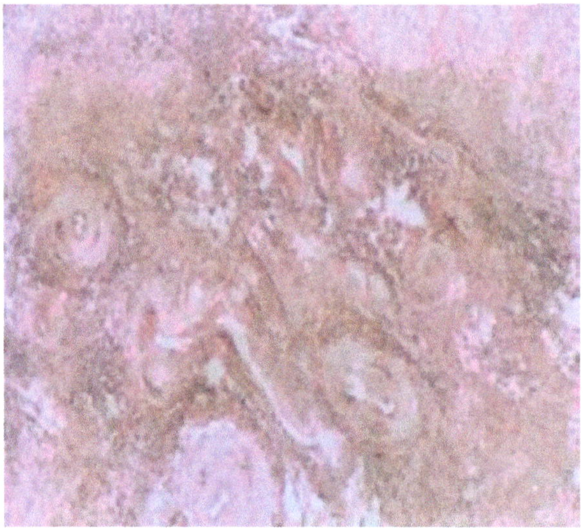

Figure 7: Proliferation of Connective tissue.

And also in the monthly survey, the highest rate of infection was in April (22.9%) and the lowest was in July (14.9%). Thus Blitz and Gibbs have demonstrated that transplantation of such arrested larvae into worm-free, susceptible ewes in winter did not result in the immediate maturation of the parasites. When maturation occurred, it coincided with the time that spring rise regularly takes place in this area (April), some IO-12 weeks after transplanting the arrested larvae. Moreover, numerous attempts to induce maturation of arrested larvae in sheep during the winter by administration of immunosuppressive drugs have failed [20-22]. In Macroscopic findings, petechial hemorrhage in the mucosa and severe hyperemia in mucosal folds were seen as described by McKenna PB [21]. Also eosinophilic infiltration has been observed that while corresponding to those of Nayebzadeh et al. [22]. Eosinophils are considered to be important elements in the response against Haemonchus infections Balice et al. [23]. In the study, there was an increased number of circulating blood eosinophils in the sheeps infected with Haemonchus larvae. This was in agreement with Terefe et al. [12]. There is also some evidence suggesting that eosinophils may contribute to pathogenesis during parasitic infection [13]. Moreover, it has previously been shown that a number of ovine parasitic gastrointestinal nematodes produce a factor(s) that promote eosinophil migration in vitro [24]. Yacob et al. [25] reported the presence of an early and high eosinophilia and migration of the same cellular components into the abomasal and intestinal mucosa in the absence of nematodes in the gut. Meanwhile, sometimes the focal accumulation of lymphocytes and tissue thickening were seen that is similar to that reported by Scott et al. [26]. Many studies have been done on this parasite. Ahmed Mir et al. [27], Zacharias et al. [28] and Scott et al. [26] have reviewed pathophysiology of Haemonchosis. Also Ameen et al. [29] and Wilson et al. [30] reported hematologic changes. Nayebzadeh et al. [22] and Troell et al. [31] studied at parasite growth stages and its changes. In Anderson [32] studies, weight loss is reported during the chronic infection with this parasite in sheep. Zacharias et al. [28] reported anemia in merino sheep. Also, Courtney et al. [33] and Nayebzadeh et al. [22] reported it too. Additionally in microscopic examination by Nayebzadeh et al. [22] proliferation of macrophages and fibroblasts and infiltration of lymphocytes and eosinophils have seen around the adult worms in pyloric region [22]. Moreover, in another study by Scott et al. [26], fundus region thickening was seen, that caused by mucous cells hyperplasia. Also Mir et al. [15] reported that lymphocytes from both naive lambs and immune sheep responded to a similar spectrum of molecular and also this report therefore supports the findings of Anthony et al. [34,35] who had suggested that lymphocyte proliferative responses in naive sheep were important in innate resistance to this parasite weight fraction in soluble antigen. Immunosuppresion is known to take place in some gastrointestinal nematode infection models [36-38]. These observations suggest that the chronic nature of primary H.contortus nematode infections may be due to a change in the type of immune response induced by larval and adult nematodes and that the adult nematodes may actively subvert the initial immune response induced after infection.

REFERENCES

1. Sultan K, Desoukey AY, Elsiefy MA, Elbahy NM (2010) An Abattoir Study on the Prevalence of Some Gastrointestinal Helminths of Sheep in Gharbia Governorate, Egypt. Global Veterinaria 5: 84-87.
2. Vlassoff A, Mckenna P (2010) Nematode parasites of economic importance in sheep in New Zealand. N Z J Zool 21: 1-8.
3. Lateef M, Iqbal Z, Jabba A, Khan MN, Akhtar MS (2005) Epidemiology of trichostrongylid nematode infections in sheep under raditional husbandry system in Pakistan. Int J Agric Biol 7: 596-600.
4. Onyenwe IW, Onwe C, Onyeabor A ,Onunkwo JI (2005) Abattoir-Based Study of the Susceptibility of Two Natural Infected Breeds of Goat to Haemonchus contortus in Nsukka Area of Enugu State, Nigeria. Animal Research International 2: 342-345.
5. Love SC, Hutchinson GW (2003) Pathology and diagnosis of internal parasites in Ruminants. University of Sydney, Australia.
6. Sissay MM, Uggla A, Waller PJ (2007) Epidemiology and seasonal dynamics of gastrointestinal nematode infections of sheep in a semi-arid region of eastern Ethiopia. Vet Parasitol 143: 311-321.
7. Santín-Durán M, Alunda JM, Hoberg EP, de la Fuente C (2008) Age distribution and seasonal dynamics of abomasal helminths in wild red deerfrom Central Spain, J Parasitol 95: 1031-1037.
8. Ijaz M, Khan MS, Avais M, Ashraf K, Ali MM (2009) Infection rate and chemotherapy of various helminthes in diarrhoeic sheep in and around Lahore. The J Anim Plt Sci 19: 13-16.
9. Burke JM, Kaplan RM, Miller JE, Terrill TH, Getz WR (2007) Accuracy of the famach system for on-farm use by sheep and goat producers in the south eastern U.S. Vet Parasitol 147: 89-95.
10. Almazán C, Avila G, Quiroz H, Ibarra F, Ochoa P (2001) Effect of parasite burden on the detection of Fasciola hepatica antigens in sera and feces of experimentally infected sheep. Vet Parasitol 97: 101-112.
11. Ahmed OF, Mustafa SA, Omer BH (2007) Pathogenesis of Haemonchus contortus in naturally and Experimentally Infected Sudanese Desert Sheep. Global Veterinaria 5: 84-87.
12. Pathogenesis of Haemonchus contortus in naturally and Experimentally Infected Sudanese Desert Sheep.
13. Terefe G, Yacob HT, Grisez C, Prevot F, Dumas E, et al. (2005) Haemonchus contortus eggexcretion and female length reduction in sheep previously infected with Oestrusovis (Diptera:Oestridae) larvae. Vet Parasitol 128: 271-283.
14. Nickdel MB, Roberts F, Brombacher F, Alexander J, Roberts CW (2001) Counter-protective role for interleukin-5 during acuteToxoplasma gondii infection. Infect Immun 69: 1044-1052.
15. Mir RA, Chishti MA, Zargar H, Ganie SA (2007) Clinocopathological changes in sheep experimentally infected with Haemonchus contortus. World J Agric Sci 3: 562-566.
16. Urquhart GM, J Armour, JL Duncan, AM Dunn, FW Jennings (1987) Veterinary parasitology. English Language Book Society, England.
17. Petrie A, Watson P (1999) Statistics for Veterinary and Animal Sciences. Blackwell Science Ltd., London, UK.
18. Qamar MF, Maqbool A (2012) Biochemical studies and sero diagnosis of haemonchusis in sheep and goats. The Journal of Animal & Plant Sciences 22: 32-38.
19. Eslami AH, Nabavi L (1976) Species of gastro-intestinal nematodes of sheep from Iran. Bull Soc Pathol Exot Filiales 69: 92-95.
20. Brunsdon RV (1966) The immunity of sheep to trichostrongyle infestations following reduction of the circulating leucocyte count by oral administrations of chlorambucil. A further study of the spring phenomenon. N Z Vet J 14: 161-162.
21. McKenna PB (1998) The effect of previous cold storage on the subsequent recovery of infective third stage nematode larvae from sheep.Vet Parasitol 80: 167-172.
22. Nayebzadeh H, Seyfiabadshapouri M, Hoghooghi N (2005) Immunization of Arabian sheep against haemonchosis with Haemonchus contortus intestinal homogenate. 15th European Congress of Clinical Microbiology and Infectious Diseases (ECCMID). Copenhagen / Denmark.

23. Balic A, Bowles VM, Meeusen EN (2000) The immunology of gastrointestinal nematodes in ruminants. Adv Parasitol 45: 181-241.

24. Wildblood LA, Kerr K, Clark DA, Cameron A, Turner DG, et al. (2005) Production of eosinophil chemo attractant activity by ovine gastrointestinal nematodes. Vet Immunol Immunopathol 107: 57-65.

25. Yacob HT, Basazinew BK, Basu AK (2008) Experimental concurrent infection of Afar breed goats with Oestrus ovis (L1) and Haemonchus contortus (L3): interaction between parasite populations, changes in parasitological and basic haematological parameters. Exp Parasitol 120: 180-184.

26. Scott I, Dick A, Irvine J, Stear MJ, McKellar QA (1999) The distribution of pepsinogen within the abomasa of cattle and sheep infected with Ostertagia spp. and sheep infected with Haemonchus contortus. Vet Parasitol 82: 145-159.

27. Ahmed Mir M, Zahoor CM, Afzal ZM, Tak H, Ahmed SG (2007) Clinicopathological Changes in Sheep Experimentaly Infected with Haemonchus contortus. World Journal of Agricultural Science 3: 562-566.

28. Zacharias F, Guimarães JE, Araújo RR, Almeida MA, Ayres MC, et al. (2008) Effect of homeopathic medicine on helminth parasitism and resistance of Haemancus contortus infected sheep. Homeopathy 97: 145-151.

29. Ameen SA, Joshua RA, Adedeji OS, Ojedapo LO (2006) Experimental studies on Gastro-Intestinal Nematode Infection; Clinical Observations and Haematological Changes FollowingHaemonchus contortus Infection in West African Dwarf (WAD)kids. Journal of Animal and Veterinary Advance5: 511-514.

30. Wilson AG, Thake DC, Heydens WE, Brewster DW, Hotz KJ (1996) Mode of action of thyroid tumor formation in the male Long–Evans rat administered high doses of alachlor. Fundam Appl Toxicol 3: 16-23.

31. Troell K, Waller P, Höglund J (2005) The development and over winter in survival of free-living larvae of Haemonchus contortus in Sweden. J Helminthol 79: 373-379.

32. Anderson GS (2000) Minimum and maximum development rates of some forensically important Callophoridae (Diptera). J Forensic Sci 45: 824-832.

33. Courtney CH, Parker CF, McClure KE, Herd RP (1984) A comparison of the periparturient rise in fecal egg counts of exotic and domestic ewes. Int J Parasitol 14: 377-381.

34. Rowe A, McMaster K, Emery D, Sangster N (2008) Haemonchus contortus infecK.tion in sheep: Parasite fecundity correlates with worm size and host lymphocyte counts . Vet Parasitol 153: 285-293.

35. Anthony RM, Rutitzky LI, Urban JF Jr, Stadecker MJ, Gause WC (2007) Protective immune mechanisms in helminth infection. Nat Rev Immunol 7: 975-987.

36. Gibbs HC (1967) Some factors involved in the “spring rise” phenomenon in sheep. N.G. Elwert Universitatus und Verlags buch hand lung, Marburg/Lund.

37. O’Sullivan BM, Donald AD (1970) A field study of nematode parasite populations in the lactating ewe. Parasitology 61: 301-315.

38. Hayward AD, Wilson AJ, Pilkington JG, Pemberton JM, Kruuk LE (2009) Ageing in a variable habitat: environmental stress affects senescence in parasite resistance in St Kilda Soay sheep. Proc Biol Sci 276: 3477-3485.

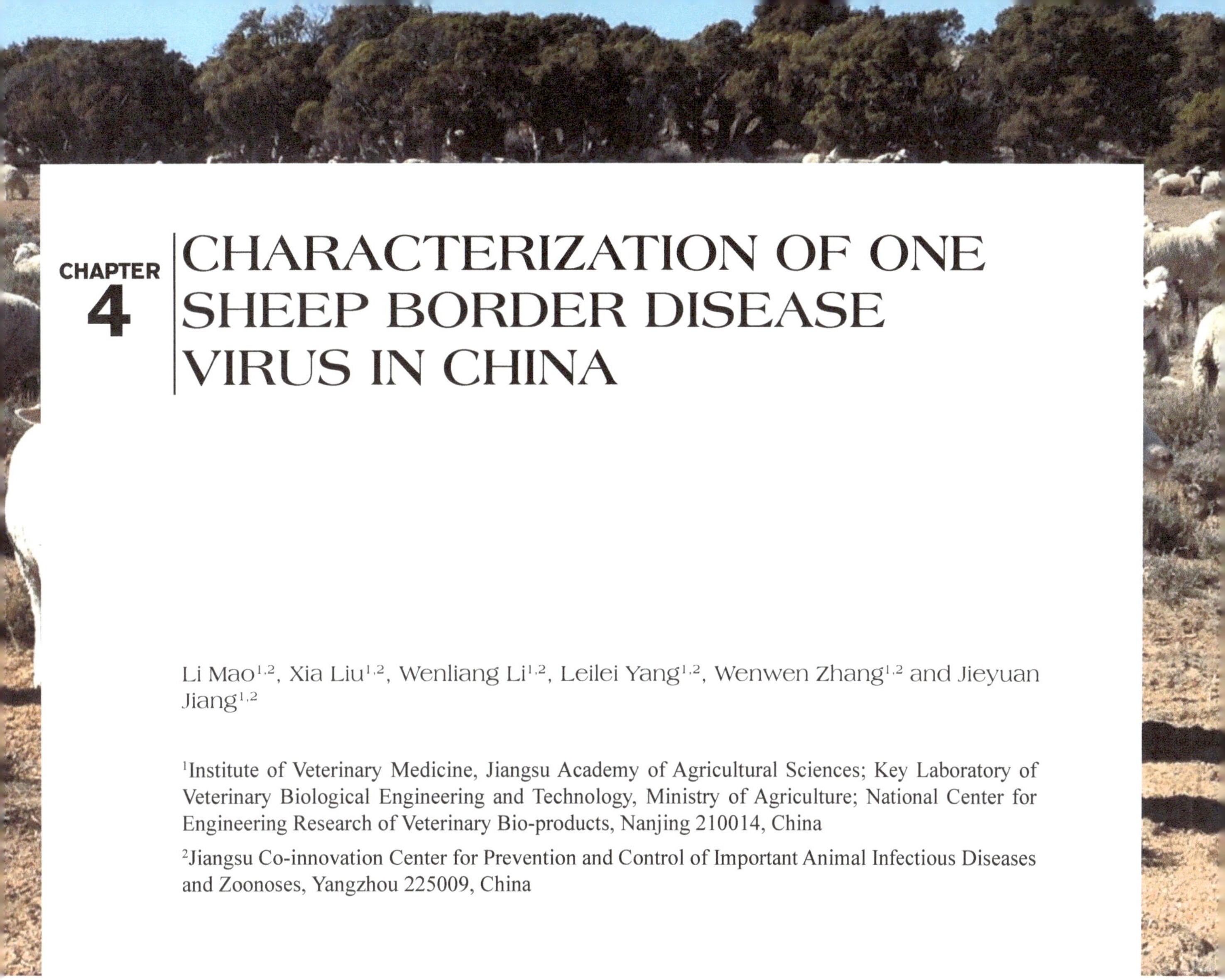

CHAPTER 4

CHARACTERIZATION OF ONE SHEEP BORDER DISEASE VIRUS IN CHINA

Li Mao[1,2], Xia Liu[1,2], Wenliang Li[1,2], Leilei Yang[1,2], Wenwen Zhang[1,2] and Jieyuan Jiang[1,2]

[1]Institute of Veterinary Medicine, Jiangsu Academy of Agricultural Sciences; Key Laboratory of Veterinary Biological Engineering and Technology, Ministry of Agriculture; National Center for Engineering Research of Veterinary Bio-products, Nanjing 210014, China

[2]Jiangsu Co-innovation Center for Prevention and Control of Important Animal Infectious Diseases and Zoonoses, Yangzhou 225009, China

ABSTRACT

Background

Border disease virus (BDV) causes border disease (BD) affecting mainly sheep and goats worldwide. BDV in goat herds suffering diarrhea was recently reported in China, however, infection in sheep was undetermined. Here, BDV infections of sheep herds in Jiangsu, China were screened; a BDV strain was isolated and identified from the sheep flocks in China. The genomic characteristics and pathogenesis of this new isolate were studied.

Results

In 2012, samples from 160 animals in 5 regions of Jiangsu province of China were screened for the presence of BDV genomic RNA and antibody by RT-PCR and ELISA, respectively. 44.4% of the sera were detected positively, and one slowly grown sheep was analyzed to be pestivirus RNA positive and antibody-negative. The sheep kept virus positive and antibody negative in the next 6 months of whole fattening period, and was defined as persistent infection (PI). The virus was isolated in MDBK cells without cytopathic effect (CPE) and named as JSLS12-01. Near-full-length genome sequenced was 12,227 nucleotides (nt). Phylogenetic analysis based on 5'-UTR and N^{pro} fragments showed that the strain belonged to genotype 3, and shared varied homology with the other 3 BDV strains previously isolated from Chinese goats. The genome sequence of JSLS12-01 also had the highest homology with genotype BDV-3 (the strain Gifhorn). Experimental infections of sheep had mild clinical signs as depression and short-period mild fever (5 days). Viremia was detected in 1–7 days post-infection (dpi), and seroconversion began after 14 dpi.

Citation: Li Mao, Xia Liu, Wenliang Li, Leilei Yang, Wenwen Zhang, and Jieyuan Jiang, Characterization of one sheep border disease virus in China, DOI: 10.1186/s12985-014-0217-9

Conclusions

This study reported the genomic and pathogenesis characterizations of one sheep BDV strain, which confirmed the occurrence of BDV infection in Chinese sheep. This sheep derived BDV strain was classified as BDV-3, together with the goat derived strains in China. These results might be helpful for further understanding of BDV infection in China and useful for prevention and control of BDV infections in the future.

BACKGROUND

Pestivirus is a genus within family *Flaviviridae*, comprises four recognized species, namely border disease virus (BDV) of small ruminants, bovine viral diarrhea viruses 1 and 2 (BVDV-1, BVDV-2) of cattle and classical swine fever virus (CSFV) of pigs, respectively [1]. Recently, new pestivirus species, such as Giraffe virus, Pronghorn virus, Bungowannah virus and HoBi-like virus have been discovered [2,3].

BDV infects small ruminants (sheep and goats) and causes border disease worldwide. Several BDV strains have been proved to infect pigs and cattle under experimental or nature conditions [4,5]. BD shares some similar characteristics with BVDV infections in cattle and goats, however, with more pronounced emphasis on a wide range of productive diseases, such as abortions, stillbirths or mummified fetuses, barren ewes, malformations and the birth of weak lambs, which leads to a considerable economic effect. The affected lambs show abnormal body conformation and "hairy-shaker" syndrome named due to the hairy fleeces and tremors of the suffered lambs [6]. Small weak lambs can be persistently infected (PI) and the virus is wide spread in all organs in infected animals. However, BDV infections in pregnant goats result exclusively in abortions and malformations in fetuses and neonates, and PI goats are rarely found out via placenta [7]. An experiment infection was carried out in pregnant ewes with BDV-4, besides a high number of stillbirths up to 32%, significantly reduced bodyweight of lambs was also observed [8]. Although severe clinical outbreaks of BD are unusual, several epizootics have been reported in sheep and goats [9-11].

The pestivirus genome consists of a positive single-stranded RNA approximately 12.3 kb in length, encoding a single open reading frame (ORF) flanked by 5'- and 3'-untranslated regions (UTR). The genome codes 4 structural proteins, the capsid (C) and three envelope proteins (E^{rns}, E1 and E2), plus seven or eight non-structural proteins [12,13]. Except the 5'-UTR region, the N^{pro} and E2 genes have also been used for genetic classification of new virus isolates [14,15]. Based on recent reports, BDV isolates have been divided into seven genotypes at least, and widely distributed in different countries, such as many European countries, Australia, New Zealand, Canada, the United States, India, Turkey, and Japan [7,16]. In 2012, BDV infections were first confirmed in several goat herds suffering serious diarrhea, and three BDV strains were isolated in China [11]. This was the first confirmed evidence of BDV genotype 3 circulations in Chinese goats, In order to further investigate the epidemic information of BDV in goats and sheep in the same regions of China, BDV sero-epidemiological survey was carried out in our lab. One BDV strain named JSLS12-01 was isolated from one slow-grown sheep. And the genomic characteristics and pathogenesis of the isolate was determined. The data might be more supplement for BDV epidemiology, pathogenicity as well as its relationship with clinical diseases in China.

RESULTS

Antibody and Viral Detection

One hundred and sixty sera from sheep and goats in five regions of Jiangsu, China were collected and detected by BDV ELISA kits (SVANOVA). The positive rate was 44.4% (71/160), with 46.3% (63/136) of goats and 33.3% (8/24) of sheep, respectively. The positive rates varied from 16.7% (2/12) to 85.7% (12/14) with the flocks (Table 1). Sero-prevalence was at least 50% in two sheep herds and one goat herd from two regions of Jiangsu (Table 1).

Table 1: Results of the diagnostic tests performed with samples using ELISA and RT-PCR

Farm	Regions	Goats/sheep	ELISA	RT-PCR
1	Suining, Xuzhou	Goats	85.7%(12/14)	1/14
2	Suining, Xuzhou	sheep	16.7%(2/12)	0/12
3	Siyang, Suqian	Goats	36%(9/25)	1/25
4	Rudong, Nantong	Goats	34.2%(13/38)	NT
5	Rudong, Nantong	sheep	50%(4/8)	0/8
6	Haian, Nantong	Goats	49.2%(29/59)	NT
7	Lishui, Nanjing	sheep	50%(2/4)	1/4

NT, Sample not tested.

In the sheep herds, an antibody-negative sheep (2 month old) from Nanjing, Jiangsu was detected positive by RT-PCR, which showed the very bright bands of 290 bp and 225 bp amplified by panpesti generic primers and BDV specific primers PBD1/PBD2, respectively. The RT-PCR products were purified and sequenced, which shared high homology with BDV strains by BLAST analysis. The RT-PCR results also showed two samples from goats were tested positive, 5'-UTR sequences were compared to sequences from GenBank, and shared 100% homology with JS12-04 strain reported previously.

Virus Isolation

The BDV RNA-positive serum was cultured and passaged in MDBK cells. After the third passage, BDV cultures have been positively detected by RT-PCR and confirmed with sequencing. However, no CPE was observed during the process of passage. The new BDV isolate was named as JSLS12-01.

Subsequent Clinical Observations and Serological Analysis

Four sampling sheep including the BDV positive were continued to rear for clinical investigation subsequently, with the same feed and management conditions. Compared to the BDV negative sheep, the infected lamb was thinner, weaker, and poorer growth, and the body weight was about 20% less at the end of fattening period (6 month long). However, no other clinical signs were observed. The four sheep were tested once 4 weeks apart, and BDV RNA was positively detected by RT-PCR and the BDV specific antibody was negative for the original BDV positive animal in the whole grown period.

Complete Genome Sequencing and Phylogenetic Analysis

RT-PCR products (Figure 1) were purified and cloned to pJET1.2 vectors for sequencing. The near full genome sequence of BDV JSLS12-01 strain was obtained and deposited in GenBank under accession number KC963426 and reported recently [17], the obtained genome of JSLS12-01 was 12, 227 nucleotides (nt) in length. The isolate shared 80.3% nucleotide homology and 89.9% amino acid homology with goat derived strain Gifhorn (a prototype of BDV-3), respectively (Table 2). It shared 72.2-77.6% homology with other BDV genotypes strains available in GenBank (Table 2). The homology with CSFV and BVDV strains were about 71% and 67%, respectively (Table 2). The whole genome sequence based phylogenetic analysis indicated that JSLS12-01 was classified into the same branch with Gifhorn with 100% bootstrap value, and matched up with the result of the Blast analysis. The isolate clearly differed from other BDV strains and other pestivirus species (CSFVs or BVDVs) (Figure 2).

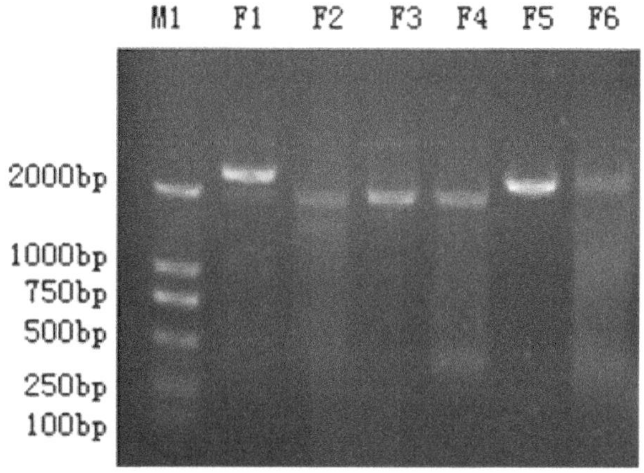

Figure 1: Six overlapping fragments covering the complete genome of JSLS12-01 (F1~F6). F1-F6 were six overlapping RT-PCR products covering the virus genome, the size of each fragment was matched sizes in the Table 1. M1: DM2000 marker.

Table 2: The homology of complete coding gene and protein sequence between JSLS12-01 and partial BDV strains

Virus strain	GenBank accession number	Pestivirus species	JSLS12-01	
			Homology of complete coding gene (%)	Homology of protein (%)
FNK2012-1	AB897785	BDV-1	77.5	86.4
BD31	U70263	BDV-1	77.0	85.6
X818	AF037405	BDV-1	76.9	85.5
Reindeer-1	AF144618	BDV-2	77.3	86.5
Gifhorn	KF925348	BDV-3	80.3	89.9
H2121	GU270877	BDV-4	77.5	87.2
Aveyron	KF918753	BDV-5	77.6	87.0
Aydin/04-TR	JX428945	BDV-7	72.2	80.1
HCLV	AF091507	CSFV	71.0	78.5
Shimen	AF092448	CSFV	71.2	79.0
KE9	EF101530	BVDV-1	67.0	72.0
6151	JN380083	BVDV-1	67.2	72.6
RNV17	JN380090	BVDV-2	67.4	72.3
XJ-04	FJ527854	BVDV-2	66.9	71.7

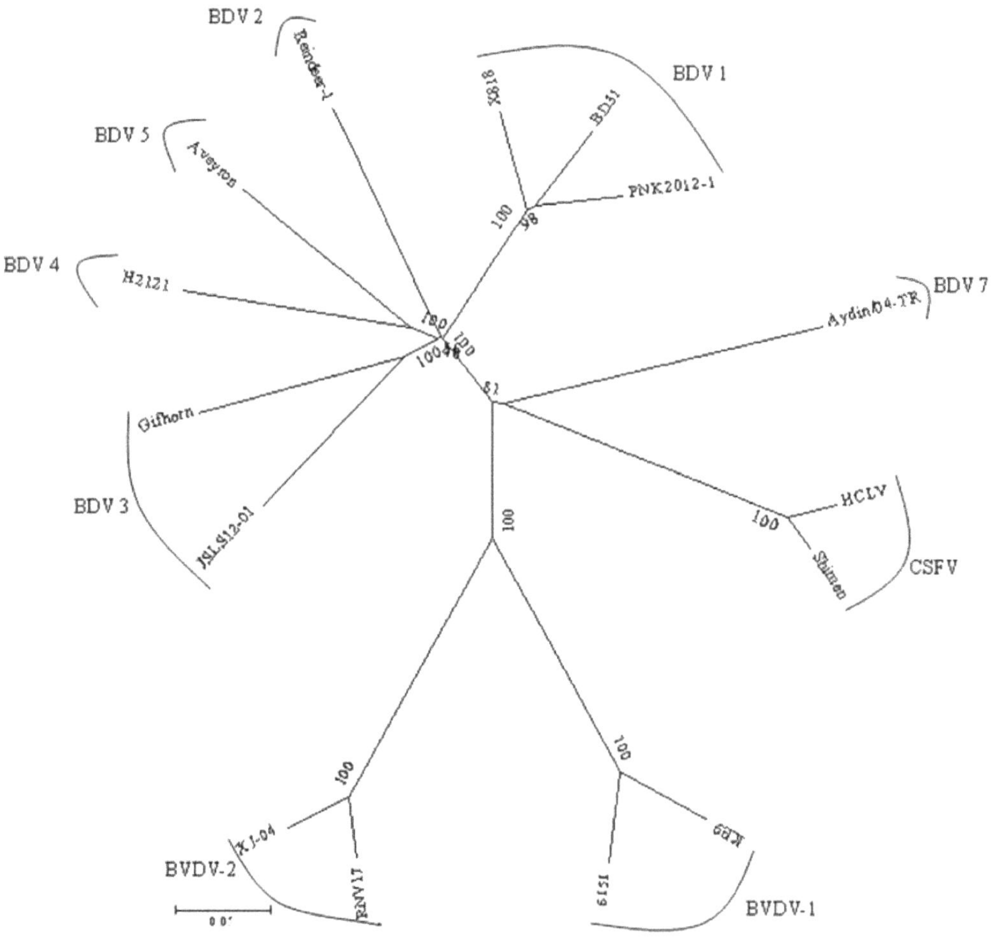

Figure 2: Phylogenetic analysis based on the complete coding sequence of BDV strains using the Neighbour-joining method. The numbers close to the major nodes indicate the bootstrap values (in %; 1000 replicates). Bar: number of substitutions per site.

5›-UTR and N^pro^ sequences of the virus were aligned with the corresponding sequences of BDV reference strains and the evolutionary relationship between these isolates was estimated by phylogenetic analysis to further characterize the JSLS12-01 isolate. The phylogenetic tree based on 5'-UTR region (225 bp) showed that the JSLS12-01 strain was grouped with BDV-3 respective strains (Figure 3). Comparison of 5›-UTR sequences revealed that BDV JSLS12-01 shared nucleotide identities of 78.6%, 83.5% and 94.4% with BDV-3 Chinese strains AH12-02, AH12-01 and JS12-04, respectively. The virus was 87.7%, 87.4% and 89.0% homology with other BDV-3 strains including Gifhorn from Spanish goats, 90-F-6338 and 90-F-6227 from sheep of France, respectively (Table 3); and also 82.5% to 85.7% with BDV-1; 84.1% with BDV-2; 76.4% to 85.1% with BDV-4; 84.2% to 85.0% with BDV-5; 86.7% with BDV- 6; 71.5% to 72.9% with BDV-7; and 70.5% to 72.6% with BDV Tunisian; respectively (Table 3). The highest identity of nucleotide sequence was 94.4% with the strain JS12-04 isolated in 2012 from Chinese goats (Table 3). JSLS12-01 shared the highest homology (73.2% to 80.7%) with other BDV-3 members on the N^{pro} sequences (Table 3). And based on the phylogenetic tree of the N^{pro}sequences also grouped the strain JSLS12-01 into BDV-3 (data not shown).

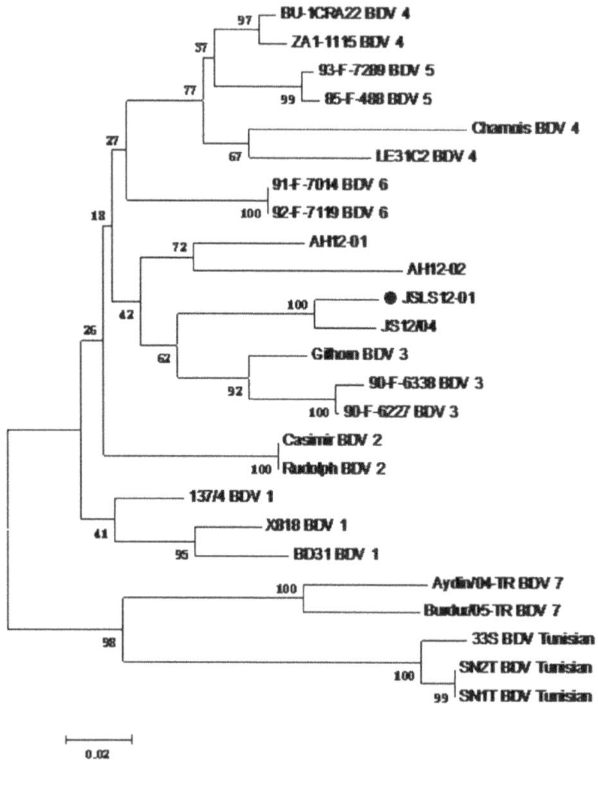

Figure 3: Neighbour-joining phylogenetic tree constructed using 225 nt 5'-UTR fragments of the pestivirus sequences found

in this study and from the GenBank. Representatives of BDV sequences have been described in Li et al. [11]. The numbers close to the major nodes indicate the bootstrap values (in %; 1000 replicates). Bar: number of substitutions per site.

Table 3: The homology of 5'-UTR and N ^{pro} genes between JSLS12-01 and partial BDV strains

Virus strain	Genotype	JSLS12-01	
		Homology of 5'-UTR gene (%)	Homology of N ^{pro} gene (%)
X818	BDV-1	82.5	64.1
BD31	BDV-1	82.6	63.7
137/4	BDV-1	85.7	66.3
Casimir	BDV-2	84.1	-
Rudolph	BDV-2	84.1	-
Gifhorn	BDV 3	87.7	73.2
AH12-01	BDV-3	83.5	75.8
AH12-02	BDV-3	78.6	73.2
JS12-04	BDV-3	94.4	80.7
90-F-6338	BDV-3	87.4	75.0
90-F-6227	BDV-3	89.0	74.6
BU-1CRA22	BDV-4	85.1	64.4
ZA1-1115	BDV-4	83.2	-
Chamois	BDV-4	76.4	-
LE31C2	BDV-4	79.3	-
85-F-488	BDV-5	84.2	70.1
93-F-7289	BDV-5	85.0	70.5
91-F-7014	BDV-6	86.7	68.1
92-F-7119	BDV-6	86.7	68.5
Burdur/05-TR	BDV-7	72.9	54.7
Aydin/04-TR	BDV-7	71.5	55.7
SN1T	BDV Tunisian	72.6	53.7
33S	BDV Tunisian	70.5	53.7
SN2T	BDV Tunisian	71.3	53.9

-: The sequence could not be obtained in GenBank.

Pathogenicity of BDV JSLS12-01

All 3 lambs (45 day old) infected with BDV JSLS12-01 cell cultures showed only moderated depression without other clinical signs. The infected animals developed high rectal temperatures (40.0-41.0°C), with peak temperatures appearing on 3–7 day-post-infection (dpi) and returned to the normal level on 8 dpi, while the control sheep kept normal during the same period (Figure 4). RT-PCR and virus isolation revealed that the virus could lead to viremia in the infected animals at 1-7dpi. The infected animals began seroconverted on 14 dpi and kept to increase in the following period (Figure 5).

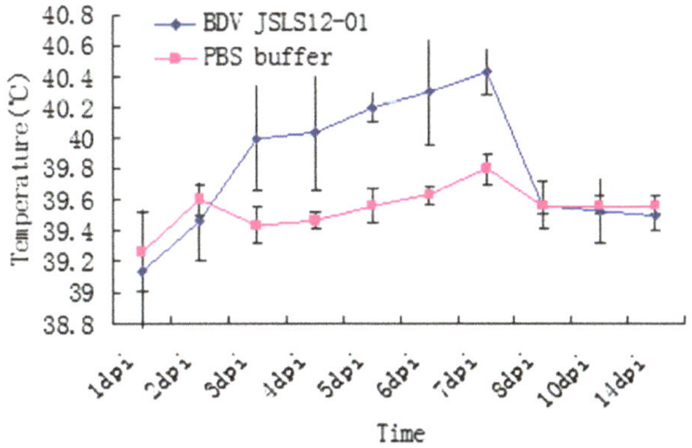

Figure 4: Body temperature observation of the experimental sheep. The body temperature of BDV JSLS12-01 infected sheep group and control group were measured at the same time during the first 14 days.

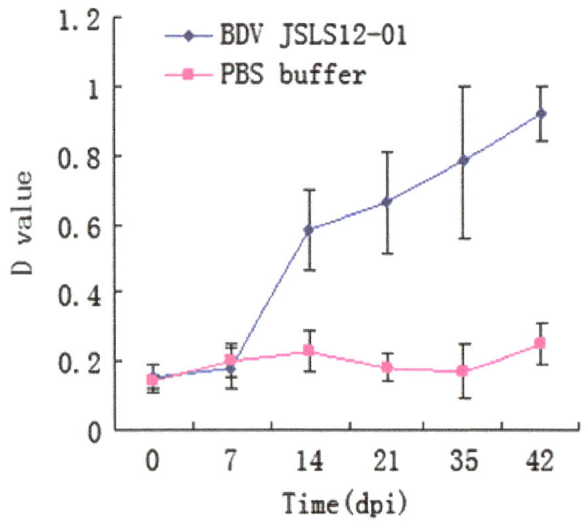

Figure 5: Antibody test of the experimental sheep. Serum samples of 0, 7, 14, 21, 35 and 42 dpi were tested for BDV specific antibodies using ELISA kit (SVANOVA).

DISCUSSION

Goats are major rearing small ruminants, and the numbers of sheep and rearing sheep farms are relative a few in Jiangsu and Anhui provinces of eastern China. BDV had been identified in Chinese diseased goats [11]. In the present study, BDV sero-epidemiological survey was carried out for goat and sheep by BDV ELISA kit and RT-PCR. Serum samples from seven flocks (4 of goats and 3 of sheep) in five regions were tested positive by ELISA (Table 1), which indicated the ubiquity of BDV infection in the small ruminant flocks. Four sheep including one was BDV RNA positive with RT-PCR were kept for the next 6 month rearing. The sheep was BDV Ab negative and viremia for the observation period; and identified as one PI animal according to the reports [7]. The PI sheep mainly showed poor-growing were agreement with BDV-4 virus infections [8]; however, classical clinical signs of BD such as paralysis and an abnormal fleece known as 'hairy shaker' were not appeared. In addition, the previous goat derived BDVs were identified from herds with diarrhea [11]. These uncharacteristic signs emphasized the difficulty of BD diagnosis based on clinical signs and the requirement for routine and accurate laboratory tests.

Phylogenetic segregations of pestiviruses into individual species and subgroups are only identified by the branching order of the phylogenetic tree [18]. The genetic diversity of BDV is greater than that of other pestivirus species. According to the molecular diversity, BDV have been divided to seven groups at least [7,19,20]. The near full sequence of the JSLS12-01 had a closer relationship with BDV-3 strains at gene level comparing with other pestivirus reference strains (BDV-1,BDV-2, BDV-3, BDV-4,BDV-5 and BDV-7). And the strain should be one new BDV-3 strain with a lot of nucleotide or amino acid variation to the respective BDV strains (Figure 2, Table 2). The isolate JSLS12-01 was the highest homology with the strain JS12-04 on the 5'-UTR and N^{pro} gene compositions, and the two viruses were isolated from sheep or goats in different regions of Jiangsu province, however, the virus JSLS12-01 had much lesser identity with the other two viruses AH12-01 and AH12-02 on the gene levels (Table 3 and Figure 3), and the late two were from Anhui province (neighborhood each other). It indicated the epidemic BDV strains in China might have complex endemic situations, and have existed for a relative long period. The BDVs in China have mutated a lot, and may form different sub-branches, such as the two strains JS12-04 and JSLS12-01 isolated in Jiangsu province formed one cluster, and the strains AH12-01 and AH12-02 from Anhui were much closed each other (Figure 3).

In addition, based on sequence alignment and phylogenetic analysis, the 4 Chinese BDV strains showed the high diversity of on the 5›-UTR compositions (Table 3) even though all of them were in BDV-3 genotype (Figure 3) [11]. The strain JSLS12-01 was only 83.5% and 78.6% homology with the strains AH12-01 and AH12-02 on 5›-UTR gene (Table 3), respectively. Furthermore, it was also found that JSLS12-01 had a very high homology of 5›-UTR sequences with other genotype viruses, such as 85.1%, 86.7% and 85% with the strains BU-1CRA22 (BDV-4), 92-F-7119 (BDV-6) and 93-F-7289 (BDV-5) (Table 3), respectively. It was true that the homology of BDV strains in the same genotype might be much less than the viruses being other genotypes. And it appeared that the BDV genotyping based on the 5›-UTR sequences could be still consummated.

Animal experiment was performed upon conventionally rearing sheep to evaluate the pathogenicity of the new BDV strain. JSLS12-01 could induce mild clinical diseases; the infected animals showed viremia at 1–7 dpi and disappeared after 7 dpi, during the same period, mild short-term pyrexia was observed (Figure 4). In addition, the infected animals seroconverted from 14 dpi (Figure 5). No other classical BD symptom was observed. The clinical symptoms of natural infected sheep mainly showed slow-growing and persisted infection. Symptoms of natural and experimental infection were very diverse, this might be related to the immune state and age of the virus infected animals and so on. To date, experimental infections of BDV have not been performed in China, the results would help to understand the pathogenicity of Chinese BDV strains in small ruminants and further systemic studies will be done in the future.

CONCLUSIONS

In conclusion, BDV infections of sheep were demonstrated in China, and the BDV JSLS12-01 strain was clustered in BDV-3 subgroups, the predominant genotype in China. The BDV infections of goats and sheep appeared with various clinical signs and epidemic information. More studies should be carried out to make sure of the virulence and biologic characteristics of BDV.

METHODS

Ethics Statement

This study was performed in strict accordance with the guidelines of Jiangsu Province Animal Regulations (Government Decree No 45). The protocol was approved by the Committee on the Ethics of Animal Experiments of the Institute of Veterinary Medicine, Jiangsu Academy of Agricultural Sciences (JAAS No 20100604).

Clinical Sampling and Observation

Serum samples were collected from 3 young sheep farms and 4 goat farms (about 2 months old) from 5 different regions in Jiangsu province of China (Table 1). A total of 24 sera from sheep and 136 sera from goats were collected. The sheep tested for BDV positive were continuously carried out for subsequent clinical observations and serological analysis in next 6 months (the fattening period) after the first sampling.

ELISA

BDV antibody detection was performed on serum samples of goats and sheep using a commercially available kit (SVANOVA BDV-Ab kit, SVANOVA Biotech, Uppsala, Sweden) according to the manufacturer's instructions.

Virus isolation

Virus isolation was carried out on the positive samples of pestivirus 5'-UTR RT-PCR as reports [16] and briefly introduced as following: the serum samples were centrifuged at 12,000 rpm for 20 min at 4°C and filtered through 0.22 μm filter, and subsequently inoculated onto confluent monolayers of Madin-Darby bovine kidney (MDBK) cells (obtained from China Institute of Veterinary Drugs Control) to culture for 96 hours with 1% FCS DMEM at 37°C and 5% CO_2 conditions. The original cells and FCS were proven to be free of pestivirus antigen and antibodies. The isolation of BDV was checked by RT-PCR as next described using Panpesti generic primers and BDV specific primers PBD1/PBD2 [21,22].

RT-PCR Detection and Complete Genomic Sequence Analysis

Sera from sheep and goats were tested for the presence of pestivirus by RT-PCR method. To detect the BDV virus, total RNA was extracted from serum samples and cell cultures by using the TRizol reagent (Invitrogen) according to the manufacturer's instruction. RT-PCR was carried out in a 50 μL reaction mixture containing 1× RT-PCR buffer (TAKARA, Bio, Inc.), 20 pM of each primer (Panpesti generic primers and BDV specific primers PBD1/PBD2 targeting 5›-UTR, with expected product sizes of 290 bp and 225 bp, respectively) [21,22], 2 U of one-step Enzyme Mix (TAKARA, Bio, Inc.) and 4 μL of RNA. The reaction was run in a thermocycler (Mjmini, BIO-RAD) according to the following program: reverse transcription at 50°C for 30 min, denaturation at 95°C for 5 min, 35 cycles at 94°C for 30 s, 54°C for 30 s and 72°C for 45 s, terminated with a final extension of 10 min at 72°C.

For the genomic long RNA RT-PCR, the extension time was 1 kb for 1 min. Amplification products were detected by electrophoresis in 1.2% agarose gels. Positive RT-PCR fragments were purified (Axygen), cloned to pJET1.2 vector (Thermo), and then transformed to *E. coli* DH5α. Positive clones, as confirmed by PCR and enzyme digestion, were sequenced. Three positive clones of each RT-PCR fragment were sequenced using the appropriate PCR primers for correct check.

Briefly, six pairs of primers were designed to amplify the 6 overlapping fragments covering the virus genome, and summarized as Table 4. The retrieved sequences were edited and assembled with SeqManTM program version 5.03 of the DNASTAR package to obtain the complete sequence of this new BDV strain.

Table 4: The primer sequence of the complete genome sequence

Amplified fragments	primer	Primer sequences(5'->3')	Location (bp)	Fragment size
F1	BVDV-F	GCCATGCCCTTAGTAGGACTAGC	1~23	2200 bp
	BDV-2300R	TATCAGGAAGGCTGTTGTCGA	2255~2273	
F2	BDV-2240 F	TTGGTGGCCATACGAGACAAC	2144~2164	1900 bp
	BDV-4140R	TGTCAAGATGAAGAATAGGGG	4023~4043	
F3	BDV-4010 F	AAGCAGTGGCTACAATCCGTG	3912~3932	1950 bp
	BDV-5960R	CATCTCTCCAATCCTCAGGTT	5865~5885	
F4	BDV-5940 F	GCAGAAGCACCCTAGCATAGC	5840~5860	2000 bp
	BDV-7940R	TATGACTACGCTCTCCAGCCG	7929~7945	
F5	BDV-7885 F	GCCTTACGCATCTCAAGCCCTC	7787~7808	2200 bp
	BDV-10110R	TGCCTCGTATGGGTGTATTTTC	10001~10022	
F6	BDV-10010 F	CAGAGCATATGGTGTCAGCATATCAG	9907~9932	2300 bp
	BDV-12326R	GGGGCTGTTAGGGTTTTTCCTTAATCC	12201~12227	

Phylogenetic Analysis

The complete coding sequence of the virus was aligned with some represented BDV, BVDV 1, BVDV 2 and CSFV strain genome sequences. The 5'-UTR and N^{pro} sequences were analyzed with sequences of BDV reference strains using 1.83 and MEGA 4.0.2, the 225 bp 5›-UTR fragments (PBD1/PBD2 product) and 487 bp N^{pro} gene (corresponding to 394-880 bp of Gifhorn genome) sequences were used for analysis, respectively. Phylogenetic analysis was carried out using the neighbor-joining (NJ) method using 1000 replicates for determination the bootstrap values.

Experimental Infection

Six one-month-old healthy sheep were tested negative for pestivirus (BDV and BVDV) infections by commercial ELISA kit (BDV: SVANOVA and BVDV: BIO-X) and RT-PCR mentioned above. They were further confirmed to be free of micoplasma infections by PCR. The sheep were randomly divided into two groups, with 3 animals in each group. Sheep of the experimental group was infected by intramuscular injection with 10^5 $TCID_{50}$ of BDV JSLS12-01 cell cultures, while the sheep in control group were inoculated with PBS buffer. All animals were monitored daily for clinical signs including depression, nasal discharge, diarrhea, coughing and rectal temperature. Serum samples were collected at day −2 to 0 prior to infection and 1, 3, 5, 7, 14, 21, 28, 35 and 42 dpi. Serum samples of days 1, 3, 5, 7, 14 and 21 were tested for viremia by RT-PCR described above. And the procedures to isolate BDV from the sera were described above. Serum samples of days 0, 7, 14, 21, 35 and 42 were tested for BDV specific antibodies using commercial ELISA kit (SVANOVA).

ACKNOWLEDGEMENTS

This work was supported by the Special Fund for Independent Innovation of Agricultural Science and Technology in Jiangsu province [CX (14)2090] and Jiangsu Provincial Natural Science Foundation of China [BK20130729].

AUTHORS' CONTRIBUTIONS

LM, XL, WL, and JJ participated in the design and conducted the majority of the experiments in the study. LM drafted the manuscript. LY and WZ contributed to the samples detection. JJ revised the manuscript. All authors read and approved the final manuscript.

REFERENCES

1. Vilcek S, Leskova V, Meyer D, Postel A, Becher P: Molecular characterization of border disease virus strain Aveyron. *Vet Microbiol* 2014, 171:87–92.
2. Liu L, Xia H, Wahlberg N, Belák S, Baule C: Phylogeny, classification and evolutionary insights into pestiviruses. *Virology* 2009, 385:351–357.
3. Mao L, Li W, Zhang W, Yang L, Jiang J: Genome sequence of a novel Hobi-like pestivirus in China. *J Virol* 2012, 86:12444.
4. Cabezón O, Rosell R, Sibila M, Lavín S, Marco I, Segalés J: Experimental infection of pigs with Border disease virus isolated from Pyrenean chamois (Rupicapra pyrenaica). *J Vet Diagn Investig* 2010, 22:360–365.
5. Sharp MW, Rawson BC: The cost of border disease infection in a commercial flock. *Vet Rec* 1986, 119:128–130.
6. Nettleton PF, Gilray JA, Russo P, Dlissi E: Border disease of sheep and goats. *Vet Res* 1998, 29:327–340.
7. Oguzoglu TC, Tan MT, Toplu N, Demir AB, Bilge-Dagalp S, Karaoglu T, Ozkul A, Alkan F, Burgu I, Haas L, Greiser-Wilke I:Border disease virus (BDV) infections of small ruminants in Turkey: A new BDV subgroup? *Vet Microbiol* 2009,135:374–379.
8. García-Pérez AL, Minguijón E, Estévez L, Barandika JF, Aduriz G, Juste RA, Hurtado A: Clinical and laboratorial findings in pregnant ewes and their progeny infected with Border disease virus (BDV-4 genotype). *Res Vet Sci* 2009, 86:345–352.
9. Mainar-Jaime RC, Vazquez-Boland JA: Associations of veterinary services and farmer characteristics with the prevalences of brucellosis and border disease in small ruminants in Spain. *Prev Vet Med* 1999, 40:193–205.
10. Valdazo-González B, Alvarez-Martinez M, Greiser-Wilke I: Genetic typing and prevalence of Border disease virus (BDV) in small ruminant flocks in Spain. *Vet Microbiol* 2006, 117:141–153.
11. Li W, Mao L, Zhao Y, Sun Y, He K, Jiang J: Detection of border disease virus (BDV) in goat herds suffering diarrhea in eastern China. *Virol J* 2013, 10:80. doi:10.1186/1743-422X-10-80.
12. Becher P, Orlich M, Thiel HJ: Complete genomic sequence of border disease virus, a pestivirus from sheep. *J Virol*1998, 72:5165–5173.
13. Collett MS, Larson R, Gold C, Strick D, Anderson DK, Purchio AF: Molecular cloning and nucleotide sequence of the pestivirus bovine viral diarrhea virus. *Virology* 1988, 165:191–199.
14. Couvreur B, Letellier C, Collard A, Quenon P, Dehan P, Hamers C, Pastoret PP, Kerkhofs P: Genetic and antigenic variability in bovine viral diarrhea virus (BVDV) isolates from Belgium. *Virus Res* 2002, 85:17–28.
15. Hurtado A, García-Pérez AL, Aduriz G, Juste RA: Genetic diversity of ruminant pestiviruses from Spain. *Virus Res* 2003,92:67–73.
16. Strong R, La Rocca SA, Ibata G, Sandvik T: Antigenic and genetic characterisation of border disease viruses isolated from UK cattle. *Vet Microbiol* 2010, 141:208–215.
17. Liu X, Mao L, Li W, Yang L, Zhang W, Wei J, Jiang J: Genome Sequence of a Border Disease Virus in China. *Genome Annouc* 2013, 1(6).
18. Becher P, Avalos Ramirez R, Orlich M, Cedillo Rosales S, König M, Schweizer M, Stalder H, Schirrmeier H, Thiel HJ: Genetic and antigenic characterization of novel pestivirus genotypes: implication for classification. *Virology* 2003, 311:96–104.
19. Dubois E, Russo P, Prigent M, Thiéry R: Genetic characterization of ovine pestiviruses isolated in France, between 1985 and 2006. *Vet Microbiol* 2008, 130:69–79.
20. Thabti F, Letellier C, Hammami S, Pépin M, Ribière M, Mesplède A, Kerkhofs P, Russo P: Detection of a novel border disease virus subgroup in Tunisian sheep. *Arch Virol* 2005, 150:215–229.
21. Albayrak H, Gumusova SO, Ozan E, Yazici Z: Molecular detection of pestiviruses in aborted foetuses from provinces in northern Turkey. *Trop Anim Health Prod* 2012, 44:677–680.
22. Vilcek S, Herring AJ, Herring JA, Nettleton PF, Lowings JP, Paton DJ: Pestiviruses isolated from pigs, cattle and sheep can be allocated into at least three genogroups using polymerase chain reaction and restriction endonuclease analysis. *Arch Virol* 1994, 136:309–323.

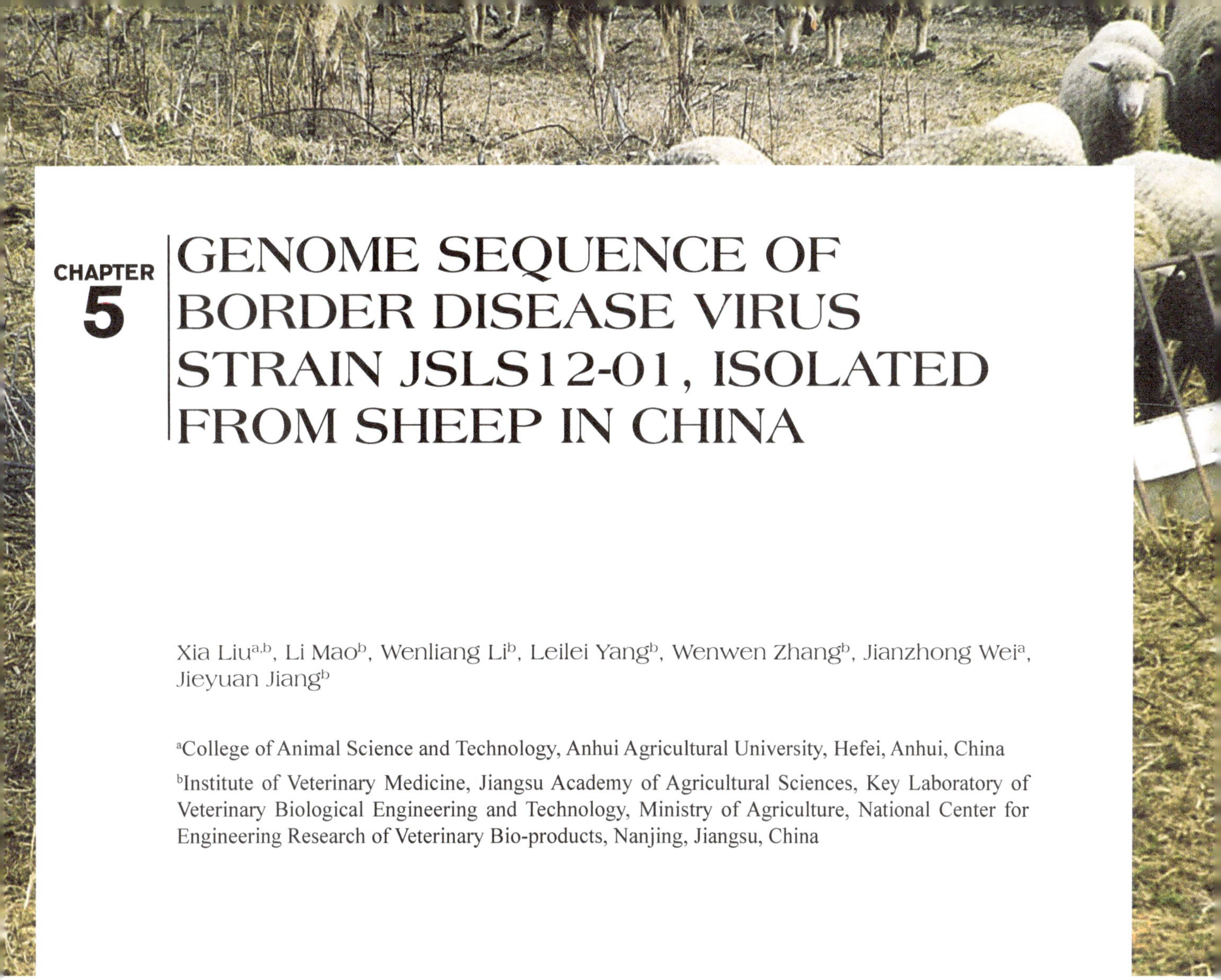

CHAPTER 5

GENOME SEQUENCE OF BORDER DISEASE VIRUS STRAIN JSLS12-01, ISOLATED FROM SHEEP IN CHINA

Xia Liu[a,b], Li Mao[b], Wenliang Li[b], Leilei Yang[b], Wenwen Zhang[b], Jianzhong Wei[a], Jieyuan Jiang[b]

[a]College of Animal Science and Technology, Anhui Agricultural University, Hefei, Anhui, China

[b]Institute of Veterinary Medicine, Jiangsu Academy of Agricultural Sciences, Key Laboratory of Veterinary Biological Engineering and Technology, Ministry of Agriculture, National Center for Engineering Research of Veterinary Bio-products, Nanjing, Jiangsu, China

ABSTRACT

Border disease virus (BDV) is a recognized virus in the genus *Pestivirus* and causes border disease (BD) in sheep and goats. Here, a novel BDV strain, JSLS12-01, was identified from sheep in Jiangsu Province, China. The complete coding sequence (CDS) was finished, which provides a better understanding of the molecular evolution of BDV isolates.

GENOME ANNOUNCEMENT

Border disease (BD) in many domestic animals, mainly sheep and goats, is caused by border disease virus (BDV), a positive-sense single-stranded RNA virus in the genus *Pestivirus* of the family *Flaviviridae*, and has substantial loss-related economic implications worldwide (**1**). The disease is basically characterized by reproductive manifestations, such as abortions, stillbirths, barren ewes, congenital disorders of lambs, and weak lambs. BDV is confirmed to persistently infect animals (2). Severe clinical outbreaks of BD are unusual, but several epizootics have been reported in sheep (3, 4). An experimental infection carried out in pregnant ewes with BDV-4 led to a high number of stillbirths, up to 32%, and significantly reduced the body weight of lambs (5). BDV infections have been reported worldwide, such as in India, Japan, Australia, Canada, the United States, and many European countries (**6**). In China, BDV was first detected from some diseased goats suffering from diarrhea in 2012, and the isolates were closely grouped with the reference Gifhorn strain of BDV-3 (7).

In this study, the complete coding sequence of BDV strain JSLS12-01 was described. It was detected and identified in a sheep blood serum sample. The total RNA extracted by using the TRIzol (Invitrogen) was reverse transcribed and amplified by PCR, and PCR fragments were cloned to pJET1.2 vector (Thermo) and sequenced. The genome was assembled using DNAStar (version 7.0).

This study was performed in strict accordance with the guidelines of Jiangsu Province Animal Regulations (government decree no. 45). The protocol was approved by the Committee on the Ethics of Animal Experiments of the Institute of Veterinary Medicine, Jiangsu Academy of Agricultural Sciences (JAAS no. 20100604).

Citation: Xia Liua, Li Mao, Wenliang Li, Leilei Yang, Wenwen Zhang, Jianzhong Wei, Jieyuan Jiang, Genome Sequence of Border Disease Virus Strain JSLS12-01, Isolated from Sheep in China, doi: 10.1128/genomeA.00502-13.

The sequenced fragment of JSLS12-01 comprising 12,227 nucleotides (nt) includes a large open reading frame of 11,694 nt, which encodes a single polyprotein flanked by near-full 5′ (278 nt) and the complete 3′ (255 nt) ends of the untranslated regions (UTRs). The 5′-UTR sequence was analyzed by ClustalX tools and MEGA 4.0.2 software with reference sequences, and phylogenetic analysis indicated that the current isolate was a newly isolated branch belonging to BDV-3 together with respective strains. Compared with the BDV strains available in GenBank, the genome sequence of JSLS12-01 has 80%, 78%, 77%, and 77% nucleotide sequence homologies with that of BDV strains Gifhorn, H2121, X818, and BD31, respectively. It displays the closest relationship to strain Gifhorn, the recognized prototype BDV-3. The amino acid sequence of the virus has 90% identity with that of Gifhorm.

BDV infection in goats occurred in China; however, no cases of BD have been reported in sheep flocks. This survey demonstrates that BDV also infected sheep in China. The results of the JSLS12-01 sequence might enhance the understanding of BDV epidemiology and evolutionary mechanisms, not only in China but also worldwide.

Nucleotide Sequence Accession Number: The complete coding sequence of BDV strain JSLS12-01 has been deposited in GenBank under the accession no.KC963426.

ACKNOWLEDGMENT

This work was supported by the Special Fund for Independent Innovation of Agricultural Science and Technology in Jiangsu province [SCX (12)3143].

REFERENCES

1. Nettleton PF, Gilray JA, Russo P, Dlissi E. 1998. Border disease of sheep and goats. Vet. Res. 29:327–340.
2. Oguzoglu TC, Tan MT, Toplu N, Demir AB, Bilge-Dagalp S, Karaoglu T, Ozkul A, Alkan F, Burgu I, Haas L, Greiser-Wilke I. 2009. Border disease virus (BDV) infections of small ruminants in Turkey: a new BDV subgroup? Vet. Microbiol. 135:374 –379.
3. Thabti F, Letellier C, Hammami S, Pépin M, Ribière M, Mesplède A, Kerkhofs P, Russo P. 2005. Detection of a novel border disease virus subgroup in Tunisian sheep. Arch. Virol. 150:215–229.
4. Cabezón O, Rosell R, Velarde R, Mentaberre G, Casas-Díaz E, Lavín S, Marco I. 2010. Border disease virus shedding and detection in naturally in fected Pyrenean chamois (Rupicapra pyrenaica). J. Vet. Diagn. Invest. 22: 744 –747.
5. García-Pérez AL, Minguijón E, Estévez L, Barandika JF, Aduriz G, Juste RA, Hurtado A. 2009. Clinical and laboratorial findings in pregnant ewes and their progeny infected with border disease virus (BDV-4 genotype). Res. Vet. Sci. 86:345–352.
6. Strong R, La Rocca SA, Ibata G, Sandvik T. 2010. Antigenic and genetic characterisation of border disease viruses isolated from UK cattle. Vet. Microbiol. 141:208 –215.
7. Li W, Mao L, Zhao Y, Sun Y, He K, Jiang J. 2013. Detection of border disease virus (BDV) in goat herds suffering diarrhea in eastern China. Virol. J. 10:80. doi:10.1186/1743-422X-10-80.

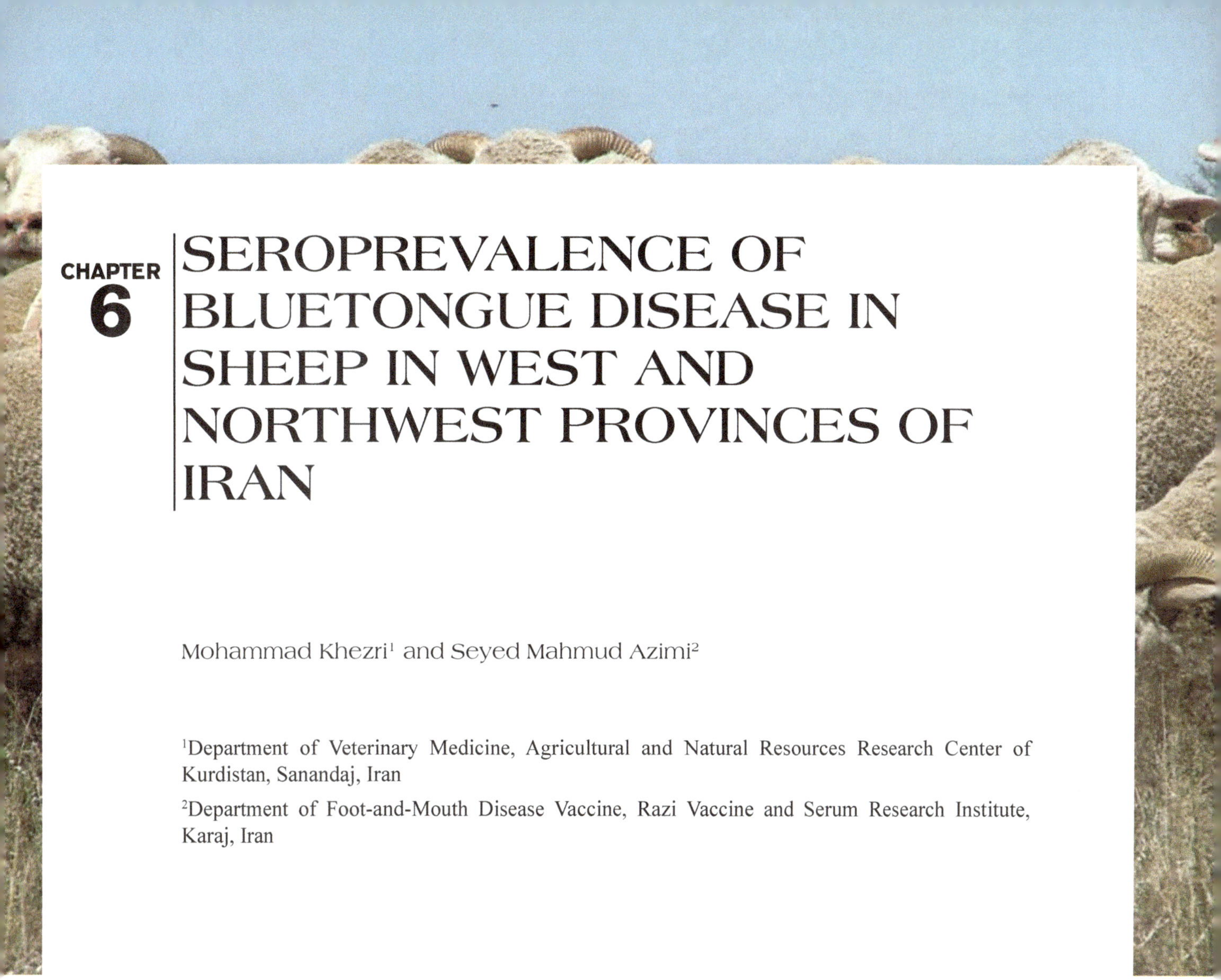

CHAPTER 6

SEROPREVALENCE OF BLUETONGUE DISEASE IN SHEEP IN WEST AND NORTHWEST PROVINCES OF IRAN

Mohammad Khezri[1] and Seyed Mahmud Azimi[2]

[1]Department of Veterinary Medicine, Agricultural and Natural Resources Research Center of Kurdistan, Sanandaj, Iran

[2]Department of Foot-and-Mouth Disease Vaccine, Razi Vaccine and Serum Research Institute, Karaj, Iran

ABSTRACT

The objective of this study was to describe the seroprevalence rates of bluetongue virus (BTV) in sheep in west and northwest provinces of Iran. Bluetongue virus, an economically important orbivirus of the*Reoviridae* family, causes a hemorrhagic disease mainly in sheep and occasionally in cattle and some species of deer. Bluetongue virus is transmitted between its mammalian hosts by certain species of biting midges (*Culicoides spp.*) and it can infect all ruminant species. Overall, 26 serotypes have been reported around the world. Due to its economic impact, bluetongue (BT) is an Office of International des Epizooties (OIE)-listed disease. A total of 756 sera samples collected during 2007-2008, were available. Sera were tested with competitive enzyme-linked immunosorbent assay (C-ELISA). The seroprevalence rate in sheep was 40.87%. The rate of positivity in sheep in west and northwest was 46.10% and 33.75%, respectively. The highest prevalence of antibodies in serum was in West Azerbaijan (64.86%), and lower was in Ardabil (23.77%).

INTRODUCTION

Bluetongue (BT) is an insect-borne viral disease to which all species of ruminants are susceptible. It occurs mostly during periods of high temperature and rainfall, and usually disappears with the first frost or severe cold weather.[1] Bluetongue virus (BTV), the causative agent of BT of ruminants, have now been identified on all continents except for Antarctica.[2,3] Bluetongue virus is transmitted between its ruminant hosts almost exclusively through the bites of the females of vector species of the *Culicoides spp.* biting midge.[4,5]Specifically, BTV exists in an extensive band that includes tropical, subtropical, and temperate regions of the world between latitudes of approximately 40° north and 35° south. Exceptions are regions of Asia and western north America, where BTV infection of ruminants occurs as far as 50° north and, recently, northern Europe.[6,7] However, the distribution of specific insect vectors and different BTV serotypes differ remarkably throughout the world, so specific vector exist with specific constellations of BTV serotypes and topotypes in relatively distinct global ecosystems.[2,8,9] Although BTV is an orbivirus, it can occasionally be transmitted via seminal fluid and across the placenta.[10] Diagnostic tests are a major component of the success in any surveillance system.

Citation: Mohammad Khezri, Seyed Mahmud Azimi, Seroprevalence of bluetongue disease in sheep in west and northwest provinces of Iran, Vet Res Forum. 2013 Summer; 4(3): 195–198.

Wide varieties of tests are capable of detecting BTV-specific anti-bodies. These include agar gel immune-diffusion (AGID), hemagglutination-inhibition (HI), complement fixation (CF) and enzyme-linked immunosorbent assay (ELISA) either blocking ELISA or competitive ELISA (C-ELISA) which are serogroup-specific and serum neutralization (SN) test which is serotype-specific.[11] Only AGID and C-ELISA are recommended as prescribed tests for international trade in the Office of International des Epizooties (OIE) Manual of Standards for Diagnostic Tests and Vaccines.[12] Reports on BT outbreaks in the second semester of 2008 in Iran,[13] sera-positive herds in Turkey,[6,14] BT infection in Saudi Arabia, and outbreaks in Oman, and the Palestinian Autonomous Territories are among the most recent incidents of the disease in the region.[15] There have been few recent published studies from the region. Thus, we designed a study to evaluate the prevalence and distribution of serum antibodies to BTV in sheep in this area of Iran (Fig. 1).

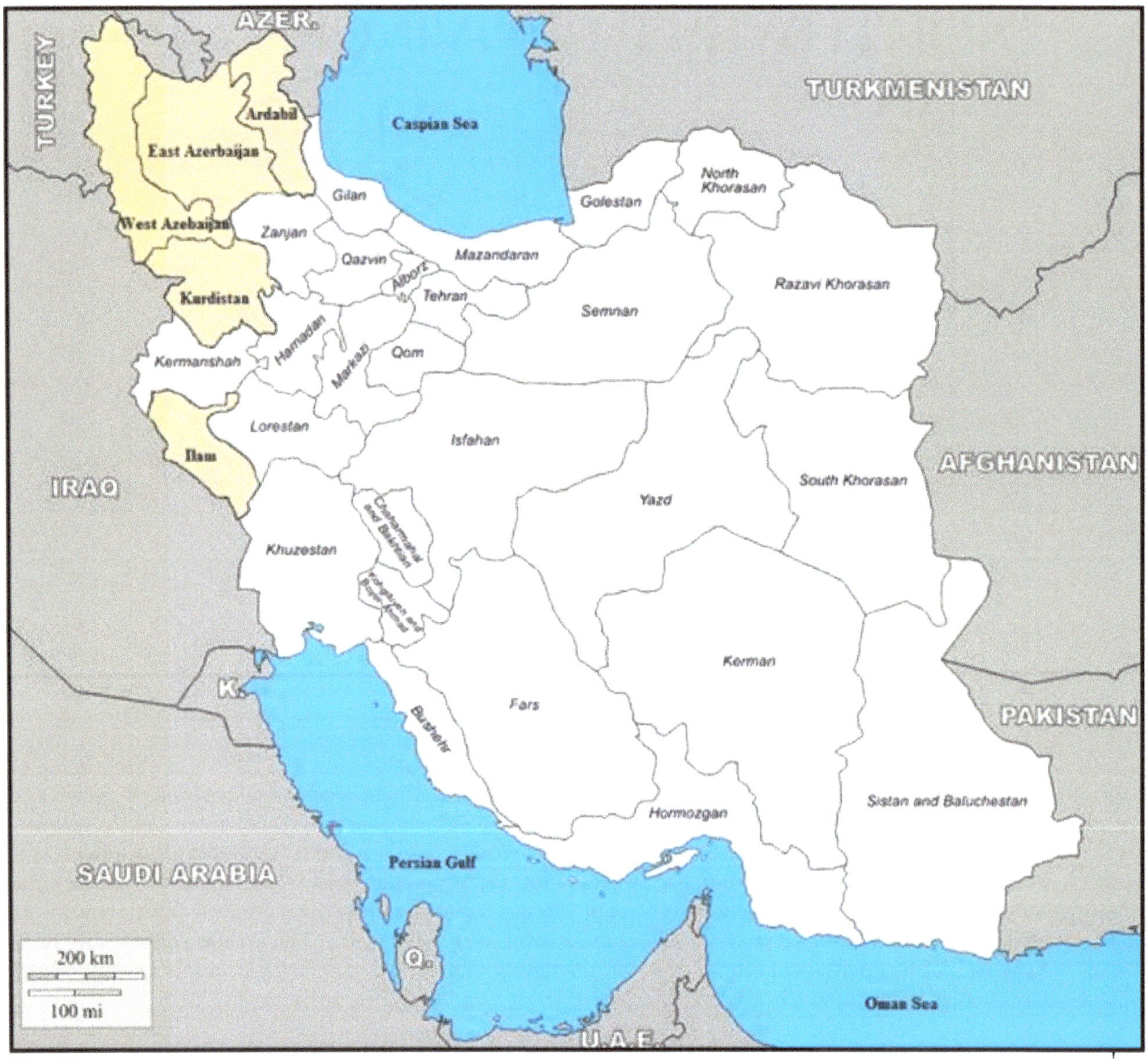

Figure 1: Map of Iran showing the location of areas where the present study was conducted.

MATERIALS AND METHODS

***Animals*:** In this study, for detection of specific antibodies to BTV in sheep blood serum samples by C-ELISA, 756 sheep blood samples collected from likely seropositive area in the west and northwest of Iran has investigated between June 2007 and September 2008.

***C-ELISA*:** Anti-BTV antibodies were detected in serum samples by group specific, C-ELISA kit (ID-Vet, Monpellier, France). The test based on competitive between test sera and an anti-VP7 for a VP7 antigen previously bound to the solid phase of ELISA plate.

RESULTS

Seroprevalence of bluetongue in west and northwest was shown in Table 1. The results showed that the seropositive rate in sheep over the whole study area was 40.87%. Presence of anti-bluetongue antibodies was found highest in west. The highest prevalence of antibodies was in West Azerbaijan (64.86%), and lower (23.77%) was in Ardabil (Table 1).

Table 1: Seroprevalence of bluetongue antibodies in sheep from the studied regions of Iran

	Number of serum samples	Number of seropositive	Positive rate (%)
Studied regions			
Northwest	320	108	33.75
West	436	201	46.10
Total	756	309	40.87
Studied Provinces			
Ardabil	122	29	23.77
East Azerbaijan	198	79	39.89
West Azerbaijan	74	48	64.86
Kurdistan	151	63	41.72
Ilam	211	90	42.65
Total	756	309	40.87

DISCUSSION

It is worth mentioning that the situation of diagnosis of this virus in neighboring countries and the Middle-East (except Turkey and Occupied Palestine) is not better than our country. In such country as Saudi Arabia, Syria, Yemen and Pakistan, the presence of virus has been documented only relying on serological tests.[6,7,16]According to recent studies, there is an evidence of occurrence of BT disease in tropical and subtropical countries (such as Iran). In such areas generally, the disease appears sub clinically and does not attract attention. In such circumstances, the presence of the virus often confirms via serological evidence. It should be mentioned that in such foci, in spite of unrevealed disease and manifestation, sometimes sudden incidence of acute forms of the disease sustain a loss.[17-19]

In Iran, identification of BTV in suspected cattle and sheep based on clinical manifestations was performed. However, there are some limitations and problems. First, it should be considered that clinical expression of BTV regarding strain and virus intensity, cattle race and environmental condition varies from per acute to subclinical. Second, symptoms of disease in sheep can be mistaken with those of other viral much diseases and even some of the non-viral diseases.[19] The objectives of the used C-ELISA test were both to confirm the BTV infected status of sheep in suspicious holdings in west and northwest of Iran (Diagnostic test). Thus, its use has been more and more often abandoned and replaced by C-ELISA tests, which are rapid and easier to use, more sensitive and specific.[20] In this study, the prevalence rate of BT antibodies in sheep was 40.87%. In other countries, the prevalence was as follows: 21.40% in Kazakhstan,[6] 29.59% in southeastern Turkey,[14]62.69% in India,[21] 54.10% in Saudi Arabia,[22] and 48.70% in Pakistan.[16] Climatic factors play an important role in the occurrence of BTV infection in animals and influence the size of vector populations and periods of their seasonal activity.[23] An analysis of climatic data was used to model the potential distribution of*Culicoides imicola* in Europe, predicting that might have spread from Spain, Greece and Italy to some areas along the Croatian coast as well as to the coastal areas of Albania, Serbia, Montenegro, Bosnia and Herzegovina.[24-27] Although more than 1000 species of *Culicoides spp.* are known worldwide, relatively few of these species have been incriminated as vectors of BTV.[28] *Culicoides* from western Turkey in relation to bluetongue disease of sheep and cattle was reported.[29] Species of vector insects that transmit BTV differ amongst regions, and are especially poorly characterized in the portions of Asia that are devoid of *C. imicola*, the traditional African-Asian vector of BTV.[2,7,29] Animals entering the western border of Iraq to Iran can be a cause of high titers of antibodies against the bluetongue virus in west of Iran. The prevalence of BT antibodies in sheep in the northwest of Iran was 33.75%. Although BTV infection of sheep is clearly widespread in northwest of Iran, the specific virus serotypes and vector insects that occur within the region remain uncharacterized, as they are in adjacent countries such as Kazakhstan.[6] The highest prevalence of BTV in sheep was in West Azerbaijan (64.86%) and Ilam (42.65%).

The results show that BTV infection is present in livestock animals in province. Some similar studies have been carried out in different area of country that mostly reported prevalence in the similar study. For example, 76.44% in East Azerbaijan,[30] 34.70% in West Azerbaijan,[7] 33.33% in Kerman,[31] 45.90% in Kurdistan, [32]53.37% in Isfahan.[33]

Furthermore, BTV infection in sheep apparently is largely subclinical.[7] During the BTV epidemics in Europe in 2008, Williamson and colleagues[34] considered clinical signs for diagnosis of the disease. The results showed low specificity of this method. These researchers believe that sometimes clinical signs of BTV in sheep are mistaken with those of such diseases as foot and mouth disease (FMD), ovine rinderpest, contagious ecthyma, and hemonchosis.[35,36] Iran located in the southeast of Europe makes it an important potential source of BTV strains and serotypes that might incur into adjacent areas.[5,37]

In conclusion, seroprevalence of BTV has been never before reported in many area of Iran (Ardabil and Ilam). As per our knowledge, this is the first study was evaluated the prevalence of antibodies to BTV in sheep in some provinces of Iran. The results showed that a high incidence rate of BT antibodies has been detected in sheep in Iran that indicate serological evidence of exposure to infection was widely distributed in some provinces. There are no restrictions on the movement of animals from one region to another within the country. Thus, outbreaks may also occur due to transportation of animals. Consequently, a well-defined control strategy for preventing and controlling the BTV may be based not only on vaccination plans and vector eradication but also restriction on the movement of animals from one region to another within the country. As a vaccination for BT is not implemented in Iran, a seropositive result indicates BT infection in domestic population.[4,31] Further researches on the isolation and identification of BT virus in sheep are encouraged.

ACKNOWLEDGEMENTS

This study was supported with a grant of Razi Vaccine and Serum Research Instituted.

REFERENCES

1. Office of International des Epizooties (OIE); [Accessed: August 23, 2006]. Bluetongue detected for the first time in Northern Europe. Available at: http://www.oie.int/en.
2. Tabachnick WJ. Culicoides and the global epidemiology of bluetongue virus infection. Vet Ital.2004;40:145–150.
3. MaclachlanNJ.Bluetongue:History,globalepidemiology, and pathogenesis. Prev Vet Med.2011;102(2):107–111.

4. Mellor PS, Widmann EJ. Bluetongue virus in the Mediterranean Basin. Vet J. 2002;164:20–37.

5. Saegerman C, Berkvens D, Mellor PS. Bluetongue epidemiology in European Union. Emerg Infect Dis.2008;14:539–544.

6. Lundervold M, Milner-Guilland EJ, O'Callaghan CJ, et al. First evidence of blue tongue virus in Kazakhstan. Vet Microbiol. 2003;92:281–287.

7. Jafari-Shoorijeh S, Ramin AG, Maclachlan NJ, et al. High seroprevalence of bluetongue virus infection in sheep flocks in West Azerbaijan, Iran. Comp Immunol Microbiol Infect Dis. 2010;33(3):243–247.

8. Maclachlan NJ, Osburn BI. Impact of bluetongue virus infection on the international movement and trade of ruminants. Am Vet Med Assoc. 2006;228:1346–1349.

9. Balasuriya UB, Nadler SA, Wilson WC, et al. The NS3 proteins of global strains of bluetongue virus evolve into regional topotypes through negative (purifying) selection. Vet Microbiol. 2008;126(1-3):91–100.

10. Schwartz-Cornil I, Mertens PPC, Contreras V, et al. Bluetongue virus: virology, pathogenesis and immunity. Vet Res. 2008;39:46–61.

11. Afshar A. Bluetongue: Laboratory diagnosis. Comp Immunol Microbiol Infect Dis. 1994;17(3-4):221–242.

12. Paris, France: Office of International des Epizooties (OIE); [Accessed: Feb 8, 2011]. Bluetongue, manual of diagnostic tests and vaccines for terrestrial animals (mammals, birds and bees) Available at:http://www.oie.int/doc/ged/D7709.

13. Office of international des epizooties (OIE); [Accessed: Feb 20, 2004]. Principles of validation of diagnostic assays for infectious diseases, manual of diagnostic tests, and vaccines for terrestrial animals (mammals, birds and bees) Available at: http://www.baphiq.gov.tw/public/Attachment/922 51 7212071.pdf.

14. Gür S. A serologic investigation of bluetongue virus in cattle, sheep and Gazella subgutturosa in south-eastern Turkey. Trop Anim Health Prod. 2008;40(3):217–221.

15. Office of international des epizooties (OIE); Final report of the 10th conference of the OIE regional commission for the middle. [Accessed: Nov 4, 2011]. Available at: http://www.oie.int/eng/session2011/A_ FR_2010PUB.pdf.

16. Akhtar S, Djallem N, Shad G, et al. Bluetongue virus seropositivity in sheep flocks in North West Frontier province, Pakistan. Prev Vet Med. 1997;29:293–298.

17. Basak AK, Grimes J, Gouet P, et al. Structures of orbivirus VP7: implications for the role of this protein in the viral life cycle. Structure. 1997;5:871–883.

18. Nikolakaki SV, Nomikou K, Koumbati M, et al. Molecular analysis of the NS3/NS3A gene of bluetongue virus isolates from the 1979 and 1998-2001 epizootics in Greece and their segregation into two distinct groups. Virus Res. 2005;114:6–14.

19. Momtaz H, Nejat S, Souod N, et al. Comparisons of competitive enzyme-linked immunosorbent assay and one step RT-PCR tests for the detection of bluetongue virus in south west of Iran. African J Biotechnol.2011;10:6857–6862.

20. Reddington JJ, Reddington GM, MacLachlan NJ. A competitive ELISA for detection of antibodies to the group antigen of bluetongue virus. J Vet Diagn Invest. 1991;3(2):144–147.

21. Sreenivasulu D, Subba Rao MV, Reddy YN, et al. Overview of bluetongue disease, viruses, vectors, surveillance and unique features: the Indian subcontinent and adjacent regions. Vet Ital. 2004;40:73–77.

22. Yousef MR, Al-Eesa AA, Al-Blowi MA. High seroprevalence of bluetongue virus antibodies in Sheep, Goats, Cattle and Camel in different districts of Saudi Arabia. Vet World. 2012;5(7):389–393.

23. Ward MP, Thurmond MC. Climatic factors associated with risk of seroconversion of cattle to bluetongue viruses in Queensland. Prev Vet Med. 1995;24(2):129–136.

24. Gloster J, Mellor PS, Manning AJ, et al. Assessing the risk of windborne spread of bluetongue in the 2006 outbreak of disease in northern Europe. Vet Rec. 2007;160:54–56.

25. Gubbins S, Carpenter S, Baylis M, et al. Assessing the risk of bluetongue to UK livestock: Uncertainty and sensitivity analysis of a temperature-dependent model for the basic reproductive number. J R Soc Interface. 2007;7:17.

26. Wilson AJ, Carpenter S, Gloster J, et al. Re-emergence of bluetongue in northern Europe in 2007. Vet Rec. 2007;161:482–486.

27. Withitann EJ, Mellor PS, Baylis M. Using climate data to map the potential distribution of Culicoides imicola (Diptera: Ceratop-ogonidae) in Europe. Rev Sci Technol Off Int Epiz. 2001;20(3):731–740.

28. Meiswinkel R, Gomulski LM, Delecolle JC, et al. The taxonomy of Culicoides vector complexes unfinished business. Vet Ital. 2004;40:151–159.

29. Maclachlan NJ. Global implications of the recent emergence of bluetongue virus in Europe. Vet Clin North Am Food Anim Pract. 2010;26:163–171.

30. Hasanpour A, Mosakhani F, Mirzaii H, et al. Seroprevalence of bluetongue virus infection in Sheep in East-Azerbaijan province in Iran . Res J Biol Sci . 2008;3:1265–1270.

31. Mozaffari AA, Khalili M, Mashayekhi M. The first survey for antibody against bluetongue virus in sheep flocks in Southeast of Iran. APJTB. 2012:S1808–S1810.

32. Khezri M. Seroprevalence of bluetongue virus antibodies in sheep in Kurdistan province in west of Ian. IJAVMS. 2012;6(3):183–188.

33. Noman V, Kargar Moakhhar R, Shah Moradi AH, et al. A seroepidemiological survey for bluetongue virus anti-body in sheep and goats of Isfahan province, Iran, Isfahan, Iran. Isfahan agricultural and natural resources research center. 2006:37.

34. Williamson S, Woodger N, Darpel K. Differential diagnosis of bluetongue in cattle and sheep. In Practice. 2008;30:242–251.

35. Elbers AR, Backx A, Ekker HM, et al. Performance of clinical signs to detect bluetongue virus serotype 8 outbreaks in cattle and sheep during the 2006-epidemic in

The Netherlands. Vet Microbiol. 2008;129:156–162.

36. Tan BH, Nason E, Staeuber N, et al. RGD tripeptide of bluetongue virus VP7 protein is responsible for core attachment to Culicoides cells. J Virol. 2001;75:3937–3947.

37. Purse BV, Mellor PS, Rogers DJ, et al. Climate change and the recent emergence of bluetongue in Europe. Nat Rev Microbiol. 2005;3:171–181.

CHAPTER 7

BRUCELLOSIS: AN ECONOMICALLY IMPORTANT INFECTION

Yasmin Bano[1], and Sajad Ahmad Lone[2]

[1]Department of Microbiology, All India Institute of Medical Sciences, Tatibandh, GE Road, Raipur, Chhattisgarh, India

[2]National Institute for Research in Tribal Health (ICMR), Nagpur Road, Jabalpur, Madhya Pradesh, India

ABSTRACT

Brucellosis is one of the world's major zoonosis, caused by bacteria of the genus Brucella. The world's most widespread zoonosis affects cattle, sheep, goats, pigs, and other animals, leading to abortion, infertility, and low milk yields. Humans acquire brucellosis from direct contact with livestock or from drinking unpasteurized milk. Brucella spp. are considered as the most common laboratory-acquired pathogens. Several serological tests have been widely used for diagnosis of Brucella such are Rose Bengal plate test (RBPT), Standard tube agglutination test (STAT), complement fixation test (CFT), enzyme linked immunosorbant assay (ELISA). Besides these, polymerase chain reaction (PCR) based identification and typing, fluorescence polarization assay (FPA) are also important diagnostic tools. The worldwide economic losses due to brucellosis are extensive. Although a number of successful vaccines are being used for immunization of animals still no satisfactory vaccine against human brucellosis is available. This review shows world literature and its impact to the history, epidemiology, virulence, diagnosis along with the control measures adopted in all over the world scenario including Indian.

INTRODUCTION

Impact on Health and Economy

Brucellosis is a highly infectious zoonotic disease and an economically important infection of humans and livestock with a worldwide distribution. It is a major veterinary and human public health problem in most parts of the world. The incidence of this disease is greatly decreased in the developed world due to effective vaccination based control programs, but remains an uncontrolled problem in regions of high endemicity such as the Mediterranean, Middle East, Africa, Latin America and parts of Asia including India [1-3]. Across the developing world, brucellosis is still a very common but often neglected disease. Brucellosis is of economic concern in many parts of the world as it results in reduced productivity, abortions, weak offspring's and major impediments for trade and export of livestock. It can also be transferred from animal to humans [4]. Brucellosis is a chronic disease with a risk of disabling consequences, but is rarely fatal in affected humans.

Citation: Yasmin Bano and Sajad Ahmad Lone, Brucellosis: An Economically Important Infection, doi:10.4172/2161-0703.1000208.

Human brucellosis is a severe debilitating disease that requires prolonged treatment with the use of several antibiotics and also involves considerable medical expenses as well as loss of working hours. Brucellosis is almost invariably transmitted to man from infected domestic animals. However, it has been documented beyond doubt, the possibility of human to human transmission of Brucella infection [5-7] i.e. humans carry the disease, but person to person transmission of brucellosis is very rare, however transmission of the disease from human to human has been reported [8-10]. Mothers who are breast-feeding may transmit the infection to their infants and sexual transmission has also been reported [10,11].

Besides a threat to human healthware brucellosis spread in livestock foci is also causing serious problems to the national economies. According to the International agreements on the veterinary regulation [12] if brucellosis is detected in at least one herd, the resettlement and sale of animals from the whole foci region should be prohibited. Such strict limitations lead to the significant brucellosis mediated economic losses.

Marston described the symptoms of brucellosis and also gave the name gastric remittent fever [13]. Brucellosis has many synonyms derived from the geographical area in which this disease is common, e.g. Mediterranean fever, Malta fever, Gibraltar fever, Cyprus fever. It was also known with the symptoms it is associated, undulant fever due its remittent character and typhomalarial fever due to its reassemble to malaria and typhoid fevers. That is why brucellosis is frequently misdiagnosed as malaria, typhoid, or venereal disease [14]. Brucellosis is also known as intermittent typhoid, bang's disease in cattle, contagious abortion, infection abortion, epizootic abortion.

This disease has been under reported from domestic animals from developing countries because of absence of national surveillance programs, diagnostic facilities and reliable data [15]. The principal symptom in all animal species is abortion or premature expulsion of the fetus. The main mode of transmission of this disease to humans is through consuming untreated milk products. Each year about a half million cases of brucellosis occurs in humans around the world [16]. There are three reports of humans infected with marine strains ofBrucella; one reported in a research laboratory worker after occupational exposure [17] and other two were community-acquired infections [18,19]. Bovine brucellosis has been eradicated in Finland, Norway, Sweden, Denmark, Belgium, Switzerland, Germany, Austria, Hungary, the former Czechoslovakia, Rumania, and Bulgaria, as well as in other developed countries [20,21].

Historical Perspective

Marston made the earliest recorded description of brucellosis in 1859 as he wrote of an illness, including his own, which differed from typhoid fever. Sir David Bruce isolated the organism from the spleen of a patient while investigating an outbreak of a fatal disease known as Mediterranean or Malta fever, affecting British soldiers stationed on the island of Malta [22]. He named the bacteria as Micrococcus melitensis due to coccoidal morphology. Hughes suggested the name undulant fever (wave like) because of characteristic fever, which rise and fall over weeks in untreated patients [23]. Write and Smith detected antibodies of M. melitensis through agglutination test in humans and explained the zoonotic potential of this disease [24] Zammit working with Mediterranean fever commission discovered the role of goats in brucellosis by isolation the organism from the milk and urine of the goats and concluded that goat was the reservoir and declared that consumption of the raw milk and cheese responsible for the human brucellosiss [25]. The report of isolation of a gram negative rod from cattle, its subsequent establishment of similarity between M. melitensis gave convincing evidence that both organisms could not be differentiated morphologically or by cultural and biochemical reactions. Both these bacteria were finally placed under one genus Brucellanamed in honour of Sir David Bruce.

CLASSIFICATION AND GENERAL CHARACTERISTICS

Scientific Classification

1. Kingdom- Bacteria
2. Phylum-Proteobacteria
3. Class-Alphaproteobacteria
4. Order-Rhizobials
5. Family-Brucellaceae
6. Genus-Brucella

The traditional taxonomy is based on phenotypic characteristics, antigenic variations and prevalence of infection in different animal hosts. The common species of Brucella associated with different animal hosts are B. melitensis (goat and sheep), B. abortus (cattle), B. suis (pig, reindeer and hare), B. ovis (sheep), B. neotomae (desert wood rat), and B. canis (dog). B. pinnipediae (seal/ otter) and B. cetaceae(porpoise/ whale) have been reported from marine mammals [26,27]. Which of them human infections are common with B. melitensis [2,26]. B. abortus as α2 proteobacteria have phylogenetic relationships with Agrobacterium, Rickettsia, Rhizobium, Rhizobacter, Ochrobacterium [28,29]. Brucella has been subdivided into biovars based on different biochemical reactions and differentiated from other related species by conventional methods such as sensitivity or tolerance to aniline dyes, production of H_2S and CO_2 requirements for growth. The taxonomy ofBrucella species is still being resolved based on 16s-rRNA gene sequence. According to the new taxonomy used by NCBI the species B. melitensis includes 5 biovars namely, abortus, canis, neotomae, ovis, and suis (Table 1).

Table 1: Taxonomic characteristics of Brucella species

Taxonomic characteristics of *Brucella* species								
			Biochemical identification					
Species	Bio- type	Host reservoir	Fuchsin	Thionin	Safranin -inhibition	H_2S production	Urease	CO_2 growth
B. mlitensis (Bruce, 1887)	1-3	Goats, sheep, camels	+	+	-	-	+ in 24 hr.	-
B. abortus (Bang, 1897)	1-6,9	Cows, camels, yaks, buffalo	+ (except biotype 2)	- (biotype 1, 2, 4)	-	+ (except biotype 5)	+ in 24 hr.	+
B. suis (Traum, 1914)	1-5	Pigs (biotypes 1-3), wild hares (biotype 2), Caribou (biotype 4), reindeer (biotype 4), wild rodents (biotype 5)	- (except biotype 3)	+	+	+ (biotype 1)	+ in 15 min.	-
B. canis (Carmichael and Bruner, 1968)	--	Canines	+ / -	+	-	-	+ in 15 min.	-
B. ovis (Van drimmelen, 1953)	--	Sheep	- for some strains		-	-	-	+
B. neotomae (Stoenner and Lackman, 1957)	--	Rodents	-		-	+	+ in 15 min.	-
B. pinnipediae* and *B. cetaceae (Ewalt et al., and Ross et al., 1994)	--	Mink whales, dolphins, porpoises (pinnipediae), seals (cetaceae)	+	+	-	-	+	- for pinnipediae and + for cetaceae.

Brucellosis in Animals

Brucellosis is a very important disease for bovines and buffaloes due to the reproductive problems it causes [30] and also the risk to public health. It is a barrier to the international trade of animals and animal products [31]. The main pathogen is B. abortus biovar 1 is universal in the presence and predominant among the seven that occurs in the world. The distribution of the different biovars varies geographically. Cattles can also become infected with B. suis, B. melitensis when they share pasture or facilities with infected pigs, goat and sheep. The infections in cattle caused by other species of Brucella are more sporadic and rarer in nature than the disease caused by B. abortus. In natural infections it is difficult to measure the incubation period (from time of infection to abortion or premature birth), as it is not possible to determine the moment of infection. Experiments have shown that the incubation period varies considerably and is inversely proportional to fetal development, i.e. the more advanced the pregnancy, the shorter the incubation period. If the female is infected orally during the breeding period, the incubation period can last up to 200 days, while if she is exposed six months after being bred, the incubation time is approximately two months. The period of "serologic incubation" (from the time of infection to the appearance of antibodies) lasts several weeks to several months. The incubation period varies according to factors such as the virulence of the strain and dose of bacteria, the route of infection and the susceptibility of the animal. In short, incubation period varying from 5 days to 5 months and can progress in various forms: acute, chronic or asymptomatic [32].

In pregnant females, abortion occurs during the second half of the pregnancy, often with retention of the placenta and resultant metritis, which may cause permanent infertility. It is estimated that the infection causes a 20% to 25% loss in milk production as a result of interrupted lactation due to abortion and delayed conception. In bulls it may become localized in the testicles and adjacent genital glands. The bacteria enter the body of animals first multiply in the regional lymph nodes and the latter carried by the lymph and blood to different organs. In experimental infection, it is possible to isolate the agent from the bloodstream after two weeks of infection. Brucella organisms are most commonly found in the lymph nodes, uterus, udder, spleen, liver, and in bulls, the genital organs. Large quantities of erythritol, a carbohydrate that stimulates the multiplication of brucellae, have been found in cow placentas and this could explain the high susceptibility of bovine fetal tissues. The virulence of Brucella in cattle is mainly due to their ability to replicate intracellularly, preferentially utilize erythritol and inhibit the mature reproductive tract, which is high in this sugar [33]. Once an infected cow aborts or gives birth normally, the pathogen does not remain long in the uterus. The infection becomes chronic and the brucellae are harboured in the cow's lymph nodes and mammary glands [34].

Cows, especially when pregnant are most susceptible, although some researchers maintain that bulls are more resistant to the infection than females. Some less susceptible cows have generalized infections and suffer losses in the reproductive system and milk production for one or more years, but then gradually recover. In such animals, the agglutination titer become negative and both the reproductive system and milk production return to normal. However, most cows become infected and their agglutination titers remain positive for many years. Brucellosis spread rapidly from animal to animal, trading and movements of animals also help maintain active infection.

Brucellosis in Humans

Brucellosis is a multi-systemic disease in human and may present with a broad spectrum of clinical manifestations and its complications can affect almost all organs and systems with varying incidence [35-37]. It is fatal in 1%–5% of untreated cases [38,39]. The symptoms and clinical signs most commonly reported are fever, fatigue, malaise, sweats, headaches, myalgia, arthalgia and weight loss [40]. Some cases have been presented with only joint pain, low back ache, and involuntary movements of limbs, burning feet or ischemic heart attacks [41]. Human brucellosis usually manifests as an acute (less than two months) or sub-acute (2-12 months) febrile illness, which may persist and progress to a chronic stage referred as chronic fatigue syndrome [42]. Complications can be different depending on the specific site of infection [43] of which meningitis and meningoencephalitis is the most common complications seen in neurobrucellosis [44]. Neurobrucellosis has been reported as an exceptional cause of transient ischemic attacks [41]. In conclusion, it should be noted that brucellosis may affect essentially any organ and that reinforces the importance of brucellosis in differential diagnosis in endemic areas [45] (Figure 1).

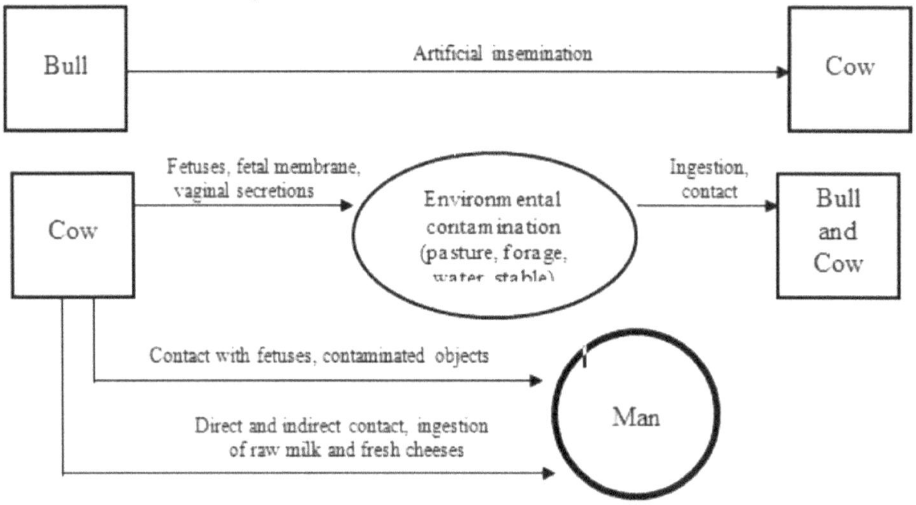

Figure 1: Brucellosis - Mode of transmission bovine brucellosis (Pedro and Boris, 2001).

Mode of Transmission

The disease is transmitted either through contaminated milk products or through direct contact with infected animals. Fresh milk and dairy products prepared from unpasteurized milk such as soft cheeses, yoghurts and ice creams may contain high amounts of the bacteria and consumption of these is an important mode of transmission to humans [46]. It is also estimated that 10-100 organisms in aerosol form constitute an infectious dose. The bacterium may enter the body through digestive tract, the lungs or mucosal layer and spread through the blood and lymphatic system to any other organ where it may infect the tissue and cause localized. This is a common laboratory transmitted infection and reported to occur in clinical, research and production laboratories [47,48]. Bacterial load in animal muscle tissue is low, but consumption of undercooked traditional delicacies such as the liver has been implicated in human infection [49]. The main sources of infection for cattle are fetus and vaginal discharges. The most common route of transmission is the gastrointestinal tract following ingestion of contaminated pasture, feed, fodder, or water. Moreover, animals customarily lick afterbirth fetuses and newborn calves, which contain a large number of the bacteria. It has been shown experimentally that the organism may penetrate broken and even intact skin, but the mode of transmission of natural infection is unknown. Vaginal route and intrauterine route used in artificial insemination are very important in transmitting the infection.

Global Scenario

The epidemiology of brucellosis is complex and Latin American countries, mainly Mexico and Peru reported a large number of cases. The same pattern holds true for Mediterranean countries like Iran, former Soviet Union and Mongolia. Seven republics of the former Soviet Union (Kyrgyzstan, Tajikistan, Kazakhstan, Azerbaijan, Turkmenistan, Armenia and Uzbekistan) are included in the 25 countries with the highest incidence of the disease worldwide, while another country of this region, Mongolia, is ranked the second. Syria has the highest annual incidence of human brucellosis worldwide [50]. Human brucellosis is found to have significant presence in rural/nomadic communities of these countries where people live in close association with animals. Worldwide, reported incidence of human brucellosis in endemic disease areas varies widely, from <0.01 to >200 per 100000 population [51] and about 500000 cases/year of human brucellosis are reported worldwide, but the estimates of the World Health Organization (WHO) suggest that, due to underreporting, the real incidence is 10–25 times higher [52]. Despite the fact that incidence of human brucellosis is unknown for most countries including India and no data are available [53].

In Saudi Arabia, 7893 human cases of brucellosis were recorded in 1987 (74 per 100000 inhabitants). In Iran, 71051 cases (13 per 100000) were recorded in 1988 and it is estimated that 80000 cases have occurred each year since 1989. In turkey 5003 cases (9 per 100000) were recorded in 1990, an incident three times higher than the period 1986-1989 (3 per 100000).

In Europe, brucellosis is declining, according to data from the European Food Safety Authority (EFSA) the number of cases decreased from 735 in 2008 to 352 in 2011 [54]. The disease affects mostly the Mediterranean countries. From 2008 to 2011 Greece, Italy, Portugal and Spain accounted for 50–80% of all the European reported cases, respectively, with B. melitensis and B. abortus being the predominant causative agents [54].

The large meat producing countries such as France, Great Britain, Australia, New Zealand, Canada and United States are free of bovine brucellosis. The three important cattle raising countries, Argentina, Brazil and Mexico, still have limited control programs. A countryby- country analysis is found in a monograph on bovine brucellosis [34]. In the rest of the world, rates of infection vary greatly from one country to another and between regions within a country. Official estimates put annual losses from bovine brucellosis in Latin America at approximately US$ 600 million [55]. A trend in the epidemiology of human brucellosis in Germany was investigated by analyzing national surveillance data (1962–2005) complemented by a questionnaire- based survey (1995–2000). The incidence decreased from 1962 to the 1980s' even though a persistent number of cases have been reported among Turkish immigrants (0.3/10000 Turks vs. 0.01/100000 in the German population [56].

Indian Scenario

India has a huge resource of livestock and dairy farming plays a substantial role in the country's rural economy [57]. The country restrains the largest buffalo population in the world (105.34 million - 57.3%) followed by the 2nd largest cattle population (199.08 million - 14.7%) [58] and highest milk production in the world, i.e. 121.8 million tonnes with per capita availability of 281 g/day [59]. Brucellosis is a highly contagious disease of dairy animals and humans in many parts of the world, including India causing significant morbidity and enormous economic losses [60,61]. The disease causes abortions in the last trimester of pregnancy, premature births followed by retention of placenta, metritis, decreased milk production and lameness as a common sequel to infection in dairy animals [62].

The occurrence of brucellosis in India was first established early in the previous century and since then has been reported from almost all states [63,64]. Many publications indicate that brucellosis is a fairly common disease in India and present in different species of mammalian farm animals including cattle, goats, buffalo, yaks, camel, horses and pigs [65-67]. A national survey in bovines a decade back indicated 5% of cattle and 3% of buffaloes of the country were infected with brucellosis [64]. The occurrence of the disease is usually high in organized farms (50%) compared to the marginal herds (10%) and this primarily associated with intensive farming practices in large organized animal farms [53,68] reported 8.5% seroprevalence of brucellosis among the dairy persons with the isolation of Brucella strain from seven cases of human brucellosis. As many as 4.2% aborted women were seropositive for disease [69].

In Gujarat, 8.5% [70] and in Hariyana, 34% human brucellosis cases were reported among veterinarians, attendants and compounders who are in contact with animals [71]. In a study conducted by Hemashettar and Patil 24 (8.2%) veterinary workers showed Brucella specific antibodies in significant titers [72]. A study by Mantur and coworkers in Bijapur reported 93 children among 5726 children as seropositive by SAT (>1:160) and confirmed it by the isolation of B. melitensis in 43 pediatric patients [73]. Handa and coworkers identified four cases with acute brucellosis in a group of 121 patients with FUO (Fever of Unknown Origin) [74].

Genome

The genome contains 2 circular chromosomes except B.suis biovar 3, which has a single chromosome. The size of the first chromosome ofB. abortus is 2,124,241 nucleotides long and codes for 2200 genes. The second chromosome is 1,162,204 nucleotides long and codes for 1156 genes. The genome has a GC content of 57%, and 81% of the genome is coding region [75]. This pathogen is different from other bacterial species as it does not contain any plasmid or genomic islands that related to pathogenicity within its genome. In addition to lacking these two features, the genome also lacks many other genes that code for common virulence factors, including "capsules, fimbriae, exotoxins, cytolysins, resistance forms, antigenic variation, plasmids, or lysogenic phages" [76]. The genes that do encode for virulence inB. abortus are being examined, but they are not well understood to say for sure the mode of the virulence of this intracellular pathogen [26].

Virulence and Pathogenicity

There are many factors which responsible for human brucellosis. The S-LPS is a major determinant of virulence and dominants the antibody response. The elimination depends on activated macrophages and hence requires the development of Th1 type cell mediated immunity.Brucella LPS is a relatively poor inducer of gamma interferon and tumor necrosis factor α, both of with are essential for the elimination of the organism [77]. The other important virulence factors include, production of inhibitory phagolysosome fusion such as adenine and guanine monophosphate levels [78]; outer membrane protein 25 which has been identified as the down regulator of TNF α [79] especially in the early stage of infection. Recently ureas enzyme has been identified as an important determinant of virulence as the areas enzyme protects bacteria in their passage through the stomach by oral route, which is the major way of infection in human brucellosis. Brucella is also considered as Class III pathogen and listed as a potential bio-threat agent that can be used in bioterrorism.

LABORATORY DIAGNOSIS

The varied symptoms which brucellosis presents make it troublesome for clinical diagnosis. The conventional diagnosis is microbiological confirmation by means of isolation of bacteria from the blood or from other body fluids. The isolation rate of Brucella is poor due to its slow growth rate, quantity of circulating viable bacteria, culture medium, blood culture techniques employed as well as presence of antibiotics that inhibits growth [80]. The demonstration of antibodies generated against Brucella by serological tests remains a viable alternative to culture and several serological tests like Standard Tube Agglutination Test (SAT) and Rose Bengal Plate Agglutination Test (RBPT) are the most popular serological tests used in the field for the diagnosis of brucellosis. Several workers have reported development of antibody detection systems based on ELISA.

Blood culture provides definite proof of brucellosis [81], but may not provide a positive result for all patients even under ideal conditions.Brucella is a slow growing organism and cultures are rarely positive and should be kept at least 45 days before the culture can be concluded negative. Many serological tests have been used for the diagnosis of brucellosis. The most commonly used tests are serum agglutination test (SAT), the coombs anti Brucella test, rose bengal plate agglutination test (RBPT, based on agglutination of colored particulate antigen (killed Brucella organisms) by the antibodies present in the patient's serum), complement fixation test (CFT), indirect heamolysis test (IHLT). Since the development of the first agglutination test of brucellosis by Wright and Smith in 1897, veterinary laboratory workers have been developing tests to improve diagnostic performance and accuracy. Among the various tests developed are rapid agglutination tests for the detection of antibodies to brucellosis in cattle sera, such as the Rose Bengal Test [82], the Card Test [83], and the Buffered Antigen Plate Agglutination Test (BPAT) [84]. These tests use acidified antigens and were developed to improve accuracy. The purpose of the acidified antigens was to reduce agglutination by IgM, thus reducing nonspecific false-positive reactions. Although rapid, these tests were largely laboratory based and subjective in the interpretation of results. With the exception of the BPAT, they did not significantly improve test accuracy [85]. The SAT detects IgG less efficiently, especially IgG1, resulting in low assay specificity [86-88]. Therefore, the SAT is generally not used as a single test, but rather in combination with other tests.

In 1897, Wright and Smith published the first description of a test for the serological diagnosis of brucellosis in man. After that, different diagnostic tests are developed and there is a need to improve them. Dotenzyme linked immunosorbent assay (dot-ELISA) for the detection of Brucella antibodies in human sera with autoclaved extract of B. abortus S99 was developed and results were compared with those of STAT, RBPT and CFT. The dot-ELISA was found to be a more sensitive and also economical and rapid test for screening of human brucellosis under field conditions [89,90] evaluated a dot-ELISA (d-ELISA) test with the serum agglutination test (SAT), micro-complement fixation test (CFT) and a plate-ELISA (p-ELISA) for field use in screening herds of goats against brucellosis and found that d-ELISA was more suitable and rapid test for screening large numbers of goats in the field. According to Shome et al., [91] the lateral flow assay (LFA) is a cost-effective and rapid technology that provides accurate detection of antibodies to B. abortus in bovine serum samples.

Brucella antibodies in bovine sera and milk was also detected using the dot-immunobinding assay (DIA), the serum agglutination test (SAT), the Rose Bengal plate test (RBPT) and the milk ring test (MRT). In DIA, B. abortus S99 antigen prepared by heat treatment was used [92].The efficiency of a single antigen as well as a combination of two antigens in the complement fixation (CF) test was determined in detecting cattle and sheep infected or vaccinated. Comparative analysis of the CF results showed that the combined S99/RB51 antigen used in the CF test increases the specificity and sensitivity and could be used in animal brucellosis surveillance [93].

The humoral immunoresponse to S brucellae is dominated by antibodies to the PS (polysaccharide) section of the Brucella S-LPS (smooth lipopolysaccharide) and it shows a typical IgM/IgG (and IgA) shift. S-LPS or PS tests proposed for the diagnosis of human brucellosis, recently include the lateral flow immunochromatography assay (LFiC) for IgM and IgG assessment, a fluorescence polarization assay, a variety of indirect ELISA, and the immunocapture Brucellacapt test [94]. In addition, a competitive ELISA (cELISA) has been proposed [95]. In acute cases (i.e., short evolution) IgM is present in the serum; then this immunoglobulin returns progressively to background levels, so that IgG (and IgA) are dominant in the sera of long evolution (i.e. chronic) patients before treatment.

TREATMENT, CONTROL AND PREVENTION

Uncomplicated acute brucellosis almost invariable responds well to appropriate antibiotic treatment [96,97]. Patients with complications, additional treatment, including in some cases surgical intervention will be necessary. To prevent disease progression and the development of complications, treatment should start as early as possible also in patients showing signs of spontaneous improvement. In all cases it is important that the patient finishes the full course of medication because the risk of incomplete recovery and relapse is otherwise increased considerably [98]. Either taking the combination of doxycycline and rifampicin (for 6 weeks), or the combination of doxycycline (100 mg twice/day orally for 6 weeks) with streptomycin (1 g/day for 2-3 weeks) is the standard treatment for brucellosis [99]. The effectiveness of the combination of streptomycin with a tetracycline has been acknowledged since the early days of antibiotic use [100], and the addition of rifampicin in treatment regimens for brucellosis also has a history of more than 30 years [101]. Treatment of complications such as spondylitis and osteomyelitis, neurobrucellosis and Brucella endocarditis may require prolonged therapy for at least 8 weeks. Other combinations such as co-trimoxazole plus doxycycline and co-trimoxazole plus rifampin have been proposed, but still need further examination [102-105]. The optimal therapy for brucellosis during pregnancy has not been established [106].

The prevention of brucellosis is mainly by control of infection in domestic livestock by mass vaccination. The use B. abortus strain S19 in cattle and B. melitensis strain Rev-1 in goat and sheep has drastically reduced its incidence in many endemic areas. Vaccination of livestock is relatively cheap and will increase the value and productivity of their animals. It is not only important to improve the health of their animals but also is an important step to reduce the risk of severe illness and disability for themselves and their family members and also reduce the transmission to the human population. India already has developed a plan for the control of bovine brucellosis3 but the non-availability of a human vaccine makes it necessary for the animal handlers, doctors and health care workers take protective measures. The avoidance of unpasteurised dairy products will prevent infection in the general population.

REFERENCES

1. Lopez M (1989) Brucellosis in Latin America. In: young EJ, Corbel MJ (Ed), Brucellosis: Clinical and Laboratory Aspects: CRC press, Boca Raton, Florida 151-161.

2. Corbel MJ (1997) Brucellosis: an overview. Emerging Infectious Diseases 3: 213-21.
3. Refai M (2002) Incidence and control of brucellosis in the Near East region. Veterinary Microbiology 90: 81-110.
4. Christopher W (2004) "Brucellosis in human". Department of Pathobiological Science, School of veterinary medicine, University of Wisconsin, Madison.
5. Naparstek E, Block CS, Slavin S (1982) Transmission of brucellosis by bone marrow transplantation. Lancet 1: 574-575.
6. Lubani MM, Dudin KI, Sharda DC, AbuSinna NM, Al-Shab T, et al. (1988) Neonatal brucellosis' European Journal of Pediatrics 147: 520-522.
7. Tikare NV, Mantur BG, Bidari LH (2008) Brucellar meningitis in an infant-evidence for human breast milk transmission. Journal of Tropical Pediatrics 54: 272-274.
8. . Mantur BG, Mangalgi SS, Mulimani M (1996) Brucellamelitensis-- a sexually transmissible agent? Lancet 347: 1763
9. Palanduz A, Palanduz S, Gruel K, Gruel N (2000) Brucellosis in a mother and her young infant: probable transmission of breast milk. International Journal of Infectious Diseases 4: 55-56.
10. Carrera AI, Lopez RMJ, Sapina AM, Lopez LA, Sacristan AR (2006) Probable transmission of brucellosis by breast milk. Journal of Tropical Pediatrics 52: 380-381.
11. Kato Y, Masuda G, Itoda I, Imamura A, Ajisawa A, et al. (2007) Brucellosis in a returned traveler and his wife: probable person-to-person transmission of Brucellamelitensis. Journal of Travel Medicine 14:343-345.
12. Office International des Épizooties (2000) "Manual of Standards for Diagnostic Tests and Vaccines," Office International des Épizooties, Paris.
13. Marston JA (1861) Report on fever (Malta).Great Britain Army Medical Department representative 3: 486.
14. McDermott JJ, Arimib SM (2002) Brucellosis in sub-Saharan Africa: epidemiology, control and impact. Veterinary Microbiology 90: 111-134.
15. Cooper CW (1992) Risk factor in transmission of brucellosis from animal to humans in Saudi Arabia. Transactions of the Royal Society of Tropical Medicine and Hygiene 86: 206-209.
16. World Health Organization (1975) Fifth report on the World Health Situation. Geneva, 1969 -1972.
17. Brew SD, Perrett LL, Stack JA, MacMillan AP, Staunton, NJ (1999) Human exposure to Brucella recovered from a sea mammal. Veterinary Record 144: 483.
18. Sohn AH, Probert WS, Glaser CA, Gupta N, Bollen AW, et al. (2003) Human neurobrocellosis with intracerebral granuloma caused by a marine mammal Brucella sp. Emerging Infectious diseases 9: 485- 488.
19. McDonald WL, Jamaludin R, Mackereth G, Hansen M, Humphrey S, et al. (2006) Characterization of Brucella sp. Strain as a marine-mammal type despite isolation from a patient with spinal osteomyelitis in New Zealand. Journal of Clinical Microbiology 44: 4363- 4370.
20. Timm BM (1982) Brucellosis. Distribution in man, domestic and wild animals. Springer, Berlin.
21. Kasyanov AN, Aslanyan RG (1982) Epizootiology and clinical appearance of animal brucellosis. In: Lesenko A, edzoonoses control Moscow, VII Centre projects.
22. Bruce Sir David (1887) Note On the Discovery of a Microorganism in Malta Fever, The Practioner 59:161-170.
23. Hughes ML (1897) Mediterranean, Malta or Undulant Fever. Macmillan London, 1-10, 28, 80, 85,148, 156, 166.
24. Wright AE, Smith F (1897)On the application of the serum test to the differential diagnosis of typhoid and Malta fever. Lancet 1: 656-9.
25. Zammit T (1905) Report of the commission on Mediterranean fever, part III. Harrison and Sons London p 83.
26. Moreno E, Cloeckaert A, Moriyon I (2002) Brucella evolution and taxonomy. Veterinary Microbiology 90: 209-277.
27. Bricker BJ, Ewalt DR, Macmillan AP, Foster G, Brew S (2000) Molecular characterization of Brucella strains isolated from marine mammals. Journal of Clinical Microbiology 38: 1258-1262.
28. Moreno E, Stackebrandt, Dorsch M, Wolters J, et al. (1990) Brucellaabortus 16s rRNA and lipid A reveal a phylogenetic relationship with members of the alpha-2 subdivision of the class proteobacteria. Journal of Bacteriology 35: 292-295.
29. Moreno E, Moriyón I (2002) Brucellamelitensis: A nasty bug with hidden credentials for virulence. Proceedings of the National Academy of Sciences 99: 1-3.
30. Nasir AA, Parveen Z, Shah A, Rashid M (2004) Seroprevalence of brucellosis in animals at government and private livestock farms in Punjab. Pakistan Veterinary Journal 24: 144-146
31. Office International des Épizooties (2009) World Organization For Animal Health. Bovine brucellosis. Article 2.4.3. In: Terrestrial Manual 2009. V.2, part 2, section 4, chapter 2.4.3.
32. CDC (2008) "Public Health Consequences of a False-Positive Laboratory Test Result for Brucella—Florida, Georgia, and Michigan, 2005," Morbidity and Mortality Weekly Report (MMWR) 57: 603-605.
33. Nicoletti P (1980) The epidemiology of bovine brucellosis. Advances in veterinary science and comparative medicine 24: 69-98.
34. Garcia-Carrillo C, Lucero NE (1993) Brucellosis bovina: Hemisferio Sur. Buenos Aires.
35. Andres MA, Burzako S, Montero GV, Franco VR (2003) Brucella endocarditis: two cases with medical treatment and successful outcome. MedicinaClínica (Barcelona) 120: 477.
36. Cesur S, Ciftci A, Sozen TH, Tekeli E (2003) A case of epididymo-orchitis and paravertebral abscess due to brucellosis. Journal of Infection 46: 251-253.

37. Gur A, Geyik MF, Dikici B, Nas K, Cevik R, et al. (2003) Complications of brucellosis in different age groups: a study of 283 cases in southeastern Anatolia of Turkey. Yonsei Medical Journal 44: 33-44.
38. Dalrymple-Champneys W (1960) Prognosis. Brucella infection and undulant fever in man. Oxford & New York: Oxford University Press 151-155.
39. Zinsstag J, Schelling E, Solera J, Blasco JM, Moriyo´n I (2011) Brucellosis. In: Palmer SR, Soulsby L, Torgeson PR, Brown DG, editors. Handbook of Zoonoses. Oxford & New York: Oxford University Press 54-62.
40. Mantur BG, Biradar MS, Bidri RC, Mulimani MS, Veerappa, et al. (2006) Protean clinical manifestations and diagnostic challenges of human brucellosis in adults: 16 years' experience in an endemic area. Journal of Medical Microbiology 55: 897-903.
41. Bingol A, Togay IC (2006) Neurobrucellosis as an exceptional cause of transient ischemic attacks. European Journal of Neurology 13: 544 -548.
42. Young EJ (1995)An overview of human brucellosis. Clinical Infectious Diseases 21: 283-289
43. HasanjaniRoushanm MR, Mohrez M, SmailnejadGangi SM, Soleimani-Amiri MJ, Hajiahmadi M (2004) Epidemiological features and clinical manifestations in 469 adult patients with brucellosis in babol, northern iran. Epidemiology & Infection 132: 1109-14.
44. Kochar DK, Kumawat BL, Agarwal N, Shubharakaran N, Aseri S, et al. (2000) Meningoencephalitis in brucellosis. Neurology India 48: 170 -3.
45. Pappas G, Akritidis N, Bosilkovski M, Tsianos E (2005) Brucellosis. The New England Journal of Medicine 352: 2325 -36.
46. Bikas C, Jelastopulu E, Leotsinidis M, Kondakis X (2003) Epidemiology of human brucellosis in a rural area of northwesternpeloponnese in Greece. European Journal of Epidemiology 18: 267 -274.
47. Arlett PR (1996) A case of laboratory acquired brucellosis. British Medical Journal 313: 1130 -1132.
48. Yagupsky P, Baron EJ (2005) Laboratory exposures to Brucellae and implications for bioterrorism. Emerging Infectious Disease journal 11: 1180 -1185
49. Malik GM (1997) A clinical study of brucellosis in the Asir region of southern Saudi Arabia.The American Journal of Tropical Medicine and Hygiene 56: 375- 377.
50. Pappas GP, Papadimitriou N, Akritidis L, Christou EV, Tsianos (2006) "The New Global Map of Human Brucellosis." Lancet Infectious Diseases 6: 91-99.
51. Boschiroli ML, Foulongne V, O'callaghan D (2001) Brucellosis: a worldwide zoonosis. Current Opinion in Microbiology 4: 58-64.
52. (1986) Joint FAO/WHO Expert Committee on Brucellosis.World Health Organization technical report series 740: 1-132.
53. Smits HL, Kadri SM (2005) Brucellosis in India: A deceptive infectious disease. Indian Journal of Medical Research 122: 375-384.
54. European Food Safety Authority (2013) The European Union summary report on trends and sources of zoonoses and zoonotic agents and food-borne outbreaks in 2011. European Food Safety Authority 11: 3129.
55. PAHO-WHO (2001) Zoonoses and Communicable disease common to man, animals and wild life, Volume I. Bacterioses and Mycoses. In: Scientific and Technical publications No.580. Pan American Health Organization Regional office of the WHO, Washington DC USA 44-67.
56. Al Dahouk S, Neubauer H, Hensel A, Schöneberg I, Nöckler K, et al. (2007) Changing epidemiology of human brucellosis, Germany, 1962-2005. Emerging Infectious Diseases 13: 1895-900.
57. Kumar R, Prabhakar RK (2013) Opportunities and challenges in Indian dairy industry supply chain: A literature review. International Journal of Logistics & Supply Chain Management Perspectives 2: 791-800.
58. (2007) Livestock Census. Department of Animal Husbandry, Dairying and Fisheries, Ministry of Agriculture, Government of India.
59. Government of India (2012) Basic Animal Husbandry Statistics. Department of Animal Husbandry, Dairying and Fisheries.
60. Singh G, Sharma DR, Sandhu KS, Dhand NK (2002) Economic losses occurring due to bovine abortions in Punjab. In: 10th International Congress of Asian-Australasian Association of Animal Production Societies, New Delhi, India 23-27.
61. McDermott J, Grace D, Zinsstag J (2013) Economics of brucellosis impact and control in low-income countries. Revue scientifiqueet technique (International Office of Epizootics) 32: 249-261.
62. Megid J, Mathias LA, Robles CA (2010) Clinical manifestations of brucellosis in domestic animals and humans. Open Veterinary Science Journal 4: 119-126.
63. Sehgal S, Bhatia R (1990) Zoonosis in India. Journal of communicable diseases 22: 227-235.
64. Renukaradhya GJ, Isloor S, Rajasekhar M (2002) Epidemiology, zoonotic aspects, vaccination and control/eradication of brucellosis in India. Veterinary Microbiology 90: 183-195.
65. Isloor S, Renukaradhya GJ, Rajasekhar M (1998) A serological survey of bovine brucellosis in India. Revue scientifiqueet technique (International Office of Epizootics) 17: 781-785.
66. Mehra KN, Dhanesar NS, Chaturvedi VK (2000) Sero-prevalence of brucellosis in bovine in Madhya Pradesh. Indian Veterinary Journal 77: 571-573.
67. Chakraborty M, Patgiri GP, Barman NN (2000) Application on delayed-type hypersensitivity test (DTH) for the diagnosis of bovine brucellosis. Indian Veterinary Journal 77: 849-851.
68. Mathur TN (1964) Brucella strains isolated from cows, buffaloes, goat, sheep and human beings at karnal: their significance with regards to the epidemiology of brucellosis. Indian Journal of Medical Research 52: 1231- 1240.

69. Randhawa AS, Karla DS, Kapur MP (1974) Someseroepidemiologic observation on brucellosis in human and animals. Indian Journal of Medical Sciences 28:133-8.

70. Panjarathinam R, Jhala CL (1986) Brucellosis in Gujarat state. Indian Journal of Pathology and Microbiology 29: 53-60.

71. Chauhan RS (1999) Brucellosis in India and its impact on export of buffalo Meat. Indian Journal of Animal Production 31: 16-17.

72. Hemashettar BM, Patil CS (1991) Brucellosis among practicing veterinarians. Indian Journal of Medical Microbiology 9: 45-47.

73. Mantur BG, Akki AS, Mangalgi SS, Patil SV, Gobbur RH, et al. (2004) Childhood brucellosis-a microbiological, epidemiological and clinical study. Journal of Tropical Pediatrics 50:153 -157.

74. Handa R, Singh S, Singh N, Wali JP (1998) Brucellosis in north India: results of a prospective study. Journal of Communicable Diseases 30: 85-87.

75. Kalasinsky KS, Hadfield T, Shea AA, Kalasinsky VF, Nelson MP, et al. (2007) "Raman chemical imaging spectroscopy reagent less detection and identification of pathogens: signature development and evaluation." Journal of Analytical Chemistry 79: 2658- 2673.

76. Detilleux PG, Billy LD, Norman FC (1990)"Penetration and intracellular growth of Brucellaabortus in non phagocytic cells in vitro." Infection and Immunity 58: 2320-2328.

77. Zhan Y, Kelso A, Cheers C (1995) Differential activation of Brucella reactive CD4+T cells by Brucella infection or immunization with antigenic extracts. Infection and Immunity 63: 969-975

78. Canning PC, Roth JA, Deyoe BL (1986) Release of 5'-guanosine monophosphate and adenine by Brucellaabortus and their role in the intracellular survival of the bacteria. Journal of Infectious Diseases 154: 464-470.

79. Jubier-Maurin V, Boigegrain RA, Cloeckert A, Gross A, Alvares-Martinez MT, et al. (2001) Major outer membrane protein Omp 25 of Brucellasuis is involved in inhibition of tumor necrosis factor alpha production during infection of human macrophages. Infection and Immunity 69: 4823-4830.

80. Yagupsky P (1999) Detection of Brucellae in blood cultures. Journal of Clinical Microbiology 37: 3437-3442

81. Al Dahouk S, Tomaso H, Nockler K, Neubauer H, Frangoulidis D (2003) Laboratory-based diagnosis of brucellosis-a review of the literature. Part I: Techniques for direct detection and identification of Brucella spp. Clinical Laboratory 49: 487-505.

82. Morgan WJ, MacKinnon DJ, Cullen GA (1969)The Rose Bengal plate agglutination test in the diagnosis of brucellosis. Veterinary Record 85: 636-s641.

83. Nicoletti P (1969) Further evaluations of serologic test procedures used to diagnose brucellosis. American Journal of Veterinary Research 30: 1811-1816.

84. Angus RD, Barton CE (1984)The production and evaluation of a buffered plate antigen for use in a presumptive test for brucellosis. In: Third International symposium on brucellosis, Algiers, Algeria, 1983. Developments in biological standardization, Basel.

85. Gall D, Nielsen K (2004) Serological diagnosis of bovine brucellosis: a review of test performance and cost comparison. Revue scientifiqueet technique (International Office of Epizootics) 23: 989-1002.

86. Corbel MJ (1972) Characterization of antibodies active in the Rose Bengal plate test for bovine brucellosis. Veterinary Record 90: 484-5.

87. Nielsen K, Heck F, Wagner G, Stiller J, Rosenbaum B, et al. (1984) Comparative assessment of antibody isotypes to Brucellaabortus by primary and secondary binding assays. Preventive Veterinary Medicine 2: 197-204.

88. Rice C, Boyes B (1971) Serum immunoglobulins in bovine brucellosis. New Zealand Veterinary Journal 19: 146-54.

89. Barbuddhe SB, Yadava VK, Singh DK (1994) Detection of IgM and IgG antibodies against Brucella by dot-ELISA in humans. Journal of Communicable Diseases 26: 1-5.

90. Singh SV, Agrawal GS, Batra HV, Gupta VK, Singh N (2000) Monitoring of Brucella infection associated with reproductive losses using multiple serological tests in organized goat and sheep flocks. The Indian journal of animal sciences 70: 154-156.

91. Shome R, Filia G, Padmashree BS, Krithiga N, Sahay S, et al. (2015) Evaluation of lateral flow assay as a field test for investigation of brucellosis outbreak in an organised buffalo farm: A pilot study. Veterinary World 8: 492-496.

92. Gurturk K, Bovnukara B, Llhan Z, Hakki EI, Gulhan T (1999) Comparison of the dot immunobinding assay with the serum agglutination test, the rose bengal plate test and the milk ring test for the detection of Brucella antibodies in bovine sera and milk. Zentralblatt fur Veterinarmedizin. Reihe B. Journal of veterinary medicine Series B 46: 279-285.

93. Adone R, Ciuchini F, Pistoia C, Pasquali P (2002) Combined S99/RB51 antigen for complement fixation test for serological diagnosis of brucellosis in cattle and sheep. Journal of Applied Microbiology 93: 872-876.

94. Franco MP, Mulder M, Gilman RH, Smits HL (2007) Human brucellosis. Lancet Infectious Diseases 7: 775-786.

95. Lucero NE, Foglia L, Ayala SM, Gall D, Nielsen KH (1999) Competitive enzyme immunoassay for diagnosis of human brucellosis. Journal of Clinical Microbiology 37: 3245-3248.

96. Solera J, Martinez-Alfaro E, Espinosa A (1997) Recognition and optimum treatment of brucellosis. Drugs 53: 245-56.

97. Solera J (2000) Treatment of human brucellosis. Le Journal medical libanais 48: 255-63.

98. Solera J, Martinez-Alfaro E, Espinosa A, Castillejos ML, Geijo P, et al. (1998) Multivariate model for predicting

relapses in human brucellosis. Journal of Infection 36: 85-92.

99. (1986) World Health Organization Joint FAO/WHO Expert Committee on Brucellosis. Sixth report. Technical Report Series 740. Geneva, Austria: WHO 1-132.

100. Spink WW (1960) Current status of therapy of brucellosis in human beings. Journal of the American Medical Association 172:697-8.

101. Philippon AM, Plommet MG, Kazmierczak A, Marly JL, Nevot PA (1977) Rifampin in the treatment of experimental brucellosis in mice and guinea pigs. Journal of Infectious Diseases 136:481-8.

102. Roushan MR, Gangi SM, Ahmadi SA (2004) Comparison of the efficacy of two months of treatment with co-trimoxazole plus doxycycline vs. co-trimoxazole plus rifampin in brucellosis. Swiss Medical Weekly 134: 564-8.

103. Solera J, Geijo P, Largo J, Rodriguez-Zapata M, Gijon J, et al. (2004) A randomized, double-blind study to assess the optimal duration of doxycycline treatment for human brucellosis. Clinical Infectious Diseases 39: 1776-82

104. El Miedany YM, El Gaafary M, Baddour M, Ahmed I (2003) Human brucellosis: do we need to revise our therapeutic policy? Journal of Rheumatology 30: 2666-72.

105. Bayindir Y, Sonmez E, Aladag A, Buyukberber N (2003) Comparison of five antimicrobial regimens for the treatment of brucellar spondylitis: a prospective, randomized study. Journal of Chemotherapy 15: 466-71.

106. Young EJ (2003) Brucella species (Brucellosis). In: Yu VL, Weber R, Raoult D (eds) Antimicrobial, therapy and vaccines. Vol. I: Microbes. New York, USA: Apple Tree Productions LLC, 121-40.

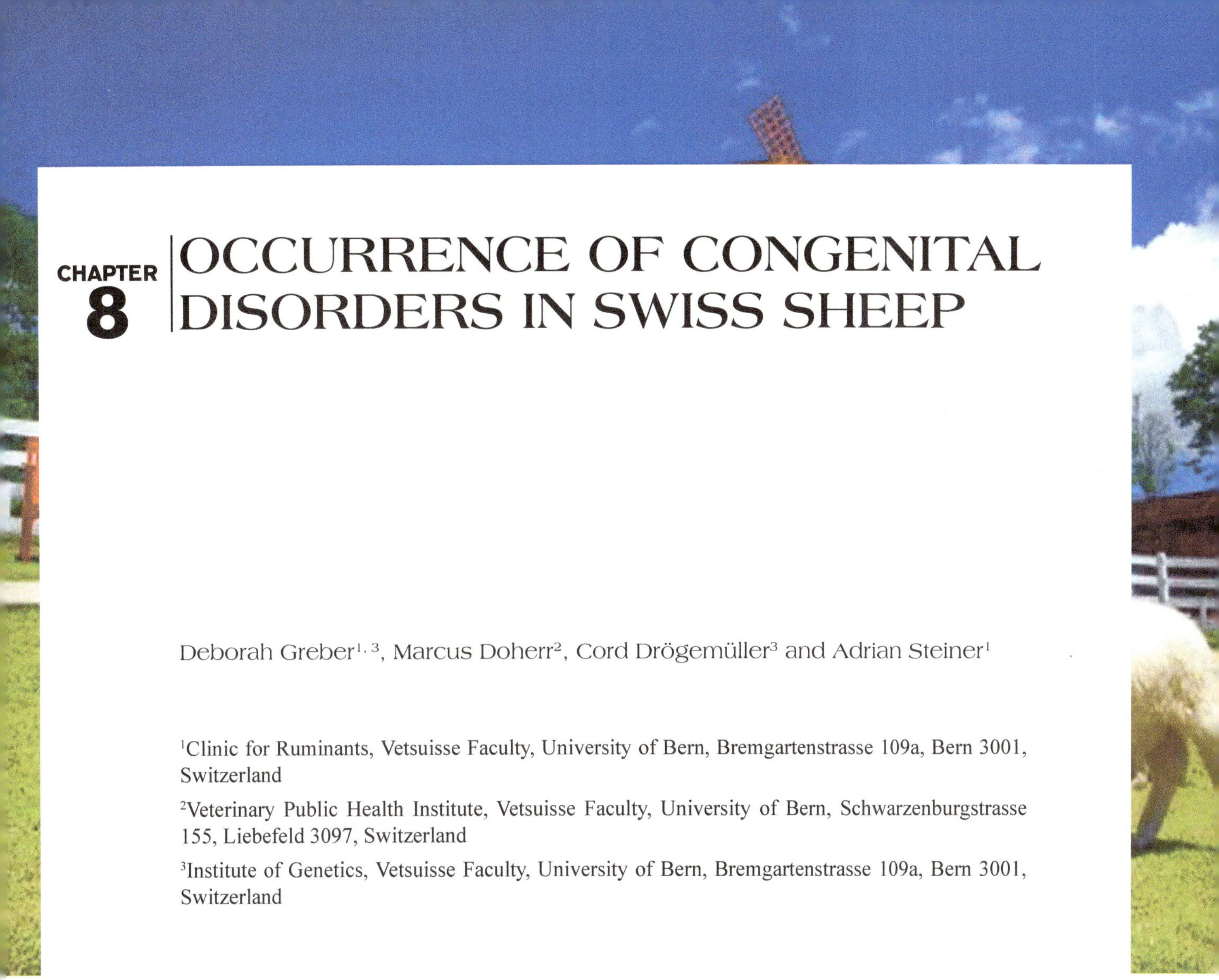

CHAPTER 8

OCCURRENCE OF CONGENITAL DISORDERS IN SWISS SHEEP

Deborah Greber[1, 3], Marcus Doherr[2], Cord Drögemüller[3] and Adrian Steiner[1]

[1]Clinic for Ruminants, Vetsuisse Faculty, University of Bern, Bremgartenstrasse 109a, Bern 3001, Switzerland

[2]Veterinary Public Health Institute, Vetsuisse Faculty, University of Bern, Schwarzenburgstrasse 155, Liebefeld 3097, Switzerland

[3]Institute of Genetics, Vetsuisse Faculty, University of Bern, Bremgartenstrasse 109a, Bern 3001, Switzerland

ABSTRACT

Background

The rates of congenital disorders in Swiss sheep were determined by a questionnaire which was sent to 3,183 members of the Swiss Sheep Breeders' Association.

Findings

A total of 993 questionnaires were returned, giving a response rate of 31.2%. Of these, 862 questionnaires originated from farms keeping one of the predominant Swiss sheep breeds: Swiss White Alpine sheep, Brown-Headed Meat sheep, Swiss Black Brown Mountain sheep and Valais Blacknose sheep. During a 10-year-period, entropion was reported in 33.6% of the farms, brachygnathia inferior in 29.5%, abdominal/umbilical hernia in 15.9%, cryptorchidism in 10.5% and torticollis in 10.5%. The most significant difference between the four breeds ($P<0.001$) occurred for entropion in Swiss White Alpine sheep and Brown-Headed Meat sheep, brachygnathia inferior in Swiss Black Brown Mountain sheep, and scrotal/inguinal hernia in Valais Blacknose sheep. The Swiss White Alpine breed showed a significantly higher animal prevalence of entropion (6.2% in 2011 and 5.5% in 2012) than other breeds ($P<0.001$).

Conclusions

These findings indicate a breed-specific necessity for action, particularly regarding Swiss animal welfare legislation, especially entropion in Swiss White Alpine sheep is concerned. In general, careful selection of breeding stock is to be recommended.

Citation: Deborah Greber, Marcus Doherr, Cord Drögemüller, and Adrian Steiner, Occurrence of congenital disorders in Swiss sheep, DOI: 10.1186/1751-0147-55-27.

BACKGROUND

Modern sheep production is primarily focused on economically important traits like meat and milk. The productivity of certain breeds has improved remarkably due to efficient breeding programs rooted in quantitative genetics. However, although stringent selection increases profitability, it may reduce effective population size, particularly when single elite rams and their progeny are used intensively. The accompanying increase in co-ancestry and inbreeding leads to the emergence of recessive genetic defects, which may cause significant economic and animal welfare concerns. For instance, in the last decade, outbreaks of arthrogryposis were reported in Suffolk sheep [1], microphthalmia in Texel sheep [2], epidermolysis bullosa in German Black-Headed Mutton [3], inherited rickets in Corriedale sheep [4], and cervical vertebral malformation in Texel sheep [5]. Long before the era of quantitative genetics such defects also emerged from time to time due to the limited availability of unrelated rams. Breeders have always tended to mate related individuals, partly due to a lack of unrelated animals, and partly in order to breed phenotypically similar animals. Nowadays this still holds true, especially in small populations e.g. of endangered breeds. It is crucial that sheep breeders implement effective strategies to control in-breeding and subsequent increased numbers of defects. A path towards that goal is to establish surveillance to detect emerging defects and collect DNA samples of defective animals. Such material can be used to study the underlying genetics of recorded defects and to develop gene tests for selection.

In the past, the occurrence of undesirable traits recognized as inherited disorders in sheep has been reported [5, 6, 7, 8]. However, a significant number of unrecorded cases is likely to have occurred have probably remained unreported [7]. Congenital disorders are not necessarily inherited as they may be due to environmental or infectious factors [7, 9, 10]. However, it is known that many congenital disorders have a genetic cause. Some of the common genetic disorders in sheep are atresia ani, arthrogryposis, brachygnathia, chondrodysplasia, cleft palate, cryptorchidism, entropion, hernia, and torticollis [5, 6]. A continuously updated database reports a total of 215 inherited ovine defects, disorders, predispositions to disease, production traits and coat colors [11]. A recent review gives an overview of predominantly recessive inherited ovine genetic traits, for which causal gene variants are known and where gene testing can be used to eliminate these undesirable mutations [12].

It is well known that the prevalence of congenital disorders varies among breeds and among lines within breeds. Once recognized, they may not be widely reported by breeders because of image damage and the financial consequences of not being able to sell potentially valuable stock. Nowadays, animal protection and welfare are of increasing importance to sheep breeders as well as to consumers. The Swiss Protection of Animals Act [13] and the Swiss Protection of Animals Ordinance [14] define that only healthy animals should be used for breeding.

Switzerland has several indigenous and locally developed breeds of sheep with unique combinations of adaptive traits to best respond to local environment pressures. In addition, several imported breeds are also established as synthetic breeds after introgression into local breeds. Presently, about 20% of Swiss sheep are registered in a herd book. The aim of this study was to describe the occurrence of congenital diseases and defects in the four main Swiss breeds of sheep, comprising more than 10,000 registered breeding animals. Therefore, we performed a survey in two certified native breeds, the Swiss Black Brown Mountain sheep (SBS) and the Valais Blacknose sheep (VBS), and two synthetic breeds, the Swiss White Alpine sheep (SWA) and the Brown-Headed Meat sheep (BHM) (Figure 1).

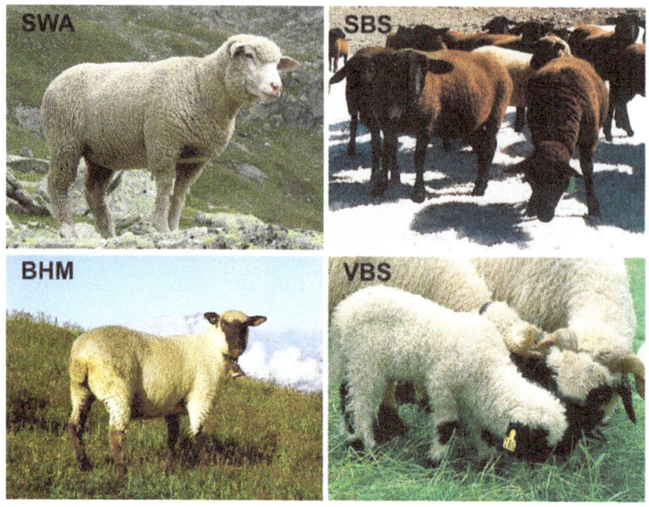

Figure 1: Representative breed individuals. (SWA=Swiss White Alpine sheep; BHM=Brown Headed Meat sheep; SBS=Swiss Black Brown Mountain sheep; VBS=Valais Blacknose sheep). Pictures were provided by the Swiss Sheep Breeders' Association.

The SBS breed was mentioned as far back as the 14th century and is a composite of different land races. Originally, it was bred for its dark, fine, high quality wool. The breed only became standardized at the beginning of the 20th century and today it accounts for about 15% of the total Swiss sheep registered. The VBS breed was first mentioned in the 15th century and today accounts for about 17% of the total sheep registered. This breed boasts exceptional characteristics which have been acquired through centuries, such as adaptability to the harsh mountain climate, good conversion of roughage, fecundity, an affable nature and loyalty to its home range.

In addition, the two predominant synthetic Swiss sheep breeds were included: SWA constitutes about 50% of total sheep registered and is a composite of several mountain breeds. Ongoing cross-breeding with foreign breeds like Merino, Texel and Ile de France has sustainably improved the meat and wool yield of the original land race sheep. The BHM breed represents one of the heaviest sheep in Switzerland and accounts for about 17% of the total sheep registered. It is the result of crossbreeding the English Oxford Downs and the German Black-Headed Mutton with the native Grabs sheep which was common to Switzerland in the 19th century. Crossbreeding with these foreign natives is still permitted to improve the breed.

This study presents the results of a questionnaire on congenital disorders sent to all members of the Swiss sheep breeders' association and attempts to estimate the occurrence of congenital disorders in the four main Swiss sheep breeds.

MATERIALS AND METHODS

The sheep owner agreed that the data from the questionnaire can be used for our study. All animal information has been obtained according to the national and international guidelines for animal welfare. There was no "animal experiment" according to the legal definitions in Switzerland.

As a first step, a questionnaire was sent to members of the Swiss sheep breeders' association that represents the herd book breeders of the four main sheep breeds included in this study. Before the questionnaire was sent to the breeders, they were informed about the common congenital disorders in a short article in a journal sent to all breeders and by oral presentations. In total, 3,183 questionnaires were sent to the breeders in early April 2012. The deadline for answers and return of the questionnaire was the 5th May 2012. As an alternative, a link to an internet-based version of the questionnaire was also provided. All answers received by the 13th May 2012 were included in the results.

The questionnaire consisted of two parts. In the first part, questions on the main breed for each flock were given: the numbers of ewes and rams on the farm at April 2012, the number of lambs in a 12-month period from January to December 2011 and in a 4-month period from January to April 2012. The breeders were also asked to report if one of the following defects had occurred during the last ten years: arthrogryposis, atresia ani, brachygnathia inferior, abdominal/umbilical hernia, scrotal/inguinal hernia, cleft palate, cryptorchidism, entropion, hydrocephalus, microphthalmia, and torticollis. We grouped the four types of hernia into two groups: abdominal/umbilical hernia and scrotal/inguinal hernia, respectively, because it may not be possible for breeders to distinguish between hernia with an almost similar appearance. In the second part, which focused on entropion, we asked for the number of affected lambs with this defect from January 2011 to December 2011 and from January to April 2012.

The results were analyzed using the statistical program NCSS 2007. The statistical significance of the difference between two independent proportions was tested with Fisher's exact and chi-square test. The *P*-value for a statistically significant difference was set at <0.05.

RESULTS AND DISCUSSION

We sent questionnaires to the 3,183 members of the Swiss sheep breeders' association, which represents about a third of all 9,428 registered sheep farmers in Switzerland in 2011 [15]. A total of 993 questionnaires were returned (31.2%), 862 of which dealt with one or more of the four breeds included: 385 flocks of SWA, 204 of BHM, 150 of SBS, and 123 of VBS, respectively. The 862 farmers corresponded to 9.1% of all sheep farmers in Switzerland.

In 2011, 68,165 animals of the four main Swiss breeds were registered in the herd book while totally 424,018 sheep were registered in the Swiss Stock Movement Database in 2011 [15]. A total of 19,982 sheep were included in the study in 2011 corresponding to 4.7% of the total registered Swiss sheep population.

As in our survey, the questionnaires were only being sent to herd book members. It can reasonably be concluded that the results tend to be at the lower limit. Herd book breeders might pay more attention to potentially congenital disorders and exclude potentially affected lambs from breeding than non-members.

Occurrence of Congenital Disorders

The proportion of farms reporting congenital disorders across the four breeds from 2002–2012 is shown in Figure 2. At farm level, the most prevalent defects were: entropion 33.6%, brachygnathia inferior 29.5%, abdominal/umbilical hernia 15.9%, cryptorchidism 10.5%, torticollis 10.5%, arthrogryposis 9%, atresia ani 7.7%, scrotal/inguinal hernia 6.9%, hydrocephalus 3.6%, cleft palate 1.7%, and microphthalmia 1.1%. Statistical analyses of the frequency of cleft palate, arthrogryposis, microphthalmia, and torticollis, showed insignificant differences among the four breeds, while significant differences were found for entropion, brachygnathia inferior, and scrotal/inguinal hernia ($P < 0.001$) (Table 1).

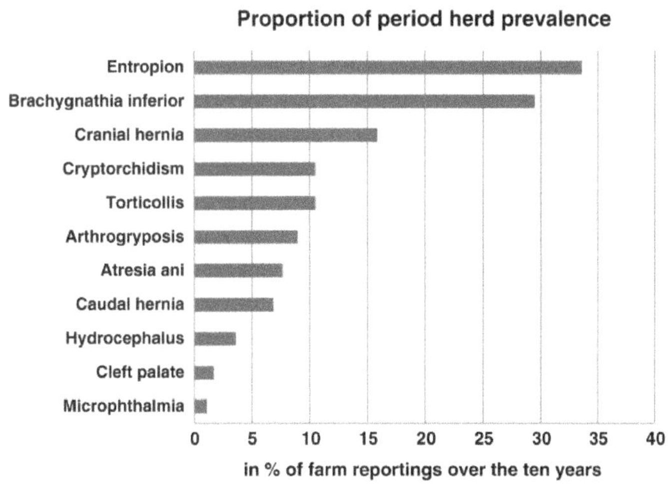

Figure 2: Proportion of farm reporting of congenital disorders of the four main Swiss sheep breeds, over a 10-year-period (2002–2012).

Table 1: Data on farm reporting congenital disorders in four Swiss sheep breeds during a 10-year-period (2002–2012)

		SWA	BHM	SBS	VBS	Total	z^2P*
Arthrogryposis	No. of farm reports	43	14	13	6	76	0.12

	Total no. of farms	380	200	148	119	847	
	Prevalence (%)	11.3	7	8.8	5	9	
Atresia ani	No. of farm reports	42	11	7	5	65	0.01
	Total no. of farms	380	199	148	119	846	
	Prevalence (%)	11.1	5.5	4.7	4.2	7.7	
Brachygnathia	No. of farm reports	131	34	66	19	250	<0.001
inferior	Total no. of farms	381	199	148	119	847	
	Prevalence (%)	34.4	17.1	44.6	16	29.5	
Cleft palate	No. of farm reports	8	1	4	1	14	0.31
	Total no. of farms	381	199	148	119	847	
	Prevalence (%)	2.1	0.5	2.7	0.8	1.7	
Cryptorchidism	No. of farm reports	46	23	17	3	89	0.02
	Total no. of farms	379	199	147	119	844	
	Prevalence (%)	12.1	11.6	11.6	2.5	10.5	
Entropion	No. of farm reports	202	74	10	3	289	<0.001
	Total no. of farms	385	203	150	123	861	
	Prevalence (%)	52.5	36.5	6.7	2.4	33.6	
Umbilical/	No. of farm reports	75	30	22	7	134	0.004
abdominal hernia	Total no. of farms	380	198	148	119	845	
	Prevalence (%)	19.7	15.2	14.9	5.9	15.9	
Scrotal/inguinal	No. of farm reports	22	4	4	28	58	<0.001
hernia	Total no. of farms	380	198	147	119	844	
	Prevalence (%)	5.8	2.0	2.7	23.5	6.9	
Hydrocephalus	No. of farm reports	22	4	3	1	30	0.015
	Total no. of farms	379	200	146	119	844	
	Prevalence (%)	5.8	2	2.1	0.8	3.6	
Microphthalmia	No. of farm reports	5	3	1	0	9	0.56
	Total no. of farms	381	199	147	119	846	
	Prevalence (%)	1.3	1.5	0.7	0	1.1	
Torticollis	No. of farm reports	48	24	9	8	89	0.07
	Total no. of farms	381	198	147	119	845	
	Prevalence (%)	12.6	12.1	6.1	6.7	10.5	

(*SWA* Swiss White Alpine sheep; *BHM* Brown Headed Meat sheep; *SBS* Swiss Black Brown Mountain sheep; *VBS* Valais Blacknose sheep).

*overall *P*-value between breeds.

A previous study on congenital disorders of sheep in Western Australia showed the occurrence of a wide range of defects: bowed forelegs, micrognathia, hermaphroditism, cryptorchidism, prognathia, atresia ani, microtia, entropion, torticollis, polythelia and arthrogryposis in order of decreasing frequency [6]. Our results are not directly comparable with these findings due to different study designs. The Australian survey identified the congenital defects commonly observed in sheep in Western Australia but gave no information on the incidence and cause of the various defects [6]. Our study reports the disorders that the breeders observed from 2002–2012 and provides estimates of the proportion of farms with particular congenital disorders. However, the two studies demonstrate that similar congenital defects occur in both regions.

The significance of the present study is limited by its design as breeders had to remember why they lost lambs in the course of the past ten years. Often, the cause of a single lost lamb remains unnoticed or forgotten while several malformed lambs are more likely to be recorded. It is likely that we have estimated the lower limit of how many farms that actually observed one of these disorders over the last ten years. On the one hand, herd book breeders probably pay more attention to congenital disorders than regular sheep farmers. In fact, we expected fewer questionnaires to be returned. On the other hand, the significant differences between the breeds indicate reliability in answering the questionnaire. We cannot rule out that reporting was biased. The study indicates that Swiss sheep breeders are interested in animal welfare and that breed-specific problems exist, especially entropion, brachygnathia inferior and hernia.

Entropion

On average, every third flock had cases of entropion during the last 10 years. Significant differences were detected between breeds as SWA had the highest proportion of farms reporting the defect (52.5%), while VBS had the lowest (2.4%). Due to rumors among breeders about a recent occurrence of this genetic defect in newborn lambs, we decided to ask for detailed data on this issue. This enabled us to give an accurate overview of the occurrence of entropion in the last two years (Table 2). The SWA breed showed a significantly higher animal prevalence (6.2% in 2011 and 5.5% in 2012) than in other breeds ($P<0.001$), while the prevalence of entropion in BHM was significantly higher than in SBS and VBS ($P<0.001$). There was no significant difference in the prevalence of entropion between SBS and VBS.

Table 2: Occurrence of entropion in 2011 (Jan to Dec) and 2012 (Jan to Apr) in the four main Swiss sheep breeds

		Number of all lambs	**Lambs affected with entropion**	**Prevalence (%)**	**Proportion (%) of farm reportings of entropion in 2011-2012**
SWA	2011	11820	737	6.2	36.9
	2012	7005	385	5.5	
BHM	2011	2618	71	2.7	19.2
	2012	2713	66	2.4	
SBS	2011	3504	7	0.2	2.7
	2012	2055	7	0.3	
VBS	2011	2215	2	0.09	1.6
	2012	1314	5	0.38	

(*SWA* Swiss White Alpine sheep; *BHM* Brown Headed Meat sheep; *SBS* Swiss Black Brown Mountain sheep; *VBS* Valais Blacknose sheep).

Table 2 clearly points out that almost every third farm keeping SWA sheep had lambs affected with entropion in the last two years. In 2011, a total of 737 out of 11,820 lambs were affected with entropion. Therefore, the study confirmed the rumors that the SWA have a higher frequency of lambs with entropion than the other breeds studied. A breed predisposition has not been reported in the literature, but a study has mentioned that entropion occurred more frequently in smaller flocks without regular exchange of the ram than in large populations [16]. Our findings show an urgent need for action against entropion in the SWA breed due to animal welfare reasons. It is advised that animals with affected offspring and the offspring itself should be excluded from breeding. However this may be complicated as successful surgery changes the phenotype as the treated animals become clinically normal. Thus, if the breeder does not accurately keep records on phenotypes, later distinguishing between normal and surgically-treated animals may be impossible. Several breeding experiments have been carried out and Littlejohn [17] claimed that the condition was not inherited as a simple Mendelian recessive defect, but that a genetic disposition existed. Taylor and Catchpole [18] stated that entropion represents an inherited disease. They postulated that the condition is caused by several recessive genes with additive effects. They showed in their experiment that the breed of the ram and the ewe influenced the probability of developing entropion. They bred three purebred Suffolk rams to purebred Scotch Half-bred ewes resulting in 10.8% of lambs with entropion, while the same Suffolk rams set to crossbreed ewes gave an incidence of 1.25% [18]. Comparable to our findings in SWA, a prevalence of 2.7 to 6.6% of entropion in lambs was recorded in three flocks in south west England over a 3 year period [19]. As we have observed in our study these authors showed that the only significant variable associated with the presence of entropion was the breed. Charolais and Texel lambs showed an increased risk of developing entropion when compared to Suffolk lambs [19]. An American study reported an overall mean incidence rate of entropion of 3.1% over a nine-year period, but the prevalence varied from 1.0 to 10.4% between different breeds [20]. Lamprecht and Pfeiffer [16] showed that female lambs are more often affected by entropion than males and observed that through the removal of the fathers of affected lambs, the frequency of the disease could be considerably decreased. Taken together, our data and the published studies on entropion show breed predispositions and indicate likely genetic causes of this disorder. Therefore, selection against this disorder might be performed in future.

Brachygnathia Inferior and Hernias

The occurrence of brachygnathia inferior and hernias showed statistically highly significant differences between breeds (Table 1). Brachygnathia inferior was the most common defect (Table 1) and 44.6% of SBS farms had recorded this defect.

Brachygnathia inferior is a common ovine defect that may be caused by recessive gene mutations, viruses, phytoteratogens or undetermined factors [7]. In some cases, brachygnathia inferior is presumably a genetic defect with a multifactorial inheritance with several genes being involved [21,22]. A recent breeding experiment showed that brachygnathia inferior in East Frisian milk sheep could not be explained by a simple monogenic Mendelian inheritance [22].

Abdominal/umbilical hernias occurred in equal frequencies in flocks of the SWA, BHM, and SBS breeds. Abdominal/umbilical hernias were significantly less common in VBS flocks ($P=0.004$) (Table 1). Birth of twins or triplets is more common in the SWA, BHM, and SBS breeds than in the VBS breed, which may affect the observed differences in prevalence among these breeds. Data on this issue was not included in the questionnaire.

Scrotal/inguinal hernia was recorded in a total of 6.9% of flocks in the last ten years. As this defect occurred in a higher proportion in the VBS than in other 3 breeds ($P<0.001$; Table 1), a breed predisposition can be assumed. Hernias are described to be either congenital or acquired and to occur as isolated defects or associated with defects of other parts of the body [23]. For scrotal hernia it was suggested that the condition has a recessive genetic character [24]. Braun and Cole [25] stated that the inheritance of inguinal and scrotal hernia in the ram is not understood; probably because their data did not fit any simple single-locus model. In the Merino breed, it is assumed, on the basis of a case report, that rams could be genetically predisposed to inguinal hernia [26].

In comparison with the other three breeds, all remaining congenital defects of interest in this survey appeared less frequently in the VBS breed. This result is somewhat surprising, because the VBS breed represents a comparatively smaller population, and it is assumed that they have a narrow gene pool. However, the data seem trustworthy as the reports of elevated numbers of scrotal/inguinal hernia for VBS indicate no concealment of disorders.

CONCLUSIONS

The survey revealed defects occurring at varying rates in four Swiss sheep breeds. There were statistically significant breed predispositions for entropion in the SWA and BHM breed, for brachygnathia inferior in the SBS breed, and for scrotal/inguinal hernia in the VBS breed. The identification of the most common defects might encourage the breeders to eliminate affected animals from their breeding program to decrease the incidence. The efficiency of this could be improved if DNA-based research was undertaken in order to develop genotyping tests.

ACKNOWLEDGMENTS

We are grateful to the team of the Swiss Sheep Breeders' Association (Schweizerischer Schafzuchtverband, SZV) and Rita Lüchinger (Beratungs- und Gesundheitsdienst für Kleinwiederkäuer, BGK).

AUTHORS' CONTRIBUTIONS

DG, CD and AS conceived and designed the study. DG conducted the survey. DG, CD and AS analyzed the data. DG and MD performed the statistical analysis. DG, CD and AS wrote the paper. All authors read and approved the final manuscript.

REFERENCES

1. Doherty ML, Kelley EP, Healy AM, Callanan JJ, Crosby TF, Skelly C, Boland MP: Congenital arthrogryposis: an inherited limb deformity in pedigree Suffolk lambs. Vet Rec. 2000, 146: 748-753. 10.1136/vr.146.26.748.
2. Becker D, Tetens J, Brunner A, Bürstel D, Ganter M, Kijas J, Drögemüller C: Microphthalmia in Texel sheep is associated with a missense mutation in the paired-like homeodomain 3 (PITX3) gene. PLoS One. 2010, 5: e8689. 10.1371/journal.pone.0008689.
3. Mömke S, Kerkmann A, Wöhlke A, Ostmeier M, Hewicker-Trautwein M, Ganter M, Kijas J, Distl O: A frameshift mutation within LAMC2 is responsible for Herlitz type junctional epidermolysis bullosa (HJEB) in black headed mutton sheep. PLoS One. 2011, 6: e18943. 10.1371/journal.pone.0018943.
4. Zhao X, Dittmer KE, Blair HT, Thompson KG, Rothschild MF, Garrick DJ: A novel nonsense mutation in the DMP1 gene identified by a genome-wide association study is responsible for inherited rickets in Corriedale sheep. PLoS One. 2011, 6: e21739. 10.1371/journal.pone.0021739.
5. Scott P: Some common genetic defects in sheep. Livestock. 2012, 17: 42-45.
6. Dennis SM: A survey of congenital defects of sheep. Vet Rec. 1974, 95: 488-490. 10.1136/vr.95.21.488.
7. Dennis SM: Congenital defects of sheep. Vet Clin N AM-Food A. 1993, 9: 203-217.
8. Saperstein G, Leipold HW, Dennis SM: Congenital defects of sheep. J Am Vet Med Assoc. 1975, 167: 314-322.
9. Distl O: Erbkrankheiten und Genveränderungen, genetische Krankheitsresistenz [in German]. Lehrbuch der Schafkrankheiten. Edited by: Behrens H, Ganter M, Hiepe T. 2001, Berlin: Blackwell, 363-384. 4
10. Angus K: Congenital malformations in sheep. In Pract. 1992, 14: 33-38. 10.1136/inpract.14.1.33.
11. Online Mendelian Inheritance in Animals, OMIA.http://omia.angis.org.au/,
12. Lühken G: Genetic testing for phenotype-causing variants in sheep and goats. Mol Cell Probe. 2012, 26: 231-237. 10.1016/j.mcp.2012.04.005.
13. Swiss Protection of Animals Act.http://www.admin.ch/ch/d/sr/455/a4.html,
14. Swiss Protection of Animals Ordinance.http://www.admin.ch/ch/d/sr/455_1/a25.html,
15. Swiss Stock Movement Database.http://www.bfs.admin.ch/bfs/portal/de/index/themen/07/03/blank/data/01/03.html,
16. Lamprecht H, Pfeiffer A: Entropion in newborn lambs. Vet Rec. 1984, 114: 251.
17. Littlejohn AI: Entropion in newborn lambs. Vet Rec. 1954, 66: 211-214.

18. Taylor M, Catchpole J: Incidence of entropion in lambs from two ewe flocks put to the same rams. Vet Rec. 1986, 118: 361.

19. Green LE, Berriatua E, Morgan KL: The prevalence and risk factors for congenital entropion in intensively reared lambs in south west England. Prev Vet Med. 1995, 24: 15-21. 10.1016/0167-5877(95)00468-C.

20. Sakul H, Kellom TR: Heritability of entropion in several US sheep breeds. Small Ruminant Res. 1996, 23: 187-190.

21. Dennis SM, Leipold H: Ovine congenital defects. Vet Bull. 1979, 49: 233-239.

22. Kerkmann A, Kuiper H, Ganter M, Distl O: Review of literature and results from test matings of East Friesian milk sheep affected with brachygnathia inferior[in German]. Berl Munch Tierarztl Wochenschr. 2008, 121: 292-305.

23. Dennis SM, Leipold HW: Congenital hernias in sheep. J Am Vet Med Assoc. 1968, 152: 999-1003.

24. Roberts SJ: Scrotal hernia in rams. A case report. Cornell Vet. 1988, 78: 351-352.

25. Braun WF, Cole WJ: Unilateral scrotal hernia repair in a ram lamb. J Am Vet Med Assoc. 1985, 187: 500.

26. Carr PM: An apparently inherited inguinal hernia in the Merino ram. Aust Vet J. 1972, 48: 126-127.

CHAPTER 9

GENOME-WIDE ASSOCIATION IDENTIFIES SLC2A9 AND NLN GENE REGIONS AS ASSOCIATED WITH ENTROPION IN DOMESTIC SHEEP

Michelle R. Mousel[1], James O. Reynolds[2], Stephen N. White[3]

[1]Range Sheep Production Efficiency Research Unit, Agricultural Research Service, Department of Agriculture, Dubois, ID, United States of America

[2]Animal Disease Research Unit, Agricultural Research Service, Department of Agriculture, Pullman, WA, United States of America

[3]Department of Veterinary Microbiology and Pathology, Washington State University, Pullman, WA, United States of America

ABSTRACT

Entropion is an inward rolling of the eyelid allowing contact between the eyelashes and cornea that may lead to blindness if not corrected. Although many mammalian species, including humans and dogs, are afflicted by congenital entropion, no specific genes or gene regions related to development of entropion have been reported in any mammalian species to date. Entropion in domestic sheep is known to have a genetic component therefore, we used domestic sheep as a model system to identify genomic regions containing genes associated with entropion. A genome-wide association was conducted with congenital entropion in 998 Columbia, Polypay, and Rambouillet sheep genotyped with 50,000 SNP markers. Prevalence of entropion was 6.01%, with all breeds represented. Logistic regression was performed in PLINK with additive allelic, recessive, dominant, and genotypic inheritance models. Two genome-wide significant (empirical $P<0.05$) SNP were identified, specifically markers in*SLC2A9* (empirical $P = 0.007$; genotypic model) and near *NLN* (empirical $P = 0.026$; dominance model). Six additional genome-wide suggestive SNP (nominal $P<1x10^{-5}$) were identified including markers in or near *PIK3CB* ($P = 2.22x10^{-6}$; additive model), *KCNB1* ($P = 2.93x10^{-6}$; dominance model), ZC3H12C ($P = 3.25x10^{-6}$; genotypic model), JPH1 ($P = 4.68x20^{-6}$; genotypic model), and *MYO3B* ($P = 5.74x10^{-6}$; recessive model). This is the first report of specific gene regions associated with congenital entropion in any mammalian species, to our knowledge. Further, none of these genes have previously been associated with any eyelid traits. These results represent the first genome-wide analysis of gene regions associated with entropion and provide target regions for the development of sheep genetic markers for marker-assisted selection.

INTRODUCTION

Entropion is an eye health problem where the eyelid rolls toward the eye, causing the hair and lashes to contact the eye and can cause blindness [1]. Blindness can occur because of corneal abrasion or secondary infections, which are common if the condition is not treated [2]. Several factors may contribute to the development of entropion, including congenital causes [3, 4], selective breeding [5, 6], scar tissue formation [7, 8], and/or age-related processes [9,10]. Congenital entropion has been identified in numerous mammals, including humans [11], horses [12], cats [13], dogs [14], rabbits [15], pigs [16], cattle [17], goats [18], and sheep [1]. In dogs, entropion has been

Citation: Mousel MR, Reynolds JO, White SN (2015) Genome-Wide Association Identifies SLC2A9 and NLN Gene Regions as Associated with Entropion in Domestic Sheep. PLoS ONE 10(6): e0128909. doi:10.1371/journal.pone.0128909.

identified as an inherited disorder of high research priority, particularly in Chinese Shar-Pei which has a frequency of 14–60% and Bulldogs with a frequency of 58% [19]. The cost of surgery in the U.S. to correct entropion ranges from $300 to $1500 in dogs [20] and in humans is at least $3000 [21], therefore, entroprion correction in the identified species costs U.S. consumers at least tens of millions of dollars per year.

There is evidence of genetic components to the development of entropion in sheep [22]. Reported worldwide frequency of entropion in lambs is quite variable from 1.1% to 80% [1, 2,4, 23, 24]. There are methods to correct entropion in lambs [25] but intervention by a veterinarian or trained personnel is costly, and untreated lambs may become blind [2]. Approximately 600,000 lambs in the U.S may be afflicted if entropion has a 10% frequency, costing about $150,000 per year to correct assuming a trained technician was paid minimum wage and could process 25 lambs per hour. These cost would increase significantly if a veterinarian was consulted for entropion correction. Heritability of entropion has been estimated to be 0.08–0.21 in Columbia, Polpay, Rambouillet, Suffolk, and Targhee breeds in the U.S. [22]. Because entropion is heritable, reduction of the condition within afflicted flocks can occur with careful selection when purchasing breeding sheep as well as culling the parents of and not breeding affected sheep. However, development of a genetic test for entropion would allow producers to more efficiently select replacement sheep without this defect.

Genotyping technologies exist which improve the probability of identifying genomic regions associated with phenotypic traits of interest in sheep. The Ovine SNP50 beadchip [26] was collaboratively, internationally developed and has been used to identify new markers associated with inherited diseases [27, 28], erythrocyte traits, [29], parasite infection [30], and other infectious disease traits [31, 32, 33]. We hypothesized that genomic regions related to development of entropion could be identified using genome-wide association using sheep as a model species. To ensure wide applicability of the findings and identify markers in more than 1 breed of sheep, 3 different breeds of sheep were evaluated in this study using genome-wide association with entropion.

MATERIALS AND METHODS

Ethics Statement

All animal care and handling procedures were reviewed and approved by the Washington State University Institutional Animal Care and Use Committee (Permit Number: 3171) and/or by the U.S. Sheep Experiment Station Animal Care and Use Committee (Permit Numbers: 10–06, 10–07). All efforts were made to minimize discomfort during collection of blood samples.

Populations and Phenotypes

At the U.S. Sheep Experiment Station (USSES), trained technicians determine entropion status within 48 hours of birth with entropion defined as the inward rolling of one or both lower eyelids in lambs. Upper eyelid entropion has never been documented is USSES lambs. All sheep born alive had entropion status recorded as either present or absent. Whole blood was collected from ewes of Rambouillet (N = 414), Polypay (N = 438), and Columbia (N = 146) breeds, ages 1–5 years. Entropion was documented in 60 of these ewes, with all breeds represented. These animals were managed in an extensive rangeland production system and bred in single sire mating pens.

Genotyping

Blood was collected by jugular venipuncture into EDTA-coated vacutainer tubes. DNA was isolated using the Invitrogen GeneCatcher gDNA 3–10 ml Blood Kit as per manufacturers' instructions (Life Technologies, Carlsbad, CA). The DNAs were checked for quality and quantity using an ND-1000 spectrophotometer (Nanodrop, Wilmington, DE) and equilibrated to 50ng/μl for genotyping. Genotyping services were provided by Geneseek Inc. (Lincoln, NE) using the OvineSNP50 Infinium BeadChip (Illumina Inc., San Diego, CA) with a set of 54,977 SNP designed by the International Sheep Genome Consortium [26].

Association Analysis

A preliminary screen for high genotype call rates (>97%) was performed to select individuals for further analysis. Multidimensional scaling analysis (MDS) of breed groups (S1 Fig [32]) and pairwise population concordance clustering were performed in PLINK v1.06 [34] as previously described [32]. Single nucleotide polymorphism inclusion screening criteria in PLINK analysis were as previously described [32]: missingness by individual (0.1), missingness by marker (0.03), minor allele frequency (0.01), and Hardy-Weinberg equilibrium (0.000001, which corresponds to P = 0.05 after Bonferroni correction for 50,000 marker tests). Four population groups were identified by population concordance clustering, including Polypay, Columbia, Rambouillet subgroup 1 and Rambouillet subgroup 2. The full model evaluated included fixed effects of population group (with 4 levels: Polypay, Columbia, Rambouillet subgroup 1, and Rambouillet subgroup 2) and SNP minor allele. Logistic regression was performed in PLINK to determine if there were genomic regions associated with presence or absence of entropion. An additional step assessed model fit for additive allelic, recessive, dominant, and genotypic inheritance models. Permutations were calculated within sire family as previously described [32]. Ten thousand permutations were performed to establish significance, and genome-wide significance was defined by empirical P<0.05. Genome-wide suggestive significance was defined by nominal P<1x10-5 per Wellcome Trust consortium guidelines [35]. PLINK only reports regression coefficients as a measure of effect size for linear regression, therefore, SAS 9.4 (SAS Institute, Cary, NC) was used to run similar genotypic models in the logistic procedure to obtain largest adjusted genotypic mean differences as a measure of effect size for entropion. An R script [36] provided by Dr. Stephen Turner (http://gettinggeneticsdone.blogspot.com/2011/04/annotated-manhattan-plots-and-qq-plots.html, viewed on 11-15-11) was used for visualization of results in Manhattan and quantile-quantile plots. Further, the top SNPs were interrogated using a threshold model similar to those described above, accounting for entropion status, breed/population cluster and genotype in the probit procedure of SAS 9.4 (SAS Inst. Inc., Cary, NC). Ensembl was used to determine the location of the SNP within genome assembly OAR_v3.1 as well as identify Ensembl annotated genes within 100 kb of the SNP. S2 Table shows the Illumina designated name of the SNP with the dbSNP rs# cluster id.

RESULTS

The total number of sheep evaluated in this genome-wide association study was 964, reduced from the original 998 due to sample quality control criteria and breed outlier status. The number of ewes per breed represented were Rambouillet (n = 399), Polypay (n = 423), and Columbia (n = 142). These included 59 sheep with entropion where all breeds were represented. The average genotyping call rate was 98.06% for the final population of sheep evaluated.

Manhattan plots showing P-values in order of chromosome position, from the genotypic and dominant analysis, are presented in Fig 1 and Fig 2, respectively. Two SNP were classified as genome-wide significant and six SNP were genome-wide suggestive (Table 1). Observed vs expected P-value distributions were visualized in quantile-quantile plots from genotypic analyses with all SNP (Fig 3) and the conditioned on the following 5 SNP, rs424438792, rs420662001, rs420083564, rs419388939, and rs405483139, (Fig 4). Fig 3 shows some of the observed P-values were divergent from the expected line indicating possible population stratification, including potentially differing frequencies of a small number of genetic mutations. Nearly all stratification is eliminated after conditioning the analysis on the 5 SNP shown above (Fig 4). This demonstrates that the apparent population stratification was due to differences in allele frequencies of SNP associated with entropion. Dominant analysis quantile-quantile plots with all SNP and conditioned on the above 5 SNP are shown in S2 Fig and S3 Fig. The genotype count for the top 8 SNP by breed and entropion status are shown in S1 Table and the raw data for these SNP may be found at:http://www.ncbi.nlm.nih.gov/projects/SNP/snp_viewBatch.cgi?ibid=1062140 orhttp://www.animalgenome.org/repository/pub/ USDA2015.0208/ Threshold analysis showed rs424438792, rs720662001, rs420083564, rs703034846, rs419388939, and rs405483139 significantly ($P < 0.04$) and rs415069937 and rs401620279 were not ($P > 0.06$) associated with entropion. The sheep genome assemble Oar_v3.1 [26] was used to determine the location of the top 8 SNP associated with entropion which were found to be located within or near the following genes: solute carrier family 2 C 9 (SLC2A9, a.k.a. GLUT9), phosphatidylinositol 4,5-bisphospate 3-kinase, catalytic subunit beta isoform (PIK3CB), myosin-IIIb (MYO3B), potassium voltage-gated channel subfamily B member 1 (KCNB1), neurolysin (NLN), zinc finger CCCH-type containing 12C (ZC3H12C), and junctophilin 1 (JPH1).

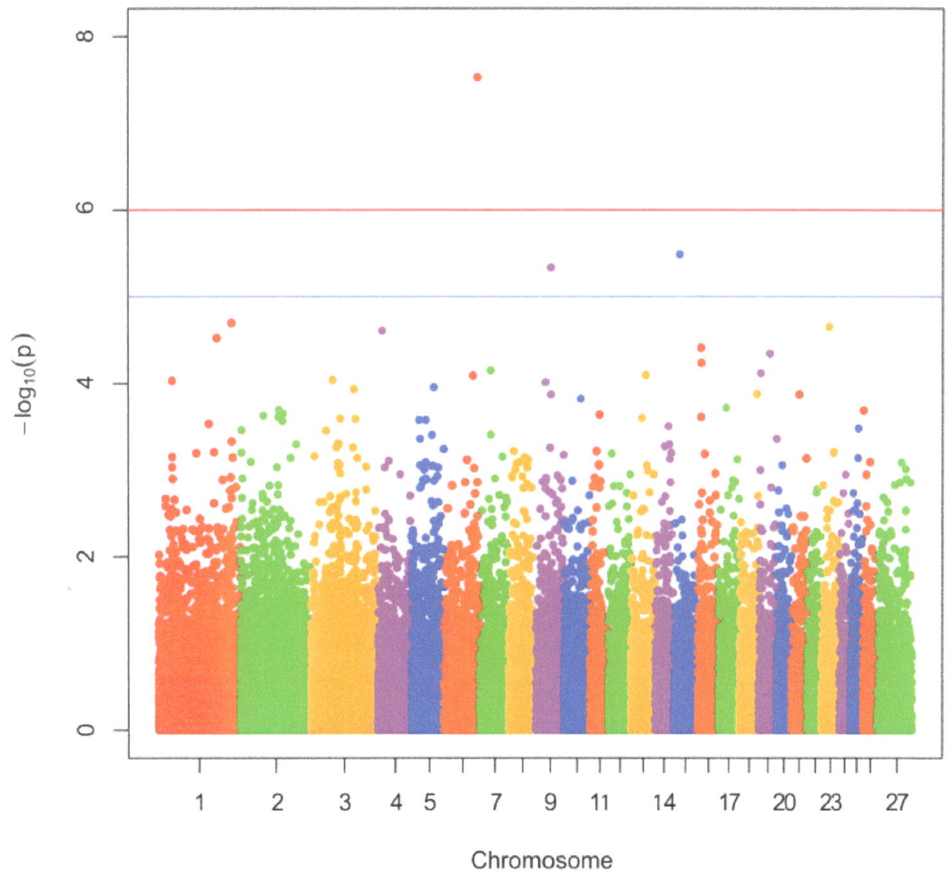

Figure 1: Genotypic Manhattan plot for entropion.

The Manhattan plot shows nominal P-values from association with entropion by chromosomal position. Data from genotypic mode of inheritance analyses. The top red line shows a genome-wide significance threshold defined by nominal P-values of 1x10-6, which is P = 0.05/50,000. The lower blue line shows a genome-wide suggestive significance threshold (1x10-5).

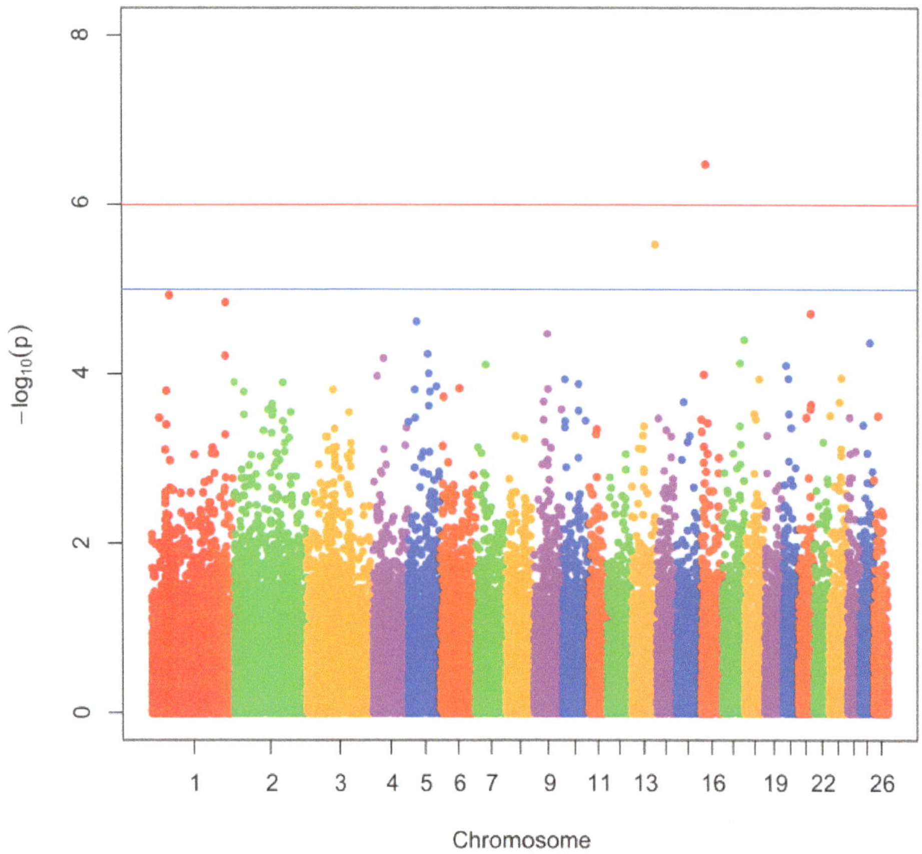

Figure 2. Dominant Manhattan plot for entropion.

The Manhattan plot shows nominal P-values from association with entropion by chromosomal position. Data from dominant mode of inheritance analyses. The top red line shows a genome-wide significance threshold defined by nominal P-values of $1x10^{-6}$, which is P = 0.05/50,000. The lower blue line shows a genome-wide suggestive significance threshold ($1x10^{-5}$).

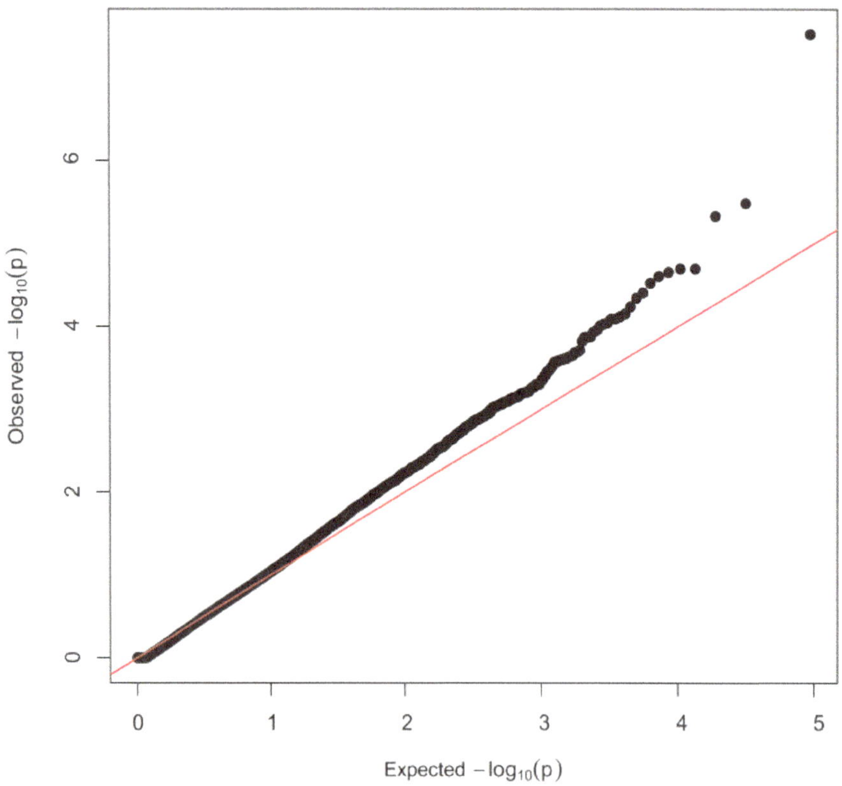

Figure 3: Quantile-quantile plots with all SNP from the genotypic analysis.

Quantile-quantile plots from association with entropion, where the expected distribution is the red line.

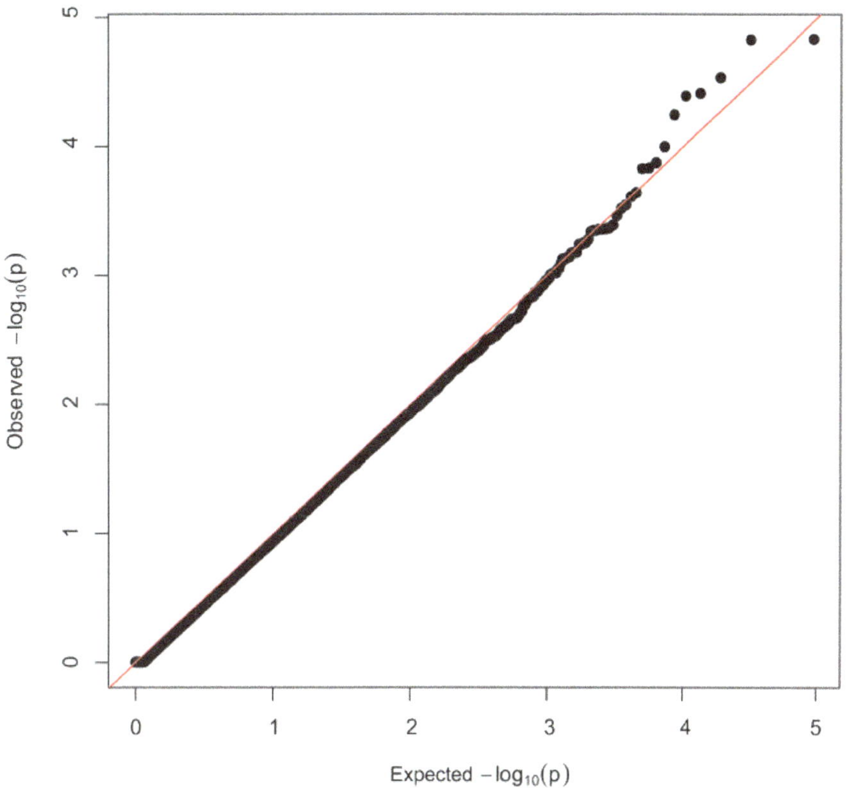

Figure 4: Quantile-quantile plots conditioned on 5 top SNP from the genotypic analysis.

Quantile-quantile plots from association with entropion, where the expected distribution is the red line. Differences in mutation allele frequency were accounted for with 5 of the top SNP in the model which eliminated apparent population stratification.

Table 1: Genomic regions associated with entropion

SNP	*Chr*	*Position (bp)*	*Best fitting model*	*Nominal P-value*	*Empirical P-value*	*Odds Ratio*	*Genes within 100 Kb on either side*
rs424438792	6	104,687,454	genotypic	2.97×10^{-8}	0.007	41.77	SLC2A9**
rs420662001	16	13,738,722	dominant	3.34×10^{-7}	0.026	11.01	NLN*, ERBB2IP
rs420083564	1	248,360,688	additive	2.22×10^{-6}	§	3.18	PIK3CB**, PRR23B
rs403034846	1	248,348,219	additive	2.22×10^{-6}	§	3.18	PIK3CB*, PRR23B
rs419388939	13	77,135,671	dominant	2.93×10^{-6}	§	4.06	KCNB1**, PTGIS
rs415069937	15	19,548,621	genotypic	3.25×10^{-6}	§	12.26	ZC3H12C
rs401620279	9	50,318,215	genotypic	4.68×10^{-6}	§	7.82	JPH1*
rs405483139	2	138,159,566	recessive	5.74×10^{-6}	§	4.27	MYO3B**

§: P>0.15
**: SNP located within gene
*: SNP located within 35 Kb of gene

DISCUSSION

Eyelid development in embryonic mammals has long been known to consist of four primary stages: specification, growth, epithelial fusion, and reopening [37, 38]. Many genes have been identified in these developmental stages using multiple phenotypes in mice including eyes-open-at-birth (EOB), and these have been grouped into two major pathways: Activin-MEKK1-JNK and TGFalpha-EGFR-ERK [38]. These pathways are required for correct eyelid development from both epithelial and mesenchymal cell layers and are important in coordinating interactions between the two [38].

However, much less is known about causes of the entropion, and especially about congenital entropion. Studies of entropion with a large infectious disease component (trachomatous entropion) have implicated contraction of the subepithelial fibrous membrane, which is formed by vertically oriented parallel collagen fibers [39]. Age-related entropion has been shown to be due largely to differences in the size of tarsal plates, the dense fibrous connective tissue that gives support and shape to the eyelid [40]. While less is known about the causes of congenital entropion, both tarsal plate problems and muscular hypertrophy have been implicated [41]. Together these results suggest fibroblasts, keratinocytes, macrophages, and myocytes, among others, may be key cell types for genetic influence on incidence of entropion [42, 43].

This is the first genome-wide association study to identify gene regions for any form of entropion in mammals, to our knowledge, and we identified two genome-wide significant and 5 genome-wide suggestive regions. None of the genes associated with the identified SNP were found directly within the Activin-MEKK1-JNK or TGFalpha-EGFR-ERK pathways [38].

The first genome-wide significant SNP (s65132) was located on chromosome 6 within *SLC2A9*. This SNP was identified in both the recessive and genotypic analysis, the genotypic model had both the smallest P-value (empirically P = 0.007) and the largest odds ratio (41.77) of any SNP in this study. The odds ratio indicated a large difference in odds of entropion by genotype, well above the odds ratio of 2 commonly used as a threshold for large effect size [44]. The*SLC2A9* gene encodes a glucose, fructose, and urate transporter with alternate splice isoforms expressed on different surfaces of polarized cells [45, 46]. In some tissues, the GLUT9 protein product of the *SLC2A9* gene is a major contributor to glucose influx [47]. Expression of*SLC2A9/GLUT9* has been shown in muscle cells at the mRNA and protein levels, and the GLUT9 protein may play a role in muscle cell proliferation [48]. Thus, it is possible that*SLC2A9* could be involved in muscle tone contributions to the development of entropion. While the *SLC2A9* gene has been most frequently associated with gout and renal disease in humans [49, 50], this is the first report of *SLC2A9* in connection to eyelid shape and positioning.

The chromosome 16 genome-wide significant SNP (OAR16_14874751), identified in both the additive and dominant analysis, had a large odds ratio of 11.01 in the dominant analysis, and was within 35Kb of *NLN* in version 3.1 of the ovine genome [51]. Neurolysin is a member of the metallopepidase M3 protein family that cleave many substrates including neurotensin and may play a role in the termination of the neurotensinergic signal in the central nervous system [52]. Neurolysin knock-out mice demonstrated that this enzyme plays a role in energy metabolism with mRNA expression differences in liver and overall increased glucose tolerance, insulin sensitivity, and gluconeogenesis [53]. In addition, NLN is part of the angiotensin-(1–7), MAS1 pathway in which genetic mutations could impact cellular development [54]. Further, active neurotensin (cleaved by neurolysin) increases epidermal growth factor expression [55], which connects NLN to the TGFalpha-EGFR-ERK pathway important for eyelid development [38]. Interestingly, neurotensin also modulates macrophage migration and inflammatory response under hyperglycemic conditions [56]. Since macrophages are one of the major cell types within eyelids [42], it is possible that *SLC2A9* might be functionally related to *NLN* in the development of entropion through the influence of sugar transport on neurotensin activity.

The other 6 genomic loci identified in this study were genome-wide suggestive. Specifically on chromosome 1, the two suggestive SNP were adjacent to one another on the Ovine SNP50 beadchip, were counted as one genomic locus, and were in the top 5 SNP of the additive and dominant analysis. This locus encompassed PIK3CB which is found on the outer membrane of eukaryotic cells and is important in many cellular pathways [57]. PIK3CB may modulate cell morphology [57], cell division, cell motility, metabolism, and apoptosis [58], thus potentially impacting neonatal development of entropion. In addition, p85α, a subunit of PIK3, has been shown to be required for mesenchymal stem cells to differentiate into osteoblasts, adipocytes, and chondrocytes in vitro [59]. The chromosome 2 genome-suggestive SNP, identified in the recessive analysis, was located within MYO3B which is a protein that mediates movement along actin filaments in the cell [60]. A GWAS evaluating adipose growth and deposition indicated that MYO3B may play a role in adipose deposition [61]. In context of this study, less adipose in the eyelid during development may play a role in entropion. The chromosome 13 genome-suggestive SNP, identified in the top 5 SNPs of both the additive and dominant analysis, was positioned within KCNB1 which plays a role in apoptosis in neurons [62] and may impact cell volume [63]. Cells with less volume within the eyelid may lead to entropion. The chromosome 15 suggestive SNP, identified in both additive and dominant analysis, had a large odds ratio of 12.26, and was within 100kb of ZC3H12C. This recently identified gene has been found to inhibit inflammation in vitro [64]. The chromosome 9 genome-suggestive SNP, located within 35 kb of JPH1, was identified in the top 5 SNPs of both the additive and dominant analysis. This gene is expressed in skeletal muscle and plays a role in intramembrane Ca2+ movement [65]. Reduced expression of JPH1 has been shown in inactive, weak skeletal muscle [66]. If the muscles underlying the eye lid were weak, this could conceivably lead to entropion.

In conclusion, we undertook the first genome-wide association study of entropion in any mammal to provide insight into genes and mechanisms influencing this condition. This research identified five chromosomal regions that were associated with entropion in three common U.S. sheep breeds, including two that were associated with very large odds ratios. Several genes have logical involvement in the development of entropion, but none had been implicated in eyelid traits previously. These results provide insight into the development of entropion in mammals, and they provide target genes and genomic regions for mutation discovery, which is ongoing. Furthermore, identifying and validating one or more markers for marker-assisted selection from future work in these genomic regions would help producers to reduce the incidence of entropion within their sheep flocks and potentially improve production.

ACKNOWLEDGMENTS

The authors gratefully acknowledge Tom Kellom, Codie Durfee, Nic Durfee, Liam Broughton-Neiswanger, Caylee Birge, David Herndon, Mike Gonzalez, Ralph Horn, James Allison, Duane Chandler, and the farm crews at Washington State University, ADRU, and USSES for technical assistance.

AUTHOR CONTRIBUTIONS

Conceived and designed the experiments: MRM SNW. Performed the experiments: MRM JOR SNW. Analyzed the data: MRM SNW. Contributed reagents/materials/analysis tools: MRM SNW. Wrote the paper: MRM JOR SNW.

REFERENCES

1. Warwick BL, Berry RO (1962) Infantile entropion in sheep. J Hered 53: 10–11. pmid:13999021

2. McManus TJ (1960) Report of entropion in newborn lambs. Aust Vet J 36: 91–92. doi: 10.1111/j.1751-

0813.1960.tb08577.x

3. Maman DY, Taub PJ (2011) Congenital entropion. Ann Plast Surg 66: 351–353. doi: 10.1097/SAP.0b013e3181e56e69. pmid:21301313
4. Greber D, Doherr M, Drögemüller C, Steiner A (2013) Occurrence of congenital disorders in Swiss sheep. Acta Veterinaria Scandinavica 55: 27–33. doi: 10.1186/1751-0147-55-27. pmid:23521894
5. Bistner S (1981) Entropion in the Shar Pei. Vet Med Small Anim Clin 76: 1246–1248. pmid:6916547
6. Allbaugh RA, Davidson HJ (2009) Surgical correction of periocular fat pads and entropion in a potbellied pig (Sus scrofa). Vet Ophthalmol 12: 115–118. doi: 10.1111/j.1463-5224.2008.00686.x. pmid:19261167
7. Guzey M, Ozardali I, Basar E, Aslan G, Satici A, Karadede S (2000) A survey of trachoma: the histopathology and mechanism of progressive cicatrization of eyelid tissues. Ophthalmologica 214: 277–284. pmid:10859511 doi: 10.1159/000027504
8. Balogun BG, Adekoya BJ, Balogun MM, Nqwu RV, Oworu O (2013) Ectropion and entropion in sub-Saharan Africa: how do we differ? Ann Afr Med 12: 193–196. doi: 10.4103/1596-3519.122682. pmid:24309406
9. Kocaoglu FA, Katircioglu YA, Tok OY, Pulat H, Omek F (2009) The histopathology of involutional ectropion and entropion. Can J Ophthalmol 44: 677–679. doi: 10.3129/i09-152. pmid:20029486
10. Michels KS, Czyz CN, Cahill KV, Foster JA, Burns JA, Everman KR (2014) Age-matched, case-controlled comparison of clinical indicators for development of entropion and ectropion. J Ophthalmol doi: 10.1155/2014/231487.
11. Zagora E (1966) Observations on trachomatous entropion and ectropoin. Ophthalmology 50: 6. doi: 10.1136/bjo.50.9.523
12. Peiffer RL Jr, Williams R, Schenk M (1977) Correction of congenital entropion in a foal. Vet Med Small Anim Clin 72: 1219–1225. pmid:587562
13. Smyth RS (1947) Entropion in the cat. Vet Rec 59: 148. pmid:20340330
14. Menges RW (1946) An operation for entropion in the dog. J Am Vet Med Assoc 109: 464. pmid:20274656
15. Fox JG, Shalev M, Beaucage CM, Smith M (1979) Congenital entropion in a litter of rabbits. Lab Anim Sci 29: 509–511. pmid:513624
16. White DG (1983) Neonatal entropion in a litter of pigs. Vet Rec 113: 542. pmid:6665961
17. Their L, Bay F (1965) Some cases of entropion in bulls. Berl Munch Tieraztl Wochenschr 78: 328–329. pmid:5858553
18. Donnelly KS, Pearce JW, Giuliano EA, Fry PR, Middleton JR (2014) Surgical correction of congenital entropion in related Boer goat kids using a combination Hotz-Celsus and lateral eyelid wedge resection procedure. Vet Ophthalmol doi: 10.1111/vop.12170.
19. Collins LM, Asher L, Summers J, McGreevy P (2011) Getting priorities straight: Risk assessment and decision-making in the improvement of inherited disorders in pedigree dogs. Vet J 189: 147–154. doi: 10.1016/j.tvjl.2011.06.012. pmid:21742521
20. Khuly P (12 October 2012) Embrace Pet Insurance, Entropion. Available:http://www.embracepetinsurance.com/health/entropion. Accessed 8 September 2014.
21. Fatwallet.com Lower eyes Entropion Repair Surgery. Available:http://www.fatwallet.com/forums/off-topic/1306349/. Accessed 9 September 2014.
22. Sakul H, Kellom TR (1996) Heritability of entropion in several US sheep breeds. Small Ruminant Res 23: 187–190. doi: 10.1016/s0921-4488(96)00911-x
23. Green LE, Berriatua E, and Morgan KL (1995) The prevalence and risk factors for congenital entropion in intensively reared lambs in south west England. Prev Vet Med 24: 15–21. doi: 10.1016/0167-5877(95)00468-c
24. Claine F, Raes M, Leemans J, Muylkens B, Kirschvink N (2013) Monitoring and management of congenital entropion in lambs: A prospective study. Small Ruminant Res 111: 1–5. doi: 10.1016/j.smallrumres.2012.11.037
25. .Sakul H, Snowder GD, Hemenway KJ (1996) Technical Note: Evaluation of techniques for correction of entropion in lambs. Small Ruminant Res 20: 187–191. doi: 10.1016/0921-4488(95)00797-0
26. Kijas JW, Lenstra JA, Hayes B, Boitard S, Porto Neto LR, San Cristobal M, et al. (2012) Geonome-wide analysis of the world's sheep breeds reveals high levels of historic mixture and strong recent selection. PLOS Biol 10: e1001258. doi: 10.1371/journal.pbio.1001258. pmid:22346734
27. Becker D, Tetens J, Brunner A, Bürstel D, Ganter M, Kijas J, et al. (2010) Microphthalmia in Texel sheep is associated with a missense mutation in the paired-like hoeodomain 3 (PITX3) gene. PLOS ONE 5: e8689. doi: 10.1371/journal.pone.0008689. pmid:20084168
28. Zhao X, Dittmer KE, Blair HT, Thompson KG, Rothschild MF, Garrick DJ (2011) A novel nonsense mutation in the DMP1 gene identified by a genome-wide association study is responsible for inherited rickets in Corriedale sheep. PLoS ONE 6(7): e21739. doi: 10.1371/journal.pone.0021739. pmid:21747952
29. Gonzalez MV, Mousel MR, Herndon DR, Jiang Y, Dalrymple BP, Reynolds JO, et al. (2013) A divergent artiodactyl *MYADAM*-like repeat is associated with erythrocyte traits and weight of lamb weaned in domestic sheep. PLOS ONE 8: e74700. doi: 10.1371/journal.pone.0074700. pmid:24023702
30. Silva MVB, Sonstegard TS, Hanotte O, Mugambi JM, Garcia JF, Nagda S, et al. (2012) Identification of quantitative trait loci affecting resistance to gastrointestinal parasites in a double backcross population of Red Maasai and Dorper sheep. Anim Genet 43: 63–71. doi: 10.1111/j.1365-2052.2011.02202.x. pmid:22221026
31. Heaton MP, Clawson ML, Chitko-Mckown CG, Leymaster KA, Smith TPL, Harhay GP, et al. (2012) Reduced lentivirus susceptibility in sheep with TMEM154 mutations. PLoS Genet 8(1): e1002467. doi: 10.1371/journal.pgen.1002467. pmid:22291605

32. White SN, Mousel MR, Herrmann-Hoesing LM, Reynolds JO, Leymaster KA, Neibergs HL, et al. (2012) Genome-wide association identifies multiple genomic regions associated with susceptibility to and control of ovine lentivirus. PLoS ONE 8(6): e65942. doi: 10.1371/journal.pone.0047829

33. White SN, Mousel MR, Reynolds JO, Herrmann-Hoesing LM, Knowles DP (2014) Variant near *ZNF389* is associated with control of ovine lentivirus in multiple flocks of sheep. Anim Genet 45: 297–300. doi: 10.1111/age.12107. pmid:24303974

34. Purcell S, Neale B, Todd-Brown K, Thomas L, Ferreira MA, Bender D, et al. (2007) PLINK: a toolset for whole-genome association and population-based linkage analysis. Am J Hum Genet 81: 559–575. pmid:17701901 doi: 10.1086/519795

35. Hindorff LA, Sethupathy P, Junkins HA, Ramos EM, Mehta JP, Collins FS, et al. (2009) Potential etiologic and functional implications of genome-wide association loci for human diseases and traits. Proc Natl Acad Sci U S A 106: 9362–9367. doi: 10.1073/pnas.0903103106. pmid:19474294

36. R Core Team (2013). R: A language and environment for statistical computing. R Foundation for Statistical Computing, Vienna, Austria. Available: http://www.R-project.org/

37. Findlater GS, McDougall RD, Kaufman MH. (1993) Eyelid development, fusion and subsequent reopening in the mouse. J Anat 183: 121–9. pmid:8270467

38. Ohuchi H (2012) Wakayama Symposium: Epithelial-mesenchymal interactions in eyelid development. Ocul Surf 10: 212–216. doi: 10.1016/j.jtos.2012.07.005. pmid:23084141

39. al-Rajhi AA, Hidayat A Nasr A, al-Faran M (1993) The histopathology and the mechanism of entropion in patients with trachoma. Ophthalmology 100:1293–1296. pmid:8371914 doi: 10.1016/s0161-6420(93)31485-5

40. Bashour M, Harvey J (2000) Causes of involutional ectropion and entropion-age-related tarsal changes are the key. Ophthal Plast Reconstr Surg 16: 131–141. pmid:10749160 doi: 10.1097/00002341-200003000-00008

41. Fox SA (1956) Primary congenital entropion. AMA Arch Ophthalmol 56: 839–842. pmid:13371990 doi: 10.1001/archopht.1956.00930040851006

42. Mohamed YH, Gong H, Amemiya T. (2003) Role of apoptosis in eyelid development. Exp Eye Res 76: 115–123. pmid:12589781 doi: 10.1016/s0014-4835(02)00269-5

43. Rice DS, Hansen GM, Liu F, Crist MJ, Newhouse MM, Potter D, et al. (2012) Keratinocyte migration in the developing eyelid requires LIMK2. PLoS One 7: e47168. doi: 10.1371/journal.pone.0047168. pmid:23071748

44. Vassy JL, Meigs JB (2012) Is genetic testing useful to predict type 2 diabetes? Best Pract Res Cl En 26: 189–201. doi: 10.1016/j.beem.2011.09.002

45. Augustin R, Carayannopoulos MO, Dowd LO, Phay JE, Moley JF, Moley KH (2004) Identification and characterization of human glucose transporter-like protein-9 (GLUT9): alternative splicing alters trafficking. J Biol Chem 279: 16229–16236. pmid:14739288 doi: 10.1074/jbc.m312226200

46. Doblado M, Moley KH (2009) Facilitative glucose transporter 9, a unique hexose and urate transporter. Am J Physiol Endocrinol Metab 297: E831–E835. doi: 10.1152/ajpendo.00296.2009. pmid:19797240

47. Takanaga H, Chaudhuri B, Frommer WB. (2008) GLUT1 and GLUT9 as major contributors to glucose influx in HepG2 cells identified by a high sensitivity intramolecular FRET glucose sensor. Biochim Biophys Acta. 1778: 1091–9. doi: 10.1016/j.bbamem.2007.11.015. pmid:18177733

48. Pyla R, Poulose N, Jun JY, Segar L. (2013) Expression of conventional and novel glucose transporters, GLUT1, -9, -10, and -12, in vascular smooth muscle cells. Am J Physiol Cell Physiol 304: C574–C589. doi: 10.1152/ajpcell.00275.2012. pmid:23302780

49. Matsuo H, Chiba T, Nagamori S, Nakayama A, Domoto H, Phetdee K, et al. (2008) Mutations in glucose transporter 9 gene SLC2A9 cause renal hypouricemia. Am J Hum Genet 83: 744–751. doi: 10.1016/j.ajhg.2008.11.001. pmid:19026395

50. Vitart V, Rudan I, Hayward C, Gray NK, Floyd J, Palmer CN, et al. (2008) SLC2A9 is a newly identified urate transporter influencing serum urate concentration, urate excretion and gout. Nat Genet 40: 437–442. doi: 10.1038/ng.106. pmid:18327257

51. Jiang Y, Xie M, Chen W, Talbot R, Maddox JF, Faraut T, et al. (2014) The sheep genome illuminates biology of the rumen and lipid metabolism. Science 344: 1168–1173. doi: 10.1126/science.1252806. pmid:24904168

52. Norman MU, Reeve SB, Dive V, Smith AI, Lew RA (2003) Endopeptidases 3.4.24.15 and 24.16 in endothelial cells: potential role in vasoactive peptide metabolism. Am J Physiol Heart Circ Physiol 284: H1978–H1984. pmid:12609826 doi: 10.1152/ajpheart.01116.2002

53. Cavalcanti DM, Castro LM, Rosa Neto JC, Seelaender M, Neves RX, Oliveira V, et al. (2014) Neurolysin knockout mice generation and initial phenotype characterization. J Biol Chem 289: 15426–15440. doi: 10.1074/jbc.M113.539148. pmid:24719317

54. Freund M, Walther T, von Bohlen Und Halbach O (2014) Effects of the angiotensin-(1–7) receptor Mas on cell proliferation and on the population of doublecortin positive cells within the dentate gyrus and piriform cortex. Eur Neuropsychopharmacol 24: 302–308. doi: 10.1016/j.euroneuro.2013.06.004. pmid:23860355

55. da Silva L, Neves BM, Moura L, Cruz MT, Carvalho E (2011) Neurotensin downregulates the pro-inflammatory properties of skin dendritic cells and increases epidermal growth factor expression. Biochim Biophys Acta 1813: 1863–1871. doi: 10.1016/j.bbamcr.2011.06.018. pmid:21767580

56. Moura LI, Silva L, Leal EC, Tellechea A, Cruz MT, Carvalho E (2013) Neurotensin modulates the migratory and inflammatory response of macrophages under hyperglycemic conditions. Biomed Res Int 2013:

941764. doi: 10.1155/2013/941764. pmid:24000330

57. Blajecka K, Marinov M, Leitner L, Uth K, Posern G, Arcaro A (2012) Phosphoinositide 3-kinase C2β regulates RhoA and the actin cytoskeleton through an interaction with Dbl. PLOS ONE 7: e44945. doi: 10.1371/journal.pone.0044945. pmid:22984590
58. Shepherd PR, Withers DJ, Siddle K (1998) Phosphoinositide 3-kinase: the key switch mechanism in insulin signalling. Biochem J 333: 471–490. pmid:9677303
59. Wu X, Chen S, Orlando SA, Yuan J, Kim ET, Munugalavadla V, et al. (2011) p85alpha regulates osteoblast differentiation by cross-talking with MAPK pathway. J Biol Chem 286: 13512–13521. doi: 10.1074/jbc.M110.187351. pmid:21324896
60. Foth BJ, Goedecke MC, Soldati D (2006) New insights into myosin evolution and classification. Proc Natl Acad Sci U S A 103: 3681–3686. pmid:16505385 doi: 10.1073/pnas.0506307103
61. Fox CS, Liu Y, White CC, Feitosa M, Smith AV, Heard-Costa N, et al. (2012) Genome-wide association for abdominal subcutaneous and visceral adipose reveals a novel locus for visceral fat in women. PLOS Genet 8: e1002695. doi: 10.1371/journal.pgen.1002695. pmid:22589738
62. Yao H, Zhou K, Yan D, Li M, Wang Y (2009) The Kv2.1 channels mediate neuronal apoptosis induced by excitotoxicity. J Neurochem 108: 909–919. doi: 10.1111/j.1471-4159.2008.05834.x. pmid:19077057
63. Walsh KB, Sweet JK, Long KJ (2001) Modulation of outward potassium currents in aligned cultures of neonatal rat ventricular myocytes during phorbol ester-induced hypertrophy. J Mol Cell Cardiol 33: 1233–1247. pmid:11444926 doi: 10.1006/jmcc.2001.1386
64. Liu L, Zhou Z, Huang S, Guo Y, Fan Y, Zhang J, et al. (2013) Zc3h12c inhibits vascular inflammation by repressing NF-kB activation and pro-inflammatory gene expression in endothelial cells. Biochem J 451:55–60. doi: 10.1042/BJ20130019. pmid:23360436
65. Golini L, Chouabe C, Berthier C, Cusimano V, Fornaro M, Bonvallet R, et al. (2011) Junctophilin 1 and 2 proteins interact with the L-type Ca2+ channel dihydrophridine recepotors (DHPRs) in skeletal muscle. J Biol Chem 286:43717–43725. doi: 10.1074/jbc.M111.292755. pmid:22020936
66. Hourdé C, Joanne P, Medja F, Mougenot N, Jacquet A, Mouisel E, et al. (2013) Voluntary physical activity protects from susceptibility to skeletal muscle contraction-induced injury but worsens heart function in mdx mice. Am J Pathol 182:1509–1518. doi: 10.1016/j.ajpath.2013.01.020. pmid:23465861

CHAPTER 10

PREVALENCE OF CRYPTOSPORIDIUM IN SMALL RUMINANTS FROM VERACRUZ, MEXICO

Dora Romero-Salas[1], Cosme Alvarado-Esquivel[2], Anabel Cruz-Romero[1], Mariel Aguilar-Domínguez[1], Nelly Ibarra-Priego[1], José O. Merino-Charrez[3], Adalberto A. Pérez de León[4] and Jesús Hernández-Tinoco[5]

[1]Laboratorio de Parasitología. UD PZTM. Facultad de Medicina Veterinaria y Zootecnia, Universidad Veracruzana, Veracruz, Mexico

[2]Laboratorio de Investigación Biomédica. Facultad de Medicina y Nutrición, Juárez University of Durango State, Avenida Universidad S/N, 34000 Durango, Mexico

[3]Facultad de Medicina Veterinaria y Zootecnia, Universidad Autónoma de Tamaulipas, Cd. Victoria, Tamaulipas, Mexico

[4]USDA-ARS Knipling-Bushland U.S. Livestock Insects Research Laboratory, and Veterinary Pest Genomics Center, Kerrville, TX, USA

[5]Institute for Scientific Research "Dr. Roberto Rivera Damm", Juárez University of Durango State, Durango, Mexico

ABSTRACT

Background

Cryptosporidiosis is a zoonotic disease caused by the protozoan parasite Cryptosporidium spp. that can affect domestic animal and human populations. In newborn ruminants, cryptosporidiosis is characterized by outbreaks of diarrhea, which can result in high morbidity and economic impact. The aim of the present study was to determine the prevalence of Cryptosporidium spp. in small ruminants from the Perote municipality in Veracruz State, Mexico. One hundred and sixty small ruminants (80 sheep and 80 goats) from eight farms located in four towns of the Perote municipality were examined following a cross-sectional study design. Stool samples were analyzed by a modification of the Faust centrifugation method, and the presence of Cryptosporidium spp. oocysts was examined using a modification of the Ziehl-Neelsen staining procedure. Bivariate and multivariate analyses were used to assess the association of Cryptosporidium infection and the general characteristics of the animals studied.

Results

Overall, 112 (70 %, 95 % CI: 62.3–76.9) of the 160 small ruminants sampled were infected with Cryptosporidiumspp. The prevalence of Cryptosporidium spp. infection in goats was 72.5 % (95 % CI: 61.4–81.9) and in sheep 67.5 % (95 % CI: 56.1–77.6). Small ruminants aged 1 month old had the highest (88.2 %; 95 % CI: 63.6–98.5) prevalence of infection. Prevalence varied from 60 % to 85 % among herds. Animal species, age, sex, breed, farm, town or cohabitation with cattle did not influence the prevalence of Cryptosporidium infection.

Citation: Dora Romero-Salas, Cosme Alvarado-Esquivel, Anabel Cruz-Romero, Mariel Aguilar-Domínguez, Nelly Ibarra-Priego, José O. Merino-Charrez, Adalberto A. Pérez de León and Jesús Hernández-Tinoco, Prevalence of Cryptosporidium in small ruminants from Veracruz, Mexico, DOI 10.1186/s12917-016-0638-3.

Conclusions

A high prevalence of infection with Cryptosporidium spp. was observed in small ruminants from the Perote municipality in Veracruz, Mexico. Infection was widely distributed among sheep and goats regardless of their age, breed or farm location. Further research is required to identify risk factors for, and to assess the veterinary public health significance of Cryptosporidium infection among sheep and goats in the Mexican state of Veracruz.

BACKGROUND

Cryptosporidium is a zoonotic protozoan parasite of the Apicomplexa phylum and the Cryptosporidiidae family [1]. *Cryptosporidium* is an important pathogen in cattle and humans [2], and infection with this parasite in cattle may lead to economic losses due to morbidity and mortality [3, 4]. *Cryptosporidium* spp. infecting sheep and goats have been found to be of public health significance [5, 6].

Cryptosporidiosis, the disease caused by *Cryptosporidium*, is characterized by diarrhea, dehydration, and weight loss [7–9]. *Cryptosporidium* affects epithelial cells of the small intestine and occasionally stomach, gall bladder, liver, trachea, and lungs in a number of mammals including humans [10, 11]. *Cryptosporidium* is a widely distributed parasite and can infect more than 170 species of vertebrates [1]. Transmission of *Cryptosporidium* occurs mainly by the fecal-oral route [7]. In sheep and goats, cryptosporidiosis is an important enteric disease resulting in diarrhea and inefficient weight gains [12], and is more severe in young than in adult animals [13, 14]. Animals infected with*Cryptosporidium* shed a large (10^8–10^9 /g) number of oocysts [15]. These oocysts are source of infection for animals and humans [16]. In humans, infection with *Cryptosporidium* causes diarrheal disease [17], and chronic and fatal disease in immunocompromised individuals [18]. Additionally, *Cryptosporidium* infection has been linked to cancer in humans [4, 19].

Infection with *Cryptosporidium* in young sheep and goats may lead to morbidity and even mortality due to diarrhea [20–22]. Effective disease prevention requires an understanding of the environmental factors predisposing animal and human populations to infectious causes of diarrhea like *Cryptosporidium* spp. [23, 24]. However, very little is known about the infection with *Cryptosporidium spp.* in sheep and goats in Mexico in general and there is a lack of information about this infection in the southern Mexican state of Veracruz in particular. Therefore, we sought to determine the prevalence of infection with *Cryptosporidium* spp. in sheep and goats in the municipality of Perote in Veracruz State, Mexico.

METHODS

Study design

This cross-sectional study was performed in the municipality of Perote in Veracruz, Mexico from July to December 2014. Perote, the capital of the municipality with the same name, is located in the central-west region of Veracruz State (19°34'N 97°15'W) at an altitude of 2400 meters above sea level and has a cold and dry climate with a mean annual temperature of 12 °C, and a mean annual rainfall of 493.6 mm.

Sheep and Goats Studied

Eighty sheep and 80 goats from the Perote municipality in Veracruz State were included in the study. Convenience sampling was applied. The small ruminant population sampled was raised in eight farms where sheep and goats herds were kept. Farms were located in four towns: 1) Perote; 2) San Antonio Limón; 3) Los Molinos; and 4) La Gloria. Ten sheep and 10 goats were sampled from each farm. Sheep and goats were young (up to 3 months old). A fecal sample from the rectum was obtained from each animal. Fecal samples were placed in a plastic bag and analyzed a day after sampling. General data of the agroecosystem and animals studied were obtained with the aid of a questionnaire. Animal data included species, age, sex, breed, presence of diarrhea, and history of deworming. Agroecosystem data collected included farm location, nearest town, sharing water with other animals, and cohabitation with dogs or cattle.

Laboratory Tests

Small ruminant fecal samples were analyzed using a modification of the centrifuge-flotation method of Faust [25]. Briefly, three grams of fecal sample were homogenized in distilled water and centrifuged at 1500 rpm for 1 min. Then supernatant was removed and the homogenization and centrifugation processes were repeated. After removing the supernatant, the sediment was resuspended in $ZnSO_4$ (44 %) and centrifuged. Finally, the supernatant was removed and sediment was examined. *Cryptosporidium* oocysts were detected by a modification of the Ziehl-Neelsen staining method [26]. Samples were examined under oil immersion objective (100x) and oocysts were identified based on morphological features.

Statistical Analysis

Results were analyzed with the aid of the software Microsoft Excel, SPSS version 15.0 (SPSS Inc. Chicago, Illinois) and STATA version 11.0. Descriptive statistics were used to determine the prevalence of *Cryptosporidium* infection in sheep and goats. We used the Pearson's chi-squared test for comparison of infection frequencies among groups. The association between *Cryptosporidium* infection, animal characteristics, and agroecosystem features was assessed by bivariate and multivariate analyses. The dependent variable was positivity to *Cryptosporidium* by Ziehl-Neelsen staining per individual animal. Independent variables included in the multivariable analysis were those with a P value ≤ 0.10 in the bivariate analysis: age, town, and farm. Odds ratio (OR) and 95 % confidence interval (CI) were calculated and statistical significance was set at a P value of<0.05.

Ethics Statement

The Bioethics and Animal Welfare Commission of the Facultad de Medicina Veterinaria y Zootecnia of Universidad Veracruzana approved this project. Owners of the sheep and goats gave their consent to study their animals. Adequate veterinary care was provided to all animals studied.

RESULTS AND DISCUSSION

Infection with *Cryptosporidium* was found in 112 (70.0 %; 95 % CI: 62.3–77.0 %) of the 160 small ruminants studied. Of the 80 sheep examined, 54 (67.5 %; 95 % CI: 56.1–77.6) were positive for *Cryptosporidium* infection. Whereas of the 80 goats studied, 58 (72.5 %; 95 % CI 61.4–81.9 %) were positive for *Cryptosporidium* infection. These results provide for the first time evidence of *Cryptosporidium spp.* infection in sheep and goats in the municipality of Perote in Veracruz, Mexico.

Information about the prevalence of infection with *Cryptosporidium* in animals in Mexico is scant. The prevalence of *Cryptosporidium* infection in sheep reported here is higher than the 34.3 % prevalence of *Cryptosporidium* infection in sheep in northern Mexico [27]. We are not aware of reports about the prevalence of *Cryptosporidium* infection in goats in Mexico. Therefore, we cannot compare our results with those in other region in the country. In an international context, the prevalence of *Cryptosporidium* infection found in sheep in Veracruz is higher than the prevalences found in sheep in Spain (31–59 %) [28, 29], Poland (10.1 %) [30], Egypt (2.5 %) [31], Iran (11.3 %) [32], Iraq (13.3 %) [33], Tunisia (11.2 %) [34], India (1.8 %) [35], and Papua New Guinea (2.2 %) [36]. Similarly, the prevalence of *Cryptosporidium* infection found in goats in Veracruz is higher than prevalences found in goats in Spain (30 %) [29], Poland (0 %) [30], Iraq (17.7 %) [33], and Papua New Guinea (4.4 %) [36]. However, comparison of prevalences of *Cryptosporidium* infection in animals among countries should be interpreted with care because matching for characteristics of animals and their raising conditions is challenging.

Sheep and goats may serve as reservoirs of *Cryptosporidium* for human infections [36]. Outbreaks of infection with *Cryptosporidium* in schoolchildren associated with contact with lamb/goat kids have been reported [37]. The occurrence of these outbreaks 3 years apart, with the same parasite in the same farm suggested that *Cryptosporidium* might establish in the environment [37]. In addition, cryptosporidiosis has been associated with consumption of unpasteurized goat milk in children [38]. Therefore, our results should alert for the risk of infection in humans in Veracruz through contact with infected sheep and goats, and consumption of unpasteurized milk from infected goats. *Cryptosporidium* infection has been reported in animals other than sheep and goat in Veracruz, Mexico. Prevalence of *Cryptosporidium* infection in cattle in several municipalities in Veracruz varied from 14.3 % to 75 % [39, 40]. Sheep, goats, and cattle are frequently raised together in Veracruz, and this interaction along with poor hygienic sanitary conditions in the agroecosystems where they are raised might account for transmission of *Cryptosporidium* infection among animal species [41]. A number of *Cryptosporidium* species/genotypes infecting sheep has been described including *C. parvum*, *C. bovis*, *C. cervine* [42–44], and *C. hominis* [42]. Whereas some *Cryptosporidium* species/genotypes infecting goats include *C. xiaoi* [36, 45], *C. parvum*, and *C. hominis* [36].

We sought to determine the association between the general characteristics of animals, their environment, and *Cryptosporidium* infection. The prevalence of *Cryptosporidium* infection did not vary significantly with small ruminant species, age, sex, or breed of the animals studied. Neonatal diarrhea in small ruminants is one of the most frequent syndromes during the first week of age and leads to important economic losses due to mortality and delayed growth. *Cryptosporidium* is a well-known cause of neonatal diarrhea in sheep [46]. However, in our study the history of diarrhea in the animals studied was not associated with *Cryptosporidium* infection. This finding agrees with that found in a study of lambs and adult sheep in Poland [30]. In the present study, the effect of dogs on *Cryptosporidium* prevalence could not be determined because all farms sampled had dogs present. We found no association between *Cryptosporidium* prevalence and a history of deworming or cohabitation with cattle. All sheep and goats studied shared water with other animals of the same farms. Table 1 shows a correlation between *Cryptosporidium* infection and general characteristics of sheep and goats and the agroecosystem where they were raised. Bivariate analysis of these characteristics showed three variables with a $P<0.10$: age, towns and farms. Multivariate analysis of the three variables with a $P<0.10$ (age, towns and farms) obtained in bivariate analysis showed no association with *Cryptosporidium* infection. The failure to find an association between the presence of infection and characteristics of the animals may have been due to the small sample size. Further studies with a larger sample size to determine the risk factors associated with *Cryptosporidium* infection in sheep and goats should be conducted to assess the veterinary public health burden of cryptosporidiosis in Mexico. In addition, further research with molecular methods to determine the *Cryptosporidium* genotypes, and subtyping of *C. parvum* or *C. ubiquitum* at the gp60 locus [47, 48] in sheep and goats in Mexico are needed.

Table 1: Correlation of *Cryptosporidium* infection with the general characteristics of the animals(sheep and goats together) and the agroecosystem where they were raised

Characteristic	No. of animals studied	*Cryptosporidium* infection No.	%	OR	95 % Confidence interval	P value
Species						
Sheep	80	54	67.5	1.00		
Goats	80	58	72.5	1.26	0.64–2.50	0.49
Age (months)						
<1	17	15	88.2	3.50	0.77–16.37	0.08
1	124	84	67.7	1.00		
2	19	13	68.4	1.03	0.36–2.91	0.95

Sex						
Male	89	58	65.2	1.00		
Female	71	54	76.1	1.69	0.84–3.41	0.13
Breed of Sheep						
Pelibuey	45	30	66.7	1.33	0.39–4.44	0.63
Dorper	20	15	75	2.00	0.47–8.49	0.34
Kathadin	15	9	60	1.00		
Breed of goats						
Mixed	46	32	69.6	1.00		
Nubian	34	26	76.5	1.42	0.51–3.90	0.49
Diarrhea						
Yes	52	33	63.5	1.00		
No	108	79	73.1	1.56	0.77–3.18	0.21
Deworming						
Yes	80	56	70	1.00		
No	80	56	70	1.00	0.50–1.96	1
Town						
Perote	40	27	67.5	1.24	0.49–3.12	0.63
San Antonio Limón	40	32	80	2.40	0.87–6.55	0.08
Los Molinos	40	28	70	1.40	0.55–3.55	0.47
La Gloria	40	25	62.5	1.00		
Farm						
1	20	14	70	1.55	0.41–5.76	0.5
2	20	13	65	1.23	0.34–4.46	0.74
3	20	15	75	2.00	0.51–7.72	0.31
4	20	17	85	3.77	0.82–17.25	0.07
5	20	14	70	1.55	0.41–5.76	0.5
6	20	14	70	1.55	0.41–5.76	0.5
7	20	12	60	1.00		
8	20	13	65	1.23	0.34–4.46	0.74
Cohabitation with cattle						
Yes	100	71	71	1.13	0.56–2.27	0.72
No	60	41	68.3	1.00		

CONCLUSIONS

The prevalence of infection with *Cryptosporidium spp* among sheep and goats in the Perote municipality in Veracruz, Mexico is relatively high. Infection was widely distributed among small ruminants regardless of their age, breed or the agroecosystem where they were raised. Further research to identify risk factors for *Cryptosporidium*infection in sheep and goats and the zoonotic potential of cryptosporidiosis in Veracruz State is needed.

ACKNOWLEDGEMENTS

This study was financially supported by Universidad Veracruzana, Veracruz, Mexico. USDA is an equal opportunity provider and employer.

AUTHORS' CONTRIBUTIONS

DRS designed the study protocol, obtained the blood samples and general data of the ruminants, analyzed the results and wrote the manuscript. CAE performed the data analysis, and wrote the manuscript. ACR, MAD, NIP, and JOMC obtained the blood samples and general data of the ruminants, and analyzed the results. AAPL and JHT analyzed the results and wrote the manuscript. All authors read and approved the final version of the manuscript.

REFERENCES

1. Romero MR, Pedrozo RH, Vera E. La Criptosporidiosis en los terneros recién nacidos. Su etiología, patogenia, síntomas, tratamiento y profilaxis. Revista de Ciencia y Tecnología dirección de investigaciones –UNA. 2001;1:1–10.

2. Bouzid M, Hunter PR, Chalmers RM, Tyler KM. *Cryptosporidium* pathogenicity and virulence. Clin Microbiol Rev. 2013;26:115–34. doi:10.1128/CMR.00076-12.

3. Casemore DP, Wright SE, Coop RL. Cryptosporidiosis: Human and animal epidemiology. In: Fayer R, editor. *Cryptosporidium* and cryptosporidiosis. Boca Raton: CRC, Press; 1997. p. 65–92.

4. Lendner M, Etzold M, Daugschies A. Cryptosporidiosis--an update. Berl Munch Tierarztl Wochenschr. 2011;124:473–84.

5. Robertson LJ, Gjerde BK, Furuseth HE. The zoonotic potential of *Giardia* and *Cryptosporidium* in Norwegian sheep: a longitudinal investigation of 6 flocks of lambs. Vet Parasitol. 2010;171(1–2):140–5. doi:10.1016/j.vetpar.2010.03.014.

6. Wang R, Li G, Cui B, Huang J, Cui Z, Zhang S, et al. Prevalence, molecular characterization and zoonotic potential of*Cryptosporidium spp.* in goats in Henan and Chongqing, China. Exp Parasitol. 2014;142:11–6. doi:10.1016/j.exppara.2014.04.001.

7. Fayer R, Morgan U, Upton SJ. Epidemiology of *Cryptosporidium*: Transmission, detection and identification. Int J Parasitol. 2000;30:1305–22.

8. Panciera RJ, Thomassen RW, Garner FM. Cryptosporidial infection in a calf. Vet Pathol. 1971;8:479–84.

9. Santín M, Trout JM, Xiao L, Zhou L, Greiner E, Fayer R. Prevalence and age-related variation of *Cryptosporidium* species and genotypes in dairy calves. Vet Parasitol. 2004;122:103–17.

10. Pilar-Izquierdo M, Ortega-Mora LM, Pereira-Bueno J, Rojo-Vázquez FA. Participación de *Cryptosporidium parvum* en brotes de diarrea en corderos en el NO de Castilla y León. Acta Parasitol Port. 1993;1:223.

11. Hunter PR, Thompson RC. The zoonotic transmission of *Giardia* and *Cryptosporidium*. Int J Parasitol. 2005;35:1181–90.

12. Foreyt WJ. Coccidiosis and cryptosporidiosis in sheep and goats. Vet Clin North Am Food Anim Pract. 1990;6:655–70.

13. Chalmers RM, Elwin K, Reilly WJ, Irvine H, Thomas AL, Hunter PR. *Cryptosporidium* in farmed animals: the detection of a novel isolate in sheep. Int J Parasitol. 2002;32:21–6.

14. de Graaf DC, Vanopdenbosch E, Ortega-Mora LM, Abbassi H, Peeters JE. A review of the importance of cryptosporidiosis in farm animals. Int J Parasitol. 1999;29:1269–87.

15. Ortegà-Mora LM, Wright SE. Age-related resistance in ovine cryptosporidiosis: patterns of infection and humoral immune response. Infect Immun. 1994;62:5003–9.

16. Lee YM, Johnson PW, Call JL, Arrowood MJ, Furness BW, Pichette SC, et al. Development and application of a quantitative, specific assay for *Cryptosporidium parvum* oocyst detection in high-turbidity environmental water samples. Am J Trop Med Hyg. 2001;65:1–9.

17. Checkley W, White Jr AC, Jaganath D, Arrowood MJ, Chalmers RM, Chen XM, et al. A review of the global burden, novel diagnostics, therapeutics, and vaccine targets for *Cryptosporidium*. Lancet Infect Dis. 2015;15:85–94. doi:10.1016/S1473-3099(14)70772-8.

18. Wilhelm CL, Yarovinsky F. Apicomplexan infections in the gut. Parasite Immunol. 2014;36:409–20. doi:10.1111/pim.12115.

19. Benamrouz S, Conseil V, Creusy C, Calderon E, Dei-Cas E, Certad G. Parasites and malignancies, a review, with emphasis on digestive cancer induced by *Cryptosporidium parvum* (Alveolata: Apicomplexa). Parasite. 2012;19:101–15.

20. Tzipori S, Angus KW, Gray EW, Campbell I, Allan F. Diarrhea in lambs experimentally infected with *Cryptosporidium* isolated from calves. Am J Vet Res. 1981;42:1400–4.

21. Kaminjolo JS, Adesiyun AA, Loregnard R, Kitson-Piggott W. Prevalence of *Cryptosporidium* oocysts in livestock in Trinidad and Tobago. Vet Parasitol. 1993;45:209–13.

22. Thompson RC, Olson ME, Zhu G, Enomoto S, Abrahamsen MS, Hijjawi NS. *Cryptosporidium* and cryptosporidiosis. Adv Parasitol. 2005;59:77–158.

23. Collinet-Adler S, Babji S, Francis M, Kattula D, Premkumar PS, Sarkar R, et al. Environmental factors associated with high fly densities and diarrhea in Vellore, India. Appl Environ Microbiol. 2015;81(17):6053–8.

24. Rossle NF, Latif B. Cryptosporidiosis as threatening health problem : a review. Asian Pac J Trop Biomed. 2013;3:916–24.

25. Leventhal R, Cheadle R. Parasitología Médica. 3ath ed. México: Ed. Interamericana, Mc Graw-Hill; 1992.

26. Casemore DP, Armstrong M, Sands RL. Laboratory diagnosis of cryptosporidiosis. J Clin Pathol. 1985;38:1337–41.

27. Alonso-Fresán MU, García-Alvarez A, Salazar-García F, Vázquez-Chagoyán JC, Pescador-Salas N, Saltijeral-Oaxaca J. Prevalence of *Cryptosporidium spp.* in asymptomatic sheep in family flocks from Mexico State. J Vet Med B Infect Dis Vet Public Health. 2005;52:482–3.

28. Causapé AC, Quílez J, Sánchez-Acedo C, del Cacho E, López-Bernad F. Prevalence and analysis of potential risk factors for *Cryptosporidium parvum* infection in lambs in Zaragoza (northeastern Spain). Vet Parasitol. 2002;104:287–98.

29. Castro-Hermida JA, González-Warleta M, Mezo M. Natural infection with *Cryptosporidium parvum* and *Giardia duodenalis*in sheep and goats in Galicia (NW, Spain). Small Rumin Res. 2007;72:96–100.

30. Majewska AC, Werner A, Sulima P, Luty T. Prevalence of *Cryptosporidium* in sheep and goats bred on five farms in west- region of Poland. Vet Parasitol. 2000;89:269–75.

31. Mahfouz ME, Mira N, Amer S. Prevalence and genotyping of *Cryptosporidium spp.* in farm animals in

Egypt. J Vet Med Sci. 2014;76:1569–75. doi:10.1292/jvms.14-0272.

32. Gharekhani J, Heidari H, Youssefi M. Prevalence of *Cryptosporidium* infection in sheep in Iran. Turkiye Parazitol Derg. 2014;38:22–5. doi:10.5152/tpd.2014.3224.

33. Mahdi NK, Ali NH. Cryptosporidiosis among animal handlers and their livestock in Basrah, Iraq. East Afr Med J. 2002;79:550–3.

34. Soltane R, Guyot K, Dei-Cas E, Ayadi A. Prevalence of *Cryptosporidium spp.* (Eucoccidiorida: Cryptosporiidae) in seven species of farm animals in Tunisia. Parasite. 2007;14:335–8.

35. Maurya PS, Rakesh RL, Pradeep B, Kumar S, Kundu K, Garg R, et al. Prevalence and risk factors associated with*Cryptosporidium spp.* infection in young domestic livestock in India. Trop Anim Health Prod. 2013;45:941–6. doi:10.1007/s11250-012-0311-1.

36. Koinari M, Lymbery AJ, Ryan UM. *Cryptosporidium* species in sheep and goats from Papua New Guinea. Exp Parasitol. 2014;141:134–7. doi:10.1016/j.exppara.2014.03.021.

37. Lange H, Johansen OH, Vold L, Robertson LJ, Anthonisen IL, Nygard K. Second outbreak of infection with a rare*Cryptosporidium parvum* genotype in schoolchildren associated with contact with lambs/goat kids at a holiday farm in Norway. Epidemiol Infect. 2014;142:2105–13. doi:10.1017/S0950268813003002.

38. Rosenthal M, Pedersen R, Leibsle S, Hill V, Carter K, Roellig DM, et al. Notes from the field: cryptosporidiosis associated with consumption of unpasteurized goat milk - Idaho, 2014. MMWR Morb Mortal Wkly Rep. 2015;64:194–5.

39. Castelán-Hernández OO, Romero-Salas D, García-Vázquez Z, Cruz-Vázquez C, Aguilar-Domínguez M, del Jesus Ibarra-Priego N, et al. Prevalence of bovine cryptosporidiosis in three ecological regions of the region of Veracruz, Mexico. Tropical and Subtropical Agroecosystems. 2011;13:461–7.

40. Romero-Salas D, Godoy-Salinas O, García-Vázquez Z, Montiel Palacios F, Chavarría-Martínez B. Prevalence of*Cryptosporidium* spp. and associated risk factors in female calves in the region of Veracruz, Mexico. Tropical and Subtropical Agroecosystems. 2012;15 Suppl 2:S89–94.

41. Sanz Ceballos L, Illescas Gómez P, Sanz Sampelayo MR, Gil Extremera F, Rodríguez OM. Prevalence of *Cryptosporidium*infection in goats maintained under semi-extensive feeding conditions in the southeast of Spain. Parasite. 2009;16:315–8.

42. Yang R, Jacobson C, Gordon C, Ryan U. Prevalence and molecular characterisation of *Cryptosporidium* and *Giardia*species in pre-weaned sheep in Australia. Vet Parasitol. 2009;161:19–24. doi:10.1016/j.vetpar.2008.12.021.

43. Mueller-Doblies D, Giles M, Elwin K, Smith RP, Clifton-Hadley FA, Chalmers RM. Distribution of *Cryptosporidium* species in sheep in the UK. Vet Parasitol. 2008;154:214–9. doi:10.1016/j.vetpar.2008.03.021.

44. Santín M, Trout JM, Fayer R. Prevalence and molecular characterization of *Cryptosporidium* and *Giardia* species and genotypes in sheep in Maryland. Vet Parasitol. 2007;146:17–24.

45. Tzanidakis N, Sotiraki S, Claerebout E, Ehsan A, Voutzourakis N, Kostopoulou D, et al. Occurrence and molecular characterization of *Giardia duodenalis* and *Cryptosporidium spp.* in sheep and goats reared under dairy husbandry systems in Greece. Parasite. 2014;21:45. doi:10.1051/parasite/2014048.

46. Quílez J, Vergara-Castiblanco C, Sánchez-Acedo C, Del Cacho E, López-Bernad F. Prevalencia de *Cryptosporidium parvum* en ganado caprino en la provincia de Zaragoza. Estudio preliminar. Acta Parasitol Port. 2001;8:167.

47. Ramo A, Quílez J, Del Cacho E, Sánchez-Acedo C. Optimization of a fragment size analysis tool for identification of*Cryptosporidium* species and Gp60 alleles infecting domestic ruminants. Vet Parasitol. 2014;205:466–71. doi:10.1016/j.vetpar.2014.08.025.

48. Connelly L, Craig BH, Jones B, Alexander CL. Genetic diversity of *Cryptosporidium spp.* within a remote population of Soay Sheep on St. Kilda Islands, Scotland. Appl Environ Microbiol. 2013;79(7):2240–6. doi:10.1128/AEM.02823-12.

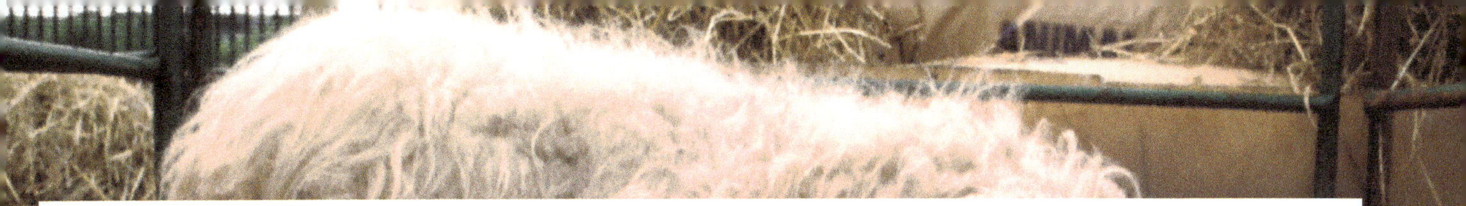

CHAPTER 11

CLINICOPATHOLOGICAL STUDIES OF GASTROINTESTINAL TRACT DISORDERS IN SHEEP WITH PARASITIC INFECTION

Sarvan Kumar[1], K. K. Jakhar[1], Satyavir Singh[2], Sandeep Potliya[3], Kailash Kumar[4] and Madan Pal[3]

[1]Department of Veterinary Pathology, Lala Lajpat Rai University of Veterinary & Animal Sciences, Hisar, Haryana, India

[2]Department of Veterinary Parasitology, Lala Lajpat Rai University of Veterinary & Animal Sciences, Hisar, Haryana, India

[3]Department of Veterinary Surgery and Radiology, Lala Lajpat Rai University of Veterinary & Animal Sciences, Hisar, Haryana, India

[4]Department of Veterinary Gynaecology and Obstetrics, Lala Lajpat Rai University of Veterinary & Animal Sciences, Hisar, Haryana, India

ABSTRACT

- **Aim: This study was envisaged to elucidate the parasitological aspects of gastrointestinal tract (GIT) disorders of sheep.**
- **Materials and Methods: Fecal, blood and serum samples collected from 31 sheep/lambs of Sheep Breeding Farm, Lala Lajpat Rai University of Veterinary & Animal Sciences, Hisar.**
- **Results: Of 25 cases, strongyle eggs (12 cases, 48%) were a major infection, followed by Strongyloides spp. (8 cases, 32%) and Moniezia spp. (5 case, 20%). In one case, massive infection of strongyle particularly Haemonchus contortus and Moniezia spp. was observed. All these animals were found negative for hemoprotozoan parasites in blood smear examination. Hematological studies revealed that significantly decreased values of hemoglobin (Hb), packed cell volume (PCV) and total erythrocytic count (TEC). Absolute leukocytic count revealed significant leukocytosis due to neutrophilia, lymphocytosis, monocytosis and eosinophilia. Serum biochemical profiles of diarrheic sheep/lambs in present study were significant decrease in values of total protein, serum globulin, glucose where as significant increase in the albumin: Globulin ratio, aspartate aminotransaminase (AST), alanine aminotransaminase (ALT), alkaline phosphatise (ALKP) and bilirubin.**
- **Conclusions: From the present study, it is reasonable to conclude that major parasitic infection of sheep/lamb observed was strongyle, followed by Strongyloides spp. and Moniezia spp. Hemato-biochemical studies revealed significant leukocytosis and increase in AST, ALT, ALKP and bilirubin.**

INTRODUCTION

Agriculture is the mainstay of Indian economy, where in agriculture and allied sector like, livestock, dairying and fisheries contribute about 15.18% of Gross Domestic Product [1]. Contribution of livestock sector to the food basket in the form of milk, egg and meat is of significance in fulfilling of animal protein requirement of ever and fast growing human population. In rural India where over 15-20% families are landless and about 80% of the land holders belong to the category of small and marginal farmers, livestock is the main source of livelihood. In the absence of fertile lands and assured irrigation which are controlled by a small population of rich farmers and lack of employment in the industrial and

Citation: Sarvan Kumar, K. K. Jakhar, Satyavir Singh, Sandeep Potliya, Kailash Kumar and Madan Pal, Clinicopathological studies of gastrointestinal tract disorders in sheep with parasitic infection, DOI: 10.14202/vetworld.2015.29-32.

service sectors, most of the rural families belonging to socio-economically weaker sections of the society maintain different species of livestock to supplement their income. Although the landowners prefer cattle and buffaloes, the landless prefer to own sheep, goat and poultry. With the policy of the State Animal Husbandry Department to extend free breeding, vaccination and veterinary services and permit free grazing on community lands, the farmers were encouraged to expand their herd size without any major financial burden [2]. This has probably been the reason for the presence of the world's largest livestock population in India. India ranks second in sheep population (71.56 million) in the world [3]. Of this 0.63 million sheep account from Haryana [4]. Although safe and effective treatment and control methods exist for the most internal and external parasites, many animals continue to suffer from preventable parasitic infections. Geographical location, housing conditions and species play a role in which parasites are likely to be a problem. Internal and external parasites can cause great discomfort, transmit disease to animals and significantly interfere with the growth and performance of animals.

Hematology and serum biochemistry of infected animals is very sensitive indicators for the degree of hepatic damage and the parasitic infection severity, in which liver damage upsets the vital metabolic processes for normal health and optimum productivity of the animal.

The purpose of this study was to overview the correlation between clinicopathology in the gastrointestinal tract (GIT) disorders due to some parasitic infection and its effect on hematology and clinical biochemistry in sheep.

MATERIALS AND METHODS

Ethical Approval

The study was conducted after the approval of the Institutional Animal Ethics Committee.

Collection of Sample

Proposed study was conducted on 31 sheep/ lambs including 6 healthy and 25 diseased sheep/ lambs affected with GIT disorders. Samples of feces, blood and serum for research was collected from Sheep Breeding Farm, Lala Lajpat Rai University of Veterinary & Animal Sciences, Hisar.

Faecal Examination for Parasitic Eggs and Ova

Fecal samples were collected directly from the rectum from clinical cases of sheep/lamb having GIT disorders. These fecal samples were examined for the presence of helminthic ova, both heavy and light, and coccidial oocysts. For examination, floatation and sedimentation methods were employed [5].

Hematological Examination

Hematological studies viz., Hb, TLC, differential leukocytic count, TEC, PCV, erythrocytic sedimentation rate (ESR), mean corpuscular volume (MCV), mean corpuscular Hb and mean corpuscular Hb concentration (MCHC) were estimated following the method of Benjamin [6] within the 6 h of blood collection.

Serum Biochemical Examination

Serum biochemical parameters were determined by using Technicon Ames RA-50 chemistry analyzer using diagnostic kits of Bayer [7]. The levels of the following plasma constituents were determined: Total protein (TP), albumin, total bilirubin and enzyme activities of alkaline phosphatase (ALKP), alanine aminotransferase (ALT) and aspartate aminotransferase (AST). The gamma-globulin levels were also measured and the albumin: Globulin ratio was calculated.

Statistical Analysis

The Student's t-test using SPSS statistics 17.0 software (IBM Corporation, New York, USA) was applied to statistically analyze the results obtained with different study groups.

RESULTS

The results of parasitic findings in 31 cases (6 healthy animals and 25 animals showing GIT disorders) of sheep/lambs are; maximum infection was in sheep of age group 2-5 months and least in age group of >1 year. Out of 25 cases, strongyle eggs (12 cases, 48%) was a major infection, followed by Strongyloides spp. (8 cases, 32%) and Moniezia spp. (5 case, 20%), respectively. In one case, mixed massive infection of strongyle particularly Haemonchus contortus, strongyloides spp. and Moniezia spp. were observed. All these animals were found negative for hemoprotozoan parasites in blood smear examination.

Hematological studies of blood collected from diarrheic sheep/lambs revealed significantly ($p \leq 0.05$) decreased values of Hb (8.184±0.194), PCV (30.40±1.146) and TEC (8.22±0.249). Absolute leukocytic count revealed significant ($p \leq 0.05$) leukocytosis (19.156±1.443) due to neutrophilia, lymphocytosis, monocytosis and eosinophilia. No effect was seen on ESR (0.14±0.004). An analysis of erythrocytic indices revealed no significant change in MCV (36.89±0.719), mean corpuscular Hb (10.22±0.463) and MCHC (27.37±0.587) as shown in Figure-1.

Serum biochemical profiles of diarrheic sheep/ lambs in present study showed significant ($p \leq 0.05$) decrease in values of TP (4.76±0.118), serum globulin (1.66±0.12030) and serum glucose (56.26±1.725) whereas significant ($p \leq 0.05$) increase in the albumin: globulin ratio (2.46±0.29345). The activity of AST (211.6±13.92), ALT (63.34±1.54) and ALKP (154.28±19.662) and total bilirubin (0.107±0.0077) were significantly ($p \leq 0.05$) increased in diarrheic sheep/lambs shown in Figures-2a and b. There was no significant difference in hemato-biochemical studies among age group.

DISCUSSION

Examination of intestinal contents/feces for parasitic isolation revealed maximum infection was in sheep of age group 2-5 months and least in age group of >1 year [8,9]. Mixed parasitic findings revealed maximum cases of mixed infection of strongyle and Strongyloides spp. and only one case of mixed infection of strongyle, Strongyloides spp. and Moniezia spp. These findings were in general, agreement with those reported by Mederos et al. and Lashari and Tasawar [10,11]. Prevailing agro-climatic conditions like overstocking of the animals, grazing of young and adult animals together with poorly drained land provide an ideal condition for the transmission of the endoparasites to build up clinical infection of the host. The overall higher incidence of nematodes infection in the areas surveyed could be attributed to lower immunity of hosts as a result of malnutrition. All the livestock in the area under investigation largely depended on grazing in deteriorated range-lands [12].

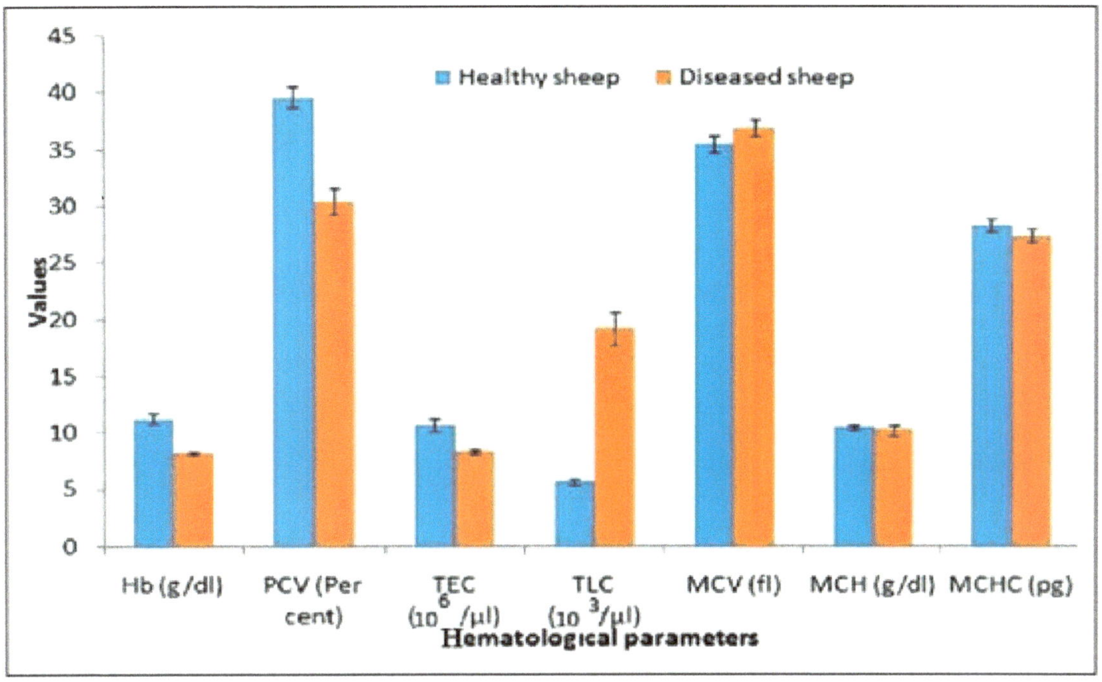

Figure-1: Histograms representing hematological parameters of healthy and diseased sheep.

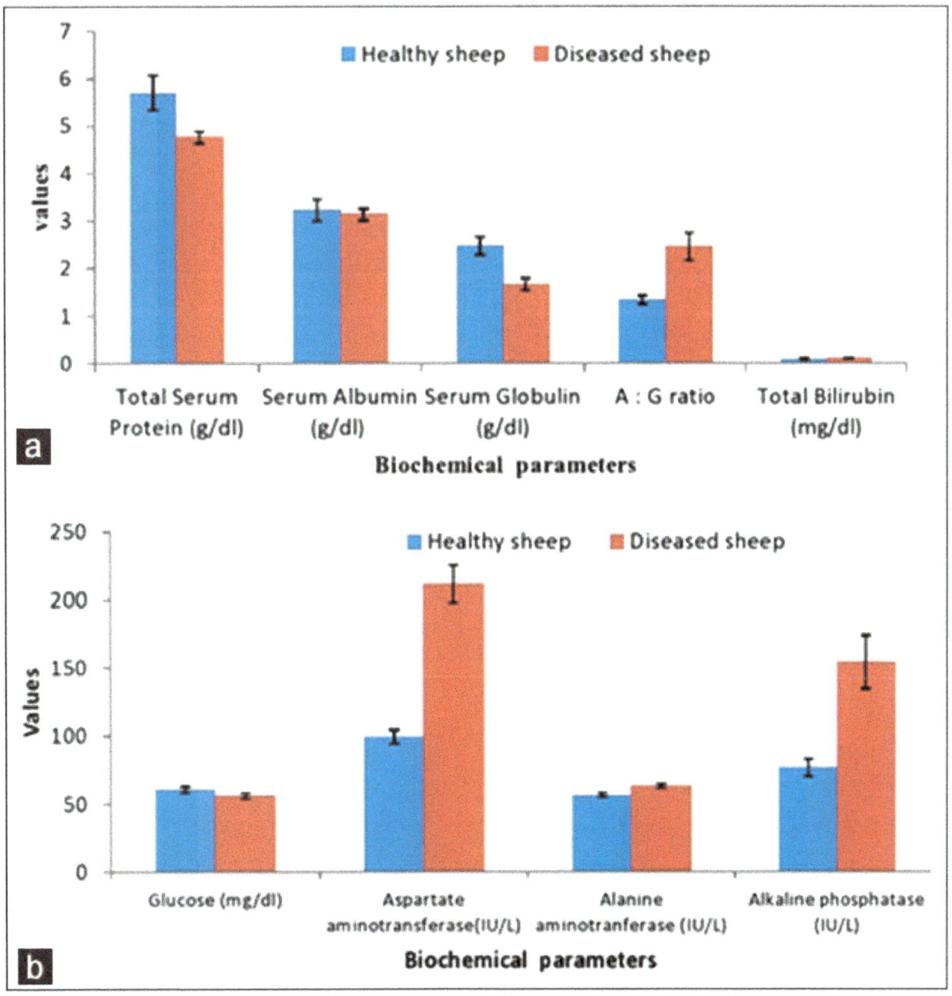

Figure-2: (a,b)Histograms representing serum biochemical parameters of healthy and diseased sheep.

Hematological studies of blood collected from diarrheic sheep/lambs revealed significantly decreased values of Hb, PCV and TEC. Amongst GI helminths of sheep. H. contortus is the predominant species. Main pathological lesion caused by H. contortus infection is anemia. Both adult and fourth stage larvae suck blood and in addition, migration of adult and larvae cause hemorrhages into the abomasum. The average blood loss due to H. contortus infection is 0.03 ml/ parasite/day [13]. The hematological studies in present investigations were in unison with the observation of Dhanlakshmi et al. [14], Zaki et al. [15] and Purohit et al. [16].

Absolute leukocytic count revealed significant leukocytosis due to neutrophilia, lymphocytosis, monocytosis and eosinophilia were in agreement with the observation of Misra et al. [17]. The decrease in value of Hb, PCV and TEC might be due to the presence of strongyle infection, which had been recognized as active blood sucker in stomach and intestine and also been observed in present studies.

Serum biochemical profiles of diarrheic sheep/ lambs in the present study were significant decrease in values of TP, serum globulin and serum glucose whereas significant increase in the albumin: globulin ratio. These results are in consonance with finding of Maiti et al. [18], Pandit et al. [19], Dhanlakshmi et al. [14] Purohit et al. [16], Bordoloi et al. [13] and Qamar and Maqbool [20]. Inappetance with the resultant reduction in dietary protein, malabsorption and plasma losses from damaged intestinal mucosa might be the main cause for marked hypoproteinemia. The inflammation of the intestine by development stages of parasites might also due to poor absorption of protein metabolites resulting low level of TP and massive ascites since ascetic fluid contains a large amount of protein [13,14]. Low serum glucose in the diarrheic sheep/ lambs might be due to decreased appetite of animals, decreased absorption into the blood stream and rapid absorption and utilization of soluble carbohydrate and lipids from the gut by parasites [21].

The activity of aspartate aminotransferase, alanine aminotransferase and alkaline phosphatase and increased total bilirubin were significantly increased in diarrheic sheep/lambs. Specific hepatic function are greatly affected by a wide variety of the pathological condition of extrahepatic origin specially GIT origin. Similar finding were also reported by Prasanthi et al. [22], Zaki et al. [15] and Bordoloi et al. [13]. Since these enzymes have their function and greatest concentration within the cell increase in enzymatic activities reflect cellular abnormalities which directly related to damage that has occurred to hepatocytes, pathological lesions of intestine and cardiac infarction [16] which were also be evidenced in presented studies. As alkaline phosphatase is widely distributed in the body and found in high concentration in bone (in oestoblast), intestinal mucosa, renal tubules cell, liver and placenta; increase in the alkaline phosphatase value in current studies suggestive to damage to mucosal cells of intestine due to parasitic pathogenesis in GIT disorders.

CONCLUSION

Parasitological findings revealed strongyle followed by Strongyloides spp. and Moniezia spp. Hematological studies evidenced that significantly decreased values of Hb, PCV and TEC. Absolute leukocytic count revealed significant leukocytosis due to neutrophilia, lymphocytosis, monocytosis and eosinophilia. There was no significant change in ESR. Serum biochemical profiles of diarrheic sheep/lambs in present study were significant decrease in values of TP, serum globulin, glucose whereas significant increase in the albumin: Globulin ratio, AST, ALT, ALKP and bilirubin.

AUTHORS' CONTRIBUTIONS

SK, KKJ and SSG have designed the study and planned the research experiments. SK performed the research experiments. SP, KK and MP help in conducting experiment. All authors read and approved the final manuscript.

ACKNOWLEDGMENTS

The authors are highly thankful to Dean, College of Veterinary Science and Animal Husbandry, LLR University of Veterinary and Animal Sciences, Hisar, India for providing necessary funds and facilities to carry out the investigation.

REFERENCES

1. Nationa l Dairy Development Board. Share of Agriculture and Livestock's Sector in Gross Domestic Products. Available from: http://www.nddb/org/. Last assessed on 20/08/2014.
2. Department of Animal Husbandry and Dairying, Haryana. Available from: http://www.pashudhanharyana.gov.in/. Last assessed on 20/08/2014.
3. Food and Agriculture Organization of The United Nations, 2010. Available from: http://www.faostat.fao.org/. Last assessed on 20/08/2014.
4. Anonymus (2012) 19th Livestock Census: All India Summary Report 2012. Department of Animal Husbandry, Ministry of Agriculture, Government of India.
5. Anonymus (1977) Manual of Veterinary Parasitological Laboratory Techniques. Ministry of Agriculture, Fishries and Food, Her Majesty's Stationary Office. Bulletin No. 18, London. p5-50.
6. Benjamin, M.M. (2008) Outline of Veterinary Clinical Pathology. 3rd ed. Reprint. The Iowa State University, Press Ames, Iowa, U.S.A. Assessed on 28/01/2013.
7. Anonymous (1990) Operating Manual of RA-50 Chemistry Analyser. Miles Diagnostic India Limited, India.
8. Kumar, S., Jakhar, K.K., Mishra, S.K. and Purohit, B.S.R. (2013) Pathology of digestive and respiratory tracts disorders in sheep. Indian J. Vet. Pathol., 37(2): 124-127.
9. Gaurav. and Jakhar K.K. (2011) Etio-pathological studies on gastrointestinal tract disorders in sheep and goat. Indian J. Vet. Pathol., 35: 116.
10. Mederos, A. Fernándezb, S., VanLeeuwenc, J., Peregrineb, A.S., Keltona, D., Menziesa, P., LeBoeufd, A. and Martine, R. (2010) Prevalence and distribution of gastrointestinal nematodes on 32 organic and conventional commercial farms in Ontario and Quebec, Canada (2006–2008). Vet. Parasitol., 170(3-4): 244-252.

11. Lashari, M.H. and Tasawar Z. (2011) Prevalence of some gastrointestinal parasites in sheep in Southern Panjab, Pakistan. Pak. Vet. J., 31(4): 295-298.

12. Gadahi, J.A., Arshed, M.J., Ali, Q., Javaid, S.B. and Shah, S.I. (2009) Prevalence of Gastrointestinal parasites of sheep and Goat in and around Rawalpindi and Islamabad, Pakistan. Vet. World, 2(2): 51-53.

13. Bordoloi G., Jas R. and Ghosh J.D. (2012) Changes in the haemato-biochemical pattern due to experimentally induced haemonchosis in Sahabadi sheep. J. Parasitol. Dis., 36(1): 101-105.

14. Dhanlakshmi, H., Jagannath, M.S. and D'Souza, P.E. (2002) Haematological and gamma globulin changes in sheep naturally infected with strongyles. Indian J. Anim. Sci., 72(12): 1094-1095.

15. Zaki, M.S., El-Shenawy, A. and El-Khateeb, R.M. (2003) Some studies on sheep naturally infested with Haemonchus contortus and some methods of treatment. Bull. Nat. Res. Cent. Cairo, 28(1): 63-71.

16. Purohit, K., Bhowmik, M.K., Roy, S., Singh, A.S. and Mukhopadhayay S.K. (2003) Some biochemical studies on Garole sheep infected with amphistome parasites. Indian J. Anim. Sci., 73(10): 1120-1122.

17. Misra, R.C., Panda, D.N. and Parida, S. (1996) Haematological and histological alteration of immature paramphistomiasis in lambs. Indian Vet. J., 73(12): 1274-1276.

18. Maiti, S.K., Rao, V.N., Pal, S. and Ali, S.L. (1999) Clinicohaematological and therapeutic studies in parasitic gastroenteritis in sheep. Indian Vet. J., 76(5): 435-437.

19. Pandit S., Jas R., Ghosh, J.D. and Moi, S. (2009) Impact of naturally occurring gastrointestinal nematodosis on serum protein concentration in Garole sheep. Environ. Ecol., 27(4): 1526-1529.

20. Qamar, M.F. and Maqbool A. (2012) Biochemical studies and serodiagnosis of haemonchosis in sheep and goats. J. Anim. Plant Sci., 22(1): 32-38.

21. Radostits, O.M., Gay, C.C., Hinchkliff, K.W. and Constable, P.D. (2007) Veterinary Medicine. 10th ed. Bailliere Tindall, London.

22. Prasanthi, B., Choudhuri, P. C. and Syaamsunder N. (1999) Biochemical observations in ovine Strongylosis. Indian Vet. J., 76(10): 892-894.

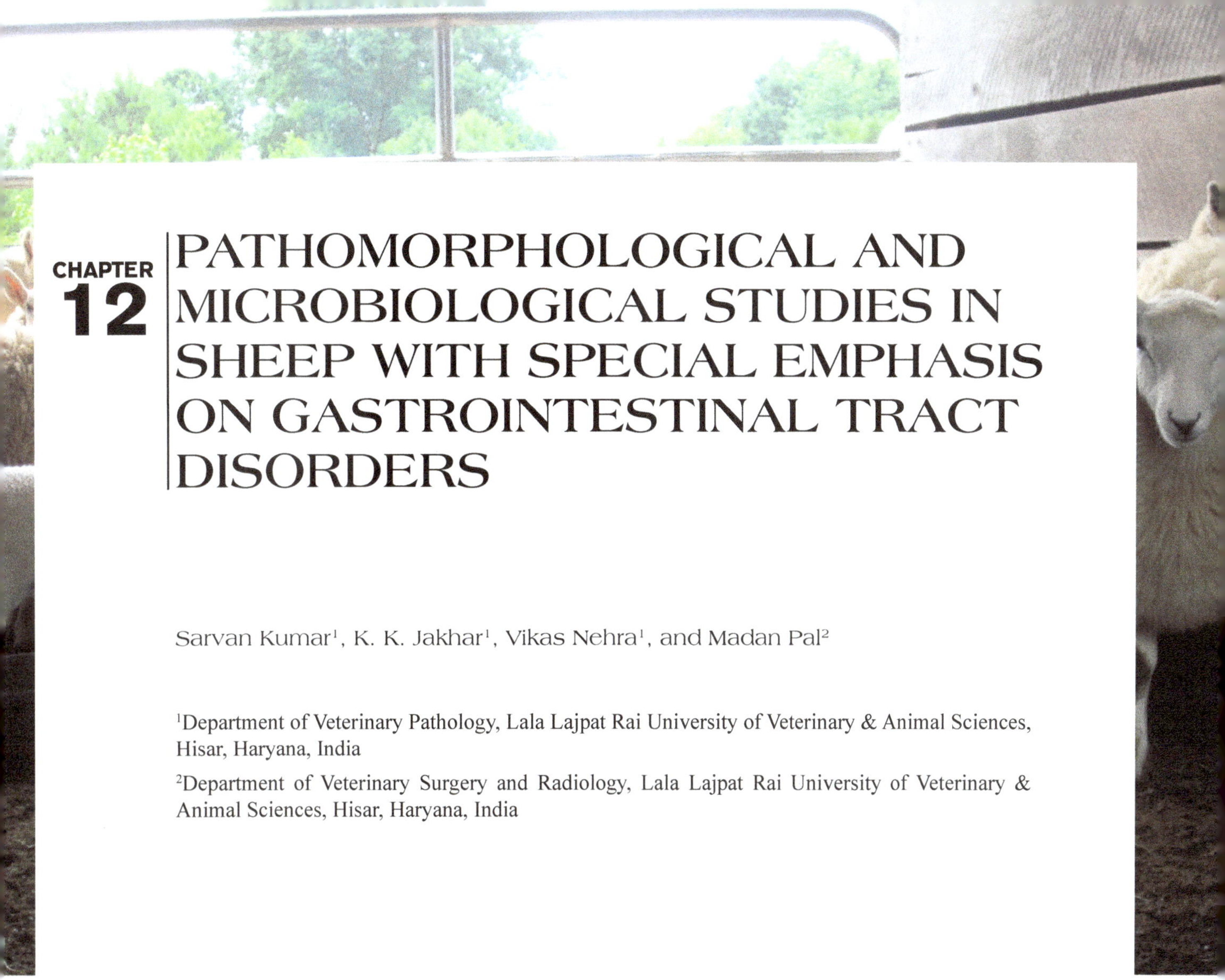

CHAPTER 12

PATHOMORPHOLOGICAL AND MICROBIOLOGICAL STUDIES IN SHEEP WITH SPECIAL EMPHASIS ON GASTROINTESTINAL TRACT DISORDERS

Sarvan Kumar[1], K. K. Jakhar[1], Vikas Nehra[1], and Madan Pal[2]

[1]Department of Veterinary Pathology, Lala Lajpat Rai University of Veterinary & Animal Sciences, Hisar, Haryana, India

[2]Department of Veterinary Surgery and Radiology, Lala Lajpat Rai University of Veterinary & Animal Sciences, Hisar, Haryana, India

ABSTRACT

- **Aim: The present study was envisaged to elucidate the pathomorphological and microbiological aspects of gastrointestinal tract (GIT) disorders of sheep/lambs.**
- **Materials and Methods: Samples for research were collected from 12 sheep died with a history of GIT disorders which were brought for post-mortem examination to the Department of Veterinary Pathology, Lala Lajpat Rai University of Veterinary and Animal Sciences, Hisar, for pathomorphological and microbiological examination.**
- **Results: Gross pathological changes in various organs noticed were abomasitis, congestion and hemorrhages in intestine; necrotic foci on liver surface; enlarged, hard, and indurated mesenteric lymph nodes, hydropericardium, congestion, hemorrhages and consolidation of lungs and congestion and soft kidneys as the major change. On histopathological examination, there were abomasitis with leukocyte infiltration, enteritis with desquamation of mucosal epithelium and goblet cell hyperplasia, lymphadenitis with depletion of lymphocytes in the germinal center of lymphoid follicle, and splenitis with depletion of lymphocytes in the white pulp. In the liver congestion, degenerative changes in hepatocytes including cloudy swelling, fatty changes, congestion in sinusoids, and dilatation of sinusoids leading to atrophy of hepatocytes. Lungs evidenced edema, congestion, emphysema, serous inflammation, thickening of interlobular septa, fibrinous pleuritis, and peribronchiolar lymphoid follicle formation. Heart revealed sarcocystosis, fibrinous pericarditis, and hyalinization of the myocardium. In kidneys, congestion, focal interstitial nephritis, hyaline degeneration, and coagulative necrosis were seen. For microbiological aspects; cultural isolation was done from samples of liver, abomasum, mesenteric lymph nodes, spleen, heart blood, lungs, and kidneys from the carcasses of sheep/lambs. *Escherichia coli* was the only bacterium isolated during present studies. *E. coli* isolates from different tissues of carcasses of sheep/lambs were subjected to *in-vitro* drug sensitivity testing. Ciprofloxacin, cefixime, polymyxin B, amoxicillin + sulbactam, and amoxicillin + clavulanic acid were the most sensitive drugs followed by amikacin, ofloxacin, ampicillin, co-trimoxazole, and amoxicillin.**

Citation: Sarvan Kumar, K. K. Jakhar, Vikas Nehral and Madan Pal, Pathomorphological and microbiological studies in sheep with special emphasis on gastrointestinal tract disorders, doi: 10.14202/vetworld.2015.1015-1020.

Conclusions: From the present study, it is reasonable to conclude that the major etiopathological cause of GIT disorders in sheep was *E. coli* infection, which causes a pathomorphological effect on various cadaver organs *viz.* abomasum, intestine, liver, mesenteric lymph nodes, lungs, spleen, kidneys, and heart followed by parasitic infection of *Haemonchus contortus*.

INTRODUCTION

Agriculture, with its allied sectors such as animal husbandry, is unquestionably the largest livelihood provider in India, more so in the vast rural areas. It also contributes about 15.18% to the gross domestic product [1]. According to the estimates of the Central Statistical Organization, the value of output from livestock and fisheries sectors together at current prices was about 31.6% of the value of output from agriculture and allied sectors. Diseases among these animals cause heavy economic loss. India ranks second in sheep population (71.56 million) in the world [2]. Of this, 0.63 million sheep account from Haryana [3].

Gastrointestinal tract (GIT) disorders are arguably the most important causes of suboptimal productivity in sheep rearing, albeit that often occurs concurrently with other problems. The principal reason for keeping farmed sheep is to convert primary forage, herbage or cereal crops into a marketable product. The efficiency of conversion of feed to meat is greater in sheep that achieve maximum growth rates than in ill-thrifty animals, because there is a daily feed requirement that must be met before the growth can occur, irrespective of the time taken to reach slaughter weight.

A number of viral, bacterial, and parasitic disease result in morbidity and mortality and decline in overall production. The diseases most commonly associated with GIT lesions are Johne's disease, *Escherichia coli*infection, Salmonellosis, enterotoxemia caused by *Clostridium perfringens* Type-B, C, and D, peste des petits ruminants, parasitism, tympany, and others diarrheic disorders. Parasitism particularly by Helminths, impairs health by causing inappetence, diarrhea, anemia, and in severe case death. Therefore, the profitability of global sheep farming is heavily influenced by the efficiency of feed conversion to meat; control of GIT disorder is a prerequisite for the economically sustainable product. To define the cause of death, complete post-mortem is a must. For this purpose, current studies were planned on the pathomorphological and microbiological investigation of GIT disorders in sheep.

MATERIALS AND METHODS

Ethical Approval

Not necessary as study based on post-mortem examination only. Samples for research were collected from the 12 sheep/lambs brought for post-mortem examination to the Department of Veterinary Pathology, Lala Lajpat Rai University of Veterinary and Animal Sciences, Hisar, for pathomorphological and microbiological examination irrespective of age, sex, and breed.

Pathomorphological Examination

Gross changes: All the tissues/organs of the carcasses were examined critically for the presence of gross pathological alterations and the lesions so detected were recorded.

Histopathology

Small piece of organs showing lesions such as abomasum, intestine, mesenteric lymph nodes, liver, spleen, heart, lungs, and kidneys were collected in 10% buffered formalin for histopathological studies. The fixed tissues were washed in running tap water overnight, dehydrated in acetone, cleared in benzene, and embedded in paraffin wax (melting point 60-62°C). Paraffin sections were cut at the thickness of 4-5 μ and staining is done using Lily Mayer's hematoxylin and 2% water soluble eosin [4].

Microbiological Examination

During post-mortem examination, tissue and heart blood samples for bacteriological studies were collected aseptically in sterile Petri dishes and sterile disposable syringe, respectively. Small pieces up to 0.5-1 cm thickness of internal organs showing lesions *viz.* liver, mesenteric lymph nodes, lungs, spleen, kidneys, and heart blood (near about 2 ml) were collected without any anticoagulant from each case for bacteriological examination. Then samples from these organs and heart blood were inoculated on nutrient agar (NA) and Mc-Conkey's lactose agar (MLA) and eosin methylene blue agar (EMB) selective media plates by streak plate technique on same day of sample collection. The plates were then incubated aerobically at 37°C for 24-48 h and examined for the presence of growth, if any. Colony characteristics were noted from NA and MLA plate. All the different type of colonies developed were obtained in pure culture. The pure cultures so obtained were subjected to a biochemical test for further characterization. Identification of all isolates was done following the procedures of Quinn *et al.* [5]. All the organisms so obtained were stained by Gram's staining and examined for their morphological characters.

In-vitro Chemotherapeutic Sensitivity

Isolates were subjected to *in-vitro* drug sensitivity testing using 10 antimicrobials by the single disc diffusion method following the method of Bauer *et al.* [6]. Ciprofloxacin (30 mcg), cefixime (5 mcg), polymyxin B (300 units/disc), amoxicillin + sulbactam (30/15 mcg), amoxicillin + clavulanic acid (20/10 mcg), amikacin (30 mcg), ofloxacin (5 mcg), ampicillin (25 mcg), co-trimoxazole (1.25 mcg), and amoxicillin (30 mcg) were used for drug sensitivity pattern. Results were recorded for the present sensitivity of microbial agent.

Parasitological Examination

During post-mortem examination; rule out every possibility of internal parasitic infection along with fecal contents of abomasum and small intestine. The severity of infection was ascertained by egg count and 150 eggs/g and more were considered as a severe infection.

RESULTS

The gross pathological changes observed in different organs were congestion, petechial to ecchymotic hemorrhage, necrotic foci, hypertrophy, catarrhal and hemorrhagic inflammation, consolidation and tubercle formation, abscess and cyst in different vital organs. In abomasum, congestion was the most prominent change (n=5). In the small intestine, major changes observed were congestion (8 cases) followed by catarrhal and hemorrhagic enteritis (n=4) as shown in Figure-1a. Major gross changes in the lymph node were enlargement, firmness, and induration (n=2). In liver, most prominent change was congestion (n=4) followed by necrotic foci (n=3), fibrinous perihepatitis (Figure-1b and c) along with enlarged gall bladder due to thick bile and abscess in liver (Figure-1d), respectively. Spleen revealed congestion (n=2) and petechial hemorrhages in parenchyma as the major change observed in case of spleen. In the heart, major changes observed were hydropericardium (n=2) followed by congestion (n=3) and hemorrhages in the endocardium. In lungs, the most prominent change was congestion (n=7) followed by emphysema (n=4) and consolidation (n=3). In two cases, formation of small tubercle was also seen in the diaphragmatic lobe. In kidneys, congestion (n=3), soft kidneys (n=3), mottled kidneys, and cyst on kidneys were the major changes observed. When fecal contents of abomasum and small intestine were observed for ruling out parasitic infection; it reveled large number of thread like organism in five cases (n=5) which were confirmed as*Haemonchus contortus*.

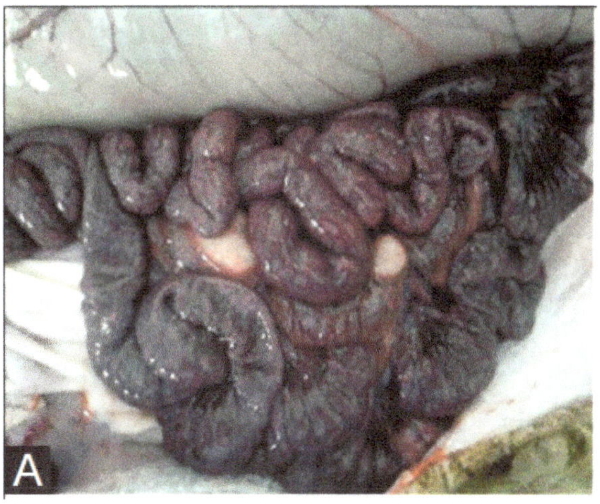

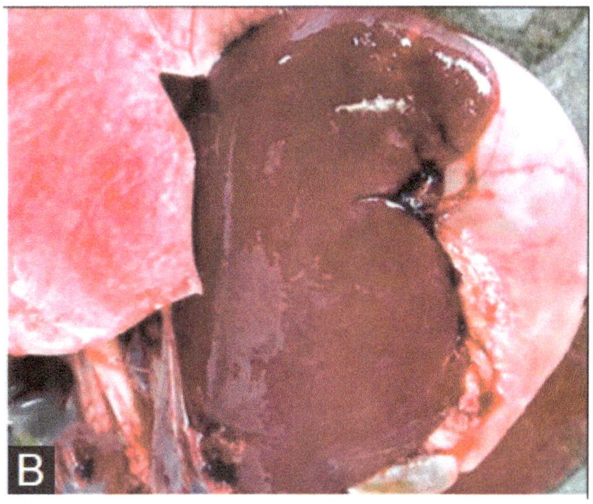

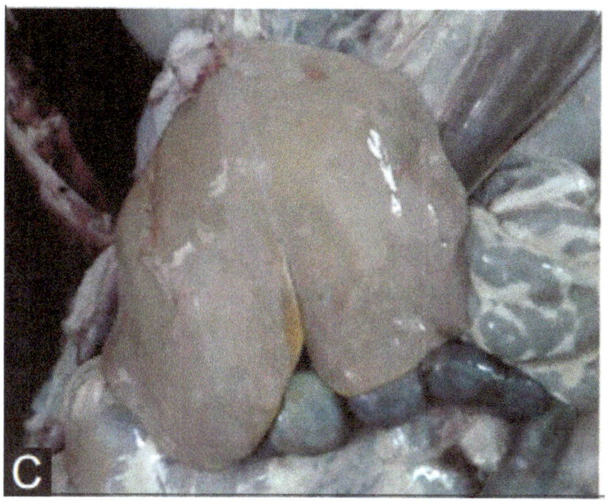

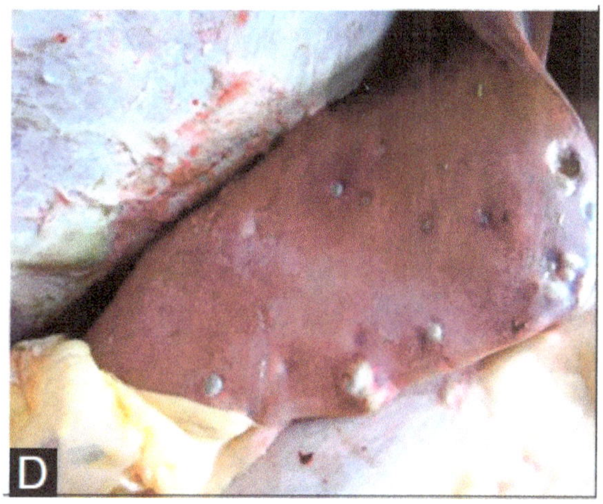

Figure-1: Haemorrhagic enteritis and enlargement of mesenteric lymph node, B: Severe congestion in liver, C: Fibrinous perihepatitis, D: Small abscess on liver.

The histopathological lesions of various organs are depicted in Figures-2-4. In abomasum, edema, congestion, and leukocytic infiltration in mucosa and submucosa with a tendency to lymphoid follicle formation were observed (Figure-2a and b). In the small intestine, major microscopic lesions were edema, mild congestion in mucosa and submucosa, and hemorrhages in the mucosa (Figure-2c and d). Other changes were goblet cell hyperplasia, necrosis and replacement of glands of Leiberkuhn's by mononuclear cells, and desquamation of mucosal epithelium. There was also depletion of lymphocytes in Payer's patches in the large intestine. In the liver, major microscopic lesions were congestion in portal triad area, leukocytic infiltration, and mild bile duct hyperplasia. Congestion of central vein with cloudy swelling and fatty changes in hepatocytes were also observed. Bacterial rods were also seen below the capsule, sinusoids with varying degree of degenerative changes in hepatocytes. Focal area of coagulative necrosis in parenchyma in the periportal area (Figure-3a) and various stages of necrosis such as pyknosis, karyorrhexis, and karyolysis were also noticed (Figure-3b). Other changes were telangiectasias along with atrophy of hepatic cords (Figure-3c). Necrosis in parenchyma and bile duct hyperplasia along with fibroblast proliferation were found. Initiation of lymphoid follicle formation along with degenerative and necrotic changes in parenchyma was seen (Figure-3d). Mesenteric lymph nodes when examined microscopically, revealed edema, congestion, and mild leukocytic infiltration in the capsule. There was depletion of lymphocytes in germinal centers of cortex (Figure-4a) and excess of mononuclear cells in medullary sinuses of the medulla. Spleen revealed mild to severe depletion of lymphocytes in white pulp area (Figure-4b) and reticulo-endothelial cell hyperplasia around the white pulp area. In the heart, edema and congestion were seen in the myocardium along with leukocytic infiltration in some cases. Severe hemorrhages in the epicardium and serous inflammation in the myocardium were evidenced. There was one case of fibrinous pericarditis and sarcocystosis in the myocardium (Figure 4c). At places, fat necrosis was seen in myocardium (Figure-4d). Hyalinization of myocardium, edema, and focal area of mild necrosis along with mononuclear cells infiltration were also observed. In lungs, histopathological lesions revealed edema, congestion, emphysematous alveoli, serous inflammation, thickened interlobular septa due to serofibrinous exudates and infiltration of mononuclear cells in the peribronchiolar area and hyperplasia bronchiolar epithelium. In the heart, there was pleuritis along with thickening of pleura and peribronchiolar lymphoid follicle formation along with serous inflammation. In kidneys, there was congestion of intertubular blood vessels and coagulative necrosis along with leukocytic infiltration. Focal areas of necrosis along with hyaline materials in tubules and interstitial nephritis with infiltration of the mononuclear cell were observed.

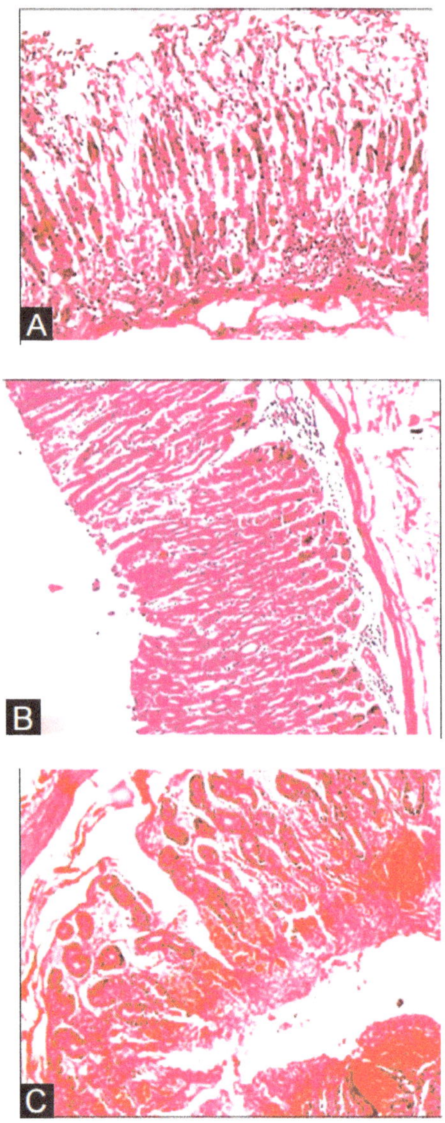

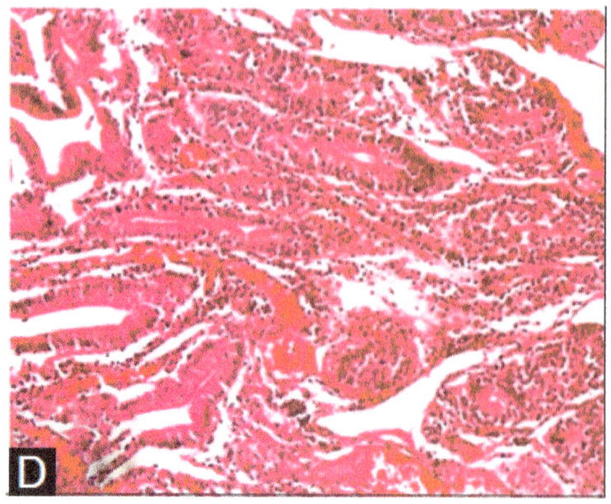

Figure-2: A: Abomasum: Leucocytic infiltration in mucosa (H. & E. × 100), B: Abomasum: Initiation of lymphoid follicle in submucosa (H. & E. × 100), C: Intestine: Severe haemorrhagic enteritis (H. & E. × 100), D: ...

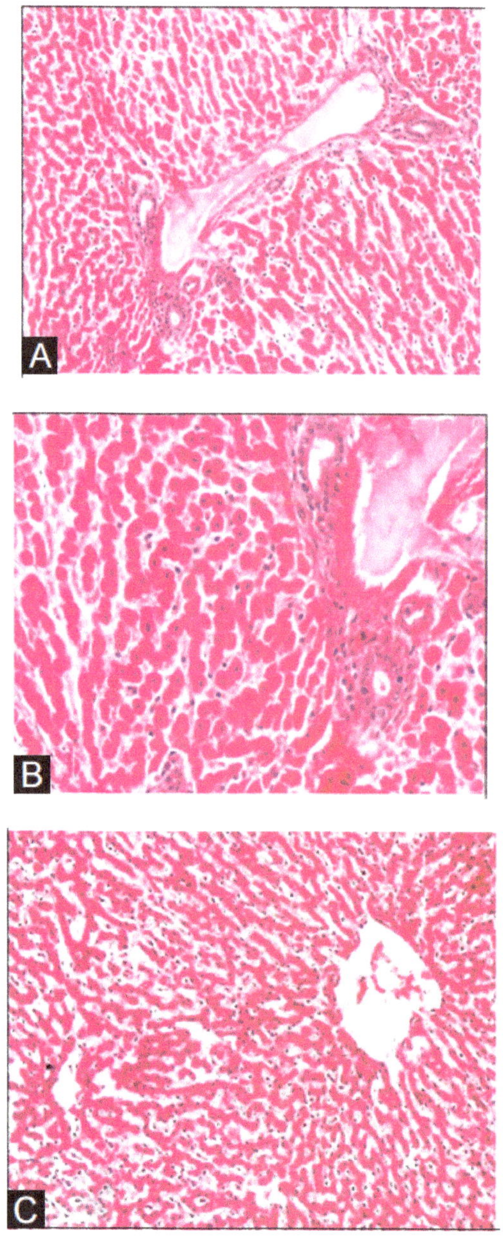

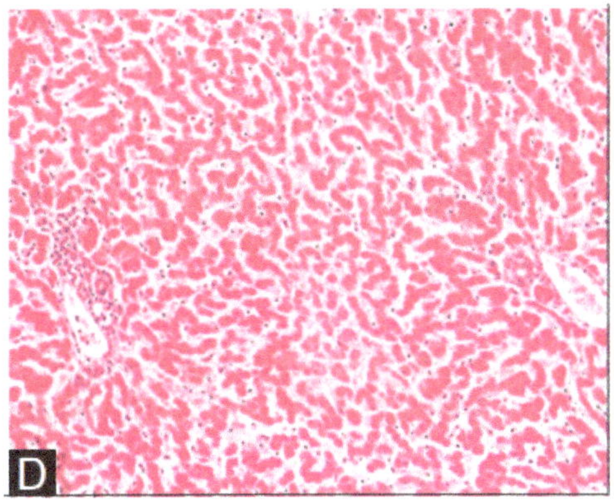

Figure-3: A: Liver: Focal area of coagulative necrosis and increased no. of bile duct in portal triad area (H. & E. × 200), B: Liver: Various stages of necrosis in hepatocytes in periportal area. (H. & E. × 400), C: Liver: Telangiectasis **...**

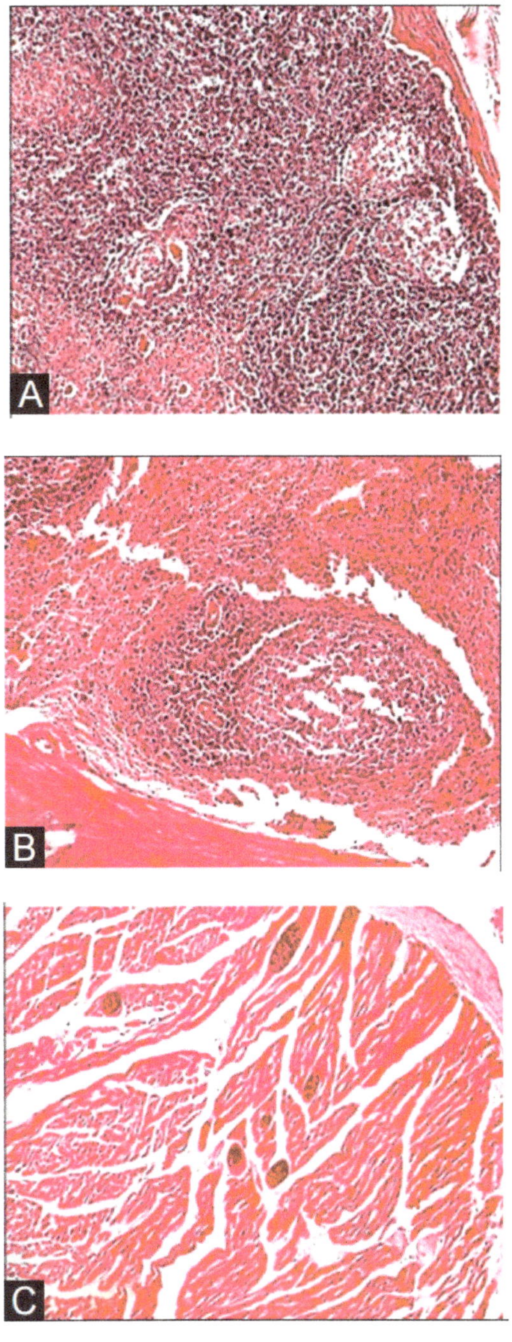

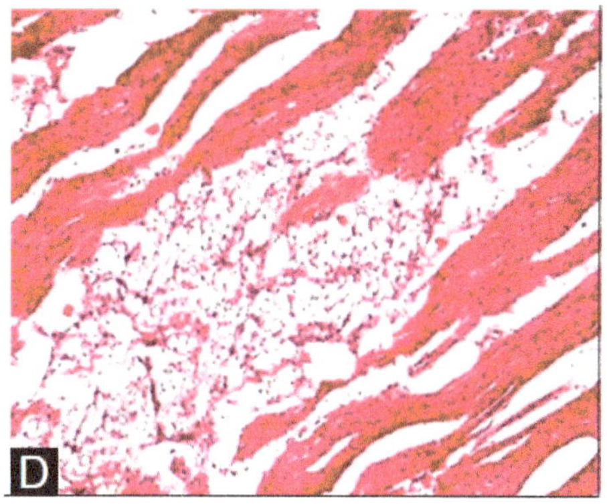

Figure-4: A: Mesentric lymph node: Depletion of lymphocytes in germinal centre in cortex of lymph node (H. & E. × 100), B: Spleen: Depletion of lymphocyte in white pulp area (H. & E. × 100), C: Heart: Pericardial fibrinous layer **...**

Out of 72 representative tissues which were collected for microbiological examination; 22 samples produced pink colonies on MLA and creamy white mucoid/non-mucoid colonies on NA. Gram-staining revealed pink colored rods and Catalase test further confirmed Gram-negative bacteria. Metallic sheen was noticed in all these cases on EMB agar. After performing biochemical tests (oxidation-fermentation test, nitrate test, H2S production on triple sugar iron medium, indole, methyl red, Voges–Proskauer, citrate utilization test, and urease test) and culture characteristics revealed isolates positive for *E. coli*. The results of *E. coli* bacteria isolated from different organs of carcasses of sheep/lambs are depicted in Figure-5. Out of 22 isolates of *E. coli*., organwise isolates were 7 from liver (31.81%), 5 from lung (22.72%), 6 from heart blood (27.27%), 3 from kidney (13.64%), and 1 from spleen (4.5%). No bacteria were isolated from mesenteric lymph nodes. All the isolates of *E. coli* showed maximum sensitivity against cefixime, ciprofloxacin, polymyxin-B, amoxicillin + sulbactam, and amoxicillin + clavulanic acid (each 100%) followed by amikacin and ofloxacin (90%). Least sensitivity was observed to ampicillin, co-trimoxazole, and amoxicillin (70%).

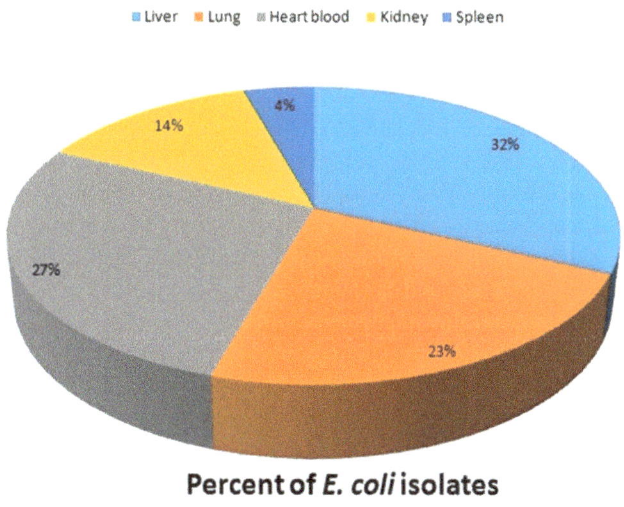

Figure-5: Organwise percent of *E. coli* isolates.

DISCUSSION

Abomasitis, catarrhal, and hemorrhagic enteritis may be due to gastrointestinal parasitism (*H. contortus*) and various bacterial and viral infections. Hemorrhagic enteritis may be because of simultaneous infection of rotavirus and *E. coli*. [7]. Rotavirus is the leading etiological agent of acute viral gastroenteritis in young ones of many species of animals. Rotavirus damages microvilli of the small intestine, which causes reduced starch digestion, results in promotion of excess bacterial (*E. coli*) growth simultaneously. It induces an osmotic effect resulting in diarrhea. In lambs, rotavirus enteritis is more severe when complicated by simultaneous infection with enterotoxigenic *E. coli*. [8]. A wide range of infectious and parasitic agents that produces myocarditis and include suppurative, necrotic, hemorrhagic, lymphocytic, and eosinophilic response. Eosinophilic myocarditis in current studies may result of sarcocystosis. Hydropericardium observed in lambs can be correlated with heavy infection of blood sucking stomach worms resulting in excessive loss of serum albumin decreasing the osmotic pressure of plasma which forces fluid to move out of blood to tissues and accumulation of fluid in pericardial sac resulting in hydropericardium [9,10]. In the present study, infection of *H. contortus* may be due to the development of resistant strain [11]. Soft kidneys may be correlated with overeating of pasture results in the accumulation of undigested starch which may enhance proliferation of*Clostridium perferingens* Type D bacteria in rapidly growing lambs. These bacteria grow in feed in upper intestine and secrete two toxins that are absorbed by the gut, alpha toxin damages gut lining, and epsilon toxin absorbed by body and causes damage to brain, heart, kidneys, and other tissues. Chronic passive congestion leads to persistent hypoxia in the centrilobular area and because of oxygen and nutrient, deprivation leads to degeneration and hepatocyte atrophy. As a result, sinusoids in these areas are dilated which leads to telangiectasias [12]. Mesenteric lymph nodes when examined microscopically, revealed edema, congestion, and mild leukocytic infiltration in capsule [13].

Microbiological finding were in consonance of studies conducted by Kumar *et al.* [14]. They concluded that out of 72 tissue samples 48 were confirmed for *E. coli*. Out of 48 isolates, only 18 were serotyped and out of these 13 belonged to 'O' serogroup whereas remaining five isolate were untypable. The most prevalent serotype were O168 (5) followed by O 60 (4), O1 (1), O91 (1), 0102 (1), and O116 (1). A relatively high rate of *E. coli* infection in sheep/lambs in the present study might be due to errors in colostrum feeding, inefficient production of antibodies, stress, and hormonal changes which enhance the growth of opportunistic bacteria and therefore, infection flare up. Sharma and Pruthi [15] reported that *E. coli* as the most predominant bacterial organism in GIT disorders of sheep carcasses followed by *Proteus* spp., *Klebsiella*spp., *Salmonella typhimurium* 4,5:i:1,2, *Staphylococcus* spp. and *Pseudomonas aeruginosa*. The *E. coli*strains belonged to 14 different serotypes, of these, 52.3% were of 7 serotypes O172 (7), O158 (14), O88 (17), O44 (7), O153 (17), O22 (11), and O25 (10). Other serotypes were O32 (1), O132 (2), O64 (1), O42 (5), O156 (5), O70 (1), and O91 (3). Three strains were rough and 21 remained untyped. More or less similar findings were revealed by Tibbo *et al.* [16] and Lashari and Tasawar [17], Sharma and Pruthi [15].

In the present investigation, anti-biogram patterns of different bacterial organisms isolated from carcasses of sheep/lambs showed varying degree of sensitivity to the chemotherapeutic agents. Ciprofloxacin, cefixime, polymyxin B, amoxicillin + sulbactam, and amoxicillin + clavulanic acid were the most sensitive drugs followed by amikacin, ofloxacin ampicillin, co-trimoxazole, and amoxicillin. Difference in antibiotic sensitivity was due to the resistance of microbe to different antibiotics and indiscriminate use of antibiotics [14]. Resistance may be due to spontaneously induced genetic mutation or the acquisition of resistance genes from other bacterial species by horizontal gene transfer via conjugation, transduction, or transformation. Many antibiotic resistance genes reside on transmissible plasmids, facilitating their transfer. Exposure to an antibiotic naturally selects for the survival of the organisms with the genes for resistance. In this way, a gene for antibiotic resistance may readily spread through an ecosystem of bacteria. Antibiotic-resistance plasmids frequently contain genes conferring resistance to several different antibiotics. Kumar *et al.* [14] also reported antibiotic resistant against different serotypes of *E. coli*. They concluded that *E. coli* strain isolated from diarrheic sheep/lambs belongs to a large number of serogroups and may be the reason for high variation in antibiotic resistance. However, present sensitivity pattern finding are not in confirmation with findings of Gaurav and Jakhar [13] and Kumar *et al.* [14] which could be ascribed to serotypes variation, acquired and genetic resistance, and selection of resistant microorganisms for different drugs.

CONCLUSION

Major etiopathological cause of GIT disorders in sheep was *E. coli* infection, which causes a pathomorphological effect on various cadaver organs *viz.* abomasum, intestine, liver, mesenteric lymph nodes along with lesions on lungs, spleen, kidneys, and heart. *Haemonchus contortus* was the second most important causative agent for GIT disorders in sheep, which was responsible for weight loss, anemia, hemorrhagic enteritis, and hydropericardium. Ciprofloxacin, cefixime, polymyxin B, amoxicillin + sulbactam, and amoxicillin + clavulanic acid were the most sensitive drugs followed by amikacin, ofloxacin ampicillin, co-trimoxazole, and amoxicillin.

AUTHORS' CONTRIBUTIONS

SK and KKJ have designed the study and planned the research experiments. SK performed the research experiment and drafted the manuscript. KKJ revised the manuscript. VN and MP helped in conducting the experiment. All authors read and approved the final manuscript.

ACKNOWLEDGMENTS

The authors are highly thankful to Dean, College of Veterinary Science and Animal Husbandry, LLR University of Veterinary and Animal Sciences, Hisar, India, for providing necessary funds and facilities to carry out the investigation.

REFERENCES

1. National Dairy Development Board. Share of Agriculture and Livestock's Sector in Gross Domestic Products. [Accessed on 20-08-2014]. Available from: http://www.nddb/org/
2. Food and Agriculture Organization of the United Nations. 2010. [Accessed on 20-08-2014]. Available from: http://www.faostat.fao.org/
3. Anonymous. 19th Livestock Census: All India Summary Report 2012. Department of Animal Husbandry, Ministry of Agriculture, Government of India; 2012.
4. Luna L.G. Manual of Histologic Staining Methods of the Armed Forces Institute of Pathology. 3rd ed. New York: McGraw Hill Book Company; 1968.
5. Quinn P.J, Carter M.E, Markey B.K, Carter G.R. Clinical Veterinary Microbiology. Edinburugh: Mosby; 1994.
6. Bauer A.W, Kirby W.M, Sherris J.C, Turck M. Antibiotic susceptibility testing by a standardised disc method. Am. J. Clin. Pathol. 1966;36:493–496.
7. Kumar S, Jakhar K.K, Mishra S.K, Purohit B.S.R. Pathology of digestive and respiratory tracts disorders in sheep. Indian J. Vet. Pathol. 2013;37(2):124–127.
8. Gazal S, Mir I.A, Iqbal A, Taku A.K, Kumar B, Bhat M.A. Ovine rotaviruses. Open Vet. J. 2011;1:50–54. [PMC free article]
9. Kumar S, Jakhar K.K, Singh S, Potliya S, Kumar K, Pal M. Clinico-pathological studies of gastrointestinal tract disorders in sheep with parasitic infection. Vet. World. 2015;8(1):29–32.
10. Kumar S, Jakhar K.K, Mishra S.K, Purohit R. Pathology of gastrointestinal tract disorders in sheep.Chennai: Paper Abstracted at XXVIII Annual Conference of Indian Association of Veterinary Pathologists from 29th and 30th December at Department of Veterinary Pathology, Madras Veterinary College; 2011. p. 63.
11. Das M, Singh S. Effect of with drawl of anthelmintics on fenbendazole and morantel resistance status of*Haemonchus contortus* in sheep and goats. Haryana Vet. 2010;49:22–24.
12. Khajuria A, Azmi S, Rahman S, Sultan Z, Sharma M. Pathomorphological changes in liver of sheep and goats due to parasitic infestation. Indian J. Vet. Pathol. 2013;37(1):1–4.
13. Gaurav , Jakhar K.K. Etio-pathological studies on gastrointestinal tract disorders in sheep and goat.Indian J. Vet. Pathol. 2011;35:116.
14. Kumar S, Jakhar K.K, Kapoor S, Sharma A. Serotyping and antimicrobial sensitivity of *Escherichia coli*isolated from gastrointestinal tract disorders in sheep. Haryana Vet. 2012;51:61–62.
15. Sharma V, Pruthi A.K. Etiopathological studies on gastrointestinal tract and liver disorders of sheep. Haryana Vet. 2008;47:98–102.
16. Tibbo M, Aragaw K, Teferi M, Haile A. Effect of strategic helminthosis control on mortality of communally grazed menz lambs of smallholders in the cool central Ethiopian highlands. Small Rumin. Res.2010;90(1-3):58–63.
17. Lashari M.H, Tasawar Z. Prevalence of some gastrointestinal parasites in sheep in Southern Punjab, Pakistan. Pak. Vet. J. 2011;31(X):XXX.

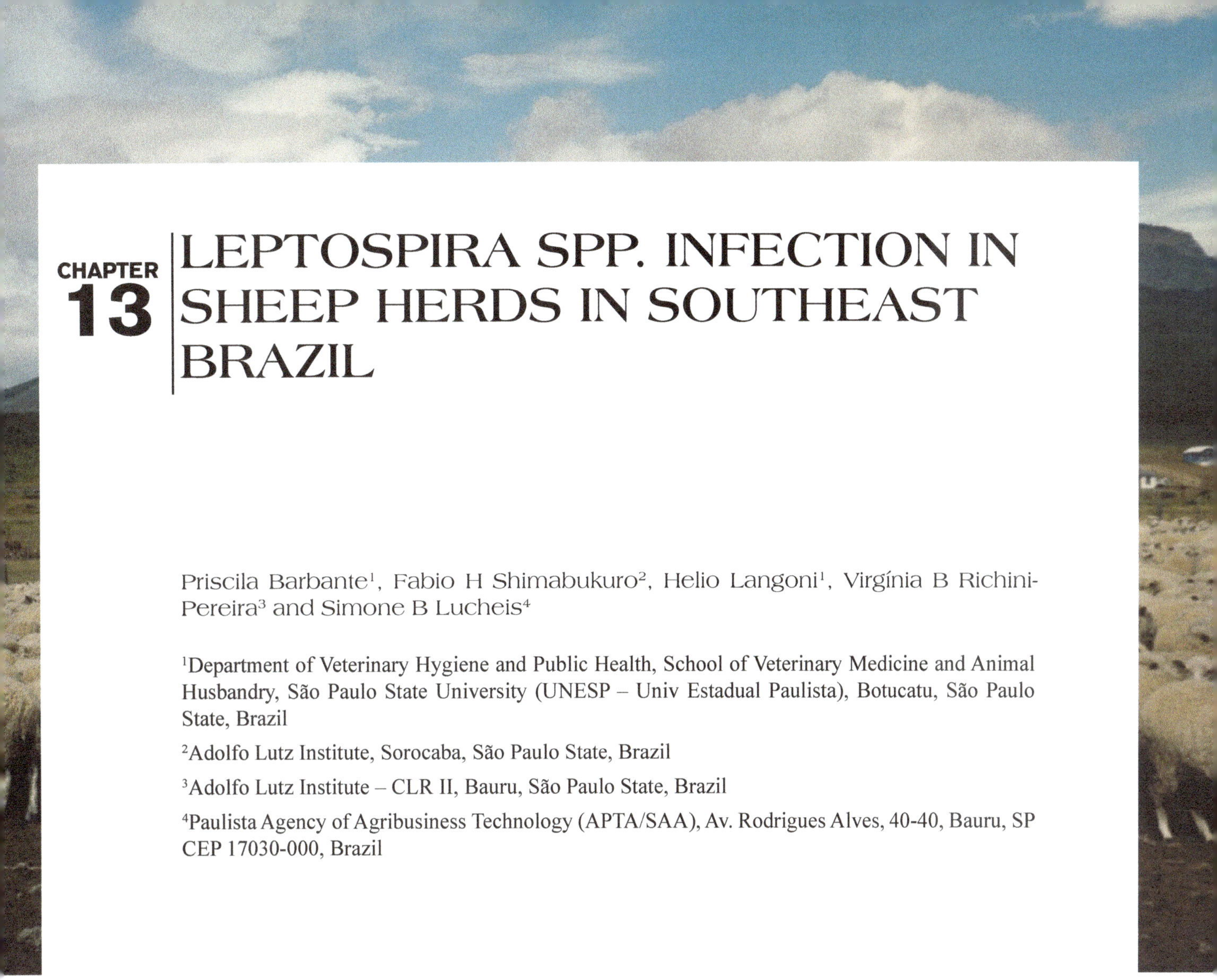

CHAPTER 13

LEPTOSPIRA SPP. INFECTION IN SHEEP HERDS IN SOUTHEAST BRAZIL

Priscila Barbante[1], Fabio H Shimabukuro[2], Helio Langoni[1], Virgínia B Richini-Pereira[3] and Simone B Lucheis[4]

[1]Department of Veterinary Hygiene and Public Health, School of Veterinary Medicine and Animal Husbandry, São Paulo State University (UNESP – Univ Estadual Paulista), Botucatu, São Paulo State, Brazil

[2]Adolfo Lutz Institute, Sorocaba, São Paulo State, Brazil

[3]Adolfo Lutz Institute – CLR II, Bauru, São Paulo State, Brazil

[4]Paulista Agency of Agribusiness Technology (APTA/SAA), Av. Rodrigues Alves, 40-40, Bauru, SP CEP 17030-000, Brazil

ABSTRACT

Background

With the aim of studying *Leptospira* spp. infection in sheep herds, blood samples and respective kidney and liver fragments were collected from 100 animals from twenty different properties during slaughter at a meat company in the Sorocaba region, São Paulo state, southeast Brazil. The microscopic agglutination test (MAT) was performed with 29 strains of *Leptospira* spp. To identify the agent in the liver and kidney, 100 samples of each tissue were submitted to culture in Fletcher medium and analyzed by the polymerase chain reaction (PCR) for *Leptospira* spp.

Results

MAT detected 23 samples serologically positive for one or more *Leptospira* spp. serovars and significantly more for Autumnalis. Eight (4%) samples were positive in culture (four kidneys and four livers), corresponding to five animals with positive serology (one animal simultaneously positive for both kidney and liver) and two negatives. PCR detected *Leptospira* spp. in 14 samples (seven kidneys and seven livers) corresponding to 12 positive animals (two animals simultaneously positive for kidney and liver), of which ten were serologically positive and two negative.

Conclusions

PCR was faster, more practical and more sensitive than culture for detecting leptospires. The results reinforce the importance of sheep in the epidemiological context of leptospirosis.

Citation: Priscila Barbante, Fabio H Shimabukuro, Helio Langoni, Virgínia B Richini-Pereira and Simone B Lucheis, Leptospira spp. infection in sheep herds in southeast Brazil, DOI: 10.1186/1678-9199-20-20.

BACKGROUND

One of the most representative zoonotic illnesses with a large economic impact on animal production is leptospirosis, an infectious disease that causes a fall in milk production, miscarriages, and low fertility. It is also a serious public health problem related to socioeconomic characteristics, floods, and occupational aspects in humans [1]. Azevedo *et al.* [2] were alerted to the transmission of the disease in slaughterhouse workers who had handled the organs and carcasses of infected animals.

Leptospira has been observed in the urine, semen and vaginal secretions of production animals, characterizing these species as susceptible to the disease from the reproductive sphere [3].

Ovine *Leptospira* spp. seems to be common in most countries, particularly in extensive flock management systems where sheep farming occurs together with cattle, allowing infection by direct contact with urine or by contaminated water in collective drinking supplies [4, 5].

Infection of sheep was first detected in Brazil by Santa Rosa and Castro [6] in animals from São Paulo state, 34% of which were found to be reactive to various *Leptospira* spp. serovars.

Later serological studies performed by Viegas *et al.* [7], found 22.8% of sheep reactive, mainly to Autumnalis, Castellonis, Grippotyphosa, and Tarassovi serovars. In another work performed in Bahia, Caldas *et al.* [8] observed 34.7% of a sample of 800 examined sheep to be reactive, most frequently to the serovars Autumnalis, Castellonis and Butembo.

Langoni *et al.* [9] studied antileptospira agglutinins in 356 ovine serum samples from different regions of São Paulo state, finding the following prevalences: Icterohaemorrhagiae (51.25%); Castellonis (20.63%), Hardjo (19.36%); Bratislava (16.25%); Andamana and Wolffi (11.88%); Copenhageni (8.75%); Grippotyphosa (4.34%); Pomona (2.5%), and Tarassovi (0.63%).

A work performed by Martins and Lilenbaum [10] in Rio de Janeiro, Brazil, reported the highest prevalence of seroreactivity in sheep (47.4%), in relation to the other species of ruminants studied, including cows and goats.

In 11 municipalities in the Presidente Dutra microregion, Maranhão state, Brazil, Carvalho *et al.* [11] analyzed 379 sheep blood serum samples using a microscopic agglutination test (MAT); of the 37 herds studied, 30 (81%) had at least one seropositive animal while the individual seroprevalence was 32%.

A study performed in the state of Rio Grande do Sul verified by MAT that from 1360 tested serum samples, 466 (34.26%) animals were reactive with antileptospira agglutinin counts varying from 100 to 3200. The main serovars encountered were: Hardjo (28.4%), Sentot (16.8%); and Hardjoprajitno (14.5%), showing that*Leptospira* spp. is spread on most farms that raise sheep in the southeast and southwest mesoregions of Rio Grande do Sul [12].

A study by Escócio *et al.* [13] analyzed the sanitary profile of sheep flocks farmed exclusively or together with cattle in the Sorocaba region of São Paulo state. High levels of leptospirosis were found and all flocks were reactive to at least one serovar of *Leptospira* spp. Autumnalis was most prevalent serovar in four sheep flocks, followed by the Pyrogenes; in seven flocks where both cattle and sheep were in the same environment, the most prevalent were the serovars Icterohaemorrhagiae, Hardjo and Javanica.

Sheep flock infection by *Leptospira* leads to serious economic losses, represented by physiological problems and reproductive alterations. In this context, the aim was to verify the occurrence of antileptospira antibodies in sheep from different municipal areas in the Sorocaba region, São Paulo state, that were slaughtered in meat plants, to study the presence of serologically positive and negative sheep as renal *Leptospira* spp. carriers (chronic phase) and detect the agent in the liver (acute phase) by culturing in Fletcher medium using the Pasteur pipette technique and by PCR.

METHODS

Animals and Samples

We sampled 100 sheep from 20 properties from different municipal areas of Sorocaba region, São Paulo state, southeast Brazil. Samples were taken at moment of slaughter, selecting five animals from each property.

During the bleeding phase, approximately 10 mL of blood was collected from each animal in a 15 mL sterile glass tube. After coagulant removal, samples were centrifuged at 3000 rpm for 15 minutes and the serum obtained was treated in a 1.5 mL microtube and frozen at –20°C for later serological testing.

Fragments from the liver and the left or right kidney were aseptically collected during the disembowelment phase. These were placed individually in plastic bags, sealed and identified, refrigerated in an isothermal box, and transferred to the laboratory.

Microscopic Agglutination Test (MAT)

MAT was performed as per Ministry of Health norms [14]. Each serum sample was initially diluted 1:100 in pH 7.2 phosphate buffered saline (PBS) as a positive cutoff point. Live cultures of 29 strains of *Leptospira* spp., used as antigens, were grown in liquid culture medium of Ellinghausen-McCullough-Johnson-Harris (EMJH), free of contamination or self-agglutination: *L. interrogans* serovars Australis, Autumnalis, Bataviae, Bratislava, Canicola, Copenhageni, Djasiman, Wolffi, Icterohaemorrhagiae, Pomona, Sentot, Hardjo, Hardjoprajitno, Hardjobovis, HardjoCTG and Hardjominiswajezak; *L. santarosai* serovar Shermani; *L. borgpetersenii* serovars Castellonis, Hebdomadis, Javanica, Pyrogenes, Tarassovi and Whitcombi; *L. kirschneri* serovars Butembo, Cynopteri and Grippotyphosa; *L. noguchi* serovar Panama and *L. biflexa* serovars Andamana and Patoc.

Considered positive were those serovars that presented 50% or more agglutination than the control. Samples found positive in the first titer were successively re-diluted at 1:2 and tested for the previously reacting serovars. The last titer was that which still presented 50% or more agglutination [15].

Leptospira spp. isolation

The liver and kidney fragments used for culture were processed as cited by Passos *et al.* [16]. The obtained material was cultivated in three tubes with Fletcher culture medium, two with an additional 100 µg 5-fluorouracil/mL and 2.5 µg neomycin, and one without antibiotics, all incubated at 29°C for 16 weeks. Readings were made fortnightly after seeding; samples were considered positive when mobile spirochetes were seen under a dark field microscope at 400×.

Polymerase Chain Reaction (PCR)

Fragments of liver and kidney weighing between 5 and 50 mg were pre-titrated with the aid of sterile pincers and bistoury and placed in sterile 1.5 mL DNAse and RNAse-free microtubes. After 1 mL of pH7.2 sterile PBS was added, the samples were centrifuged at 19,000 g for 15 minutes (kidney) and 19,000 g for 30 minutes (liver) at 4°C according to Heinemann *et al.* [17] with some modifications for tissue wash; supernatant was discarded and 50 µL of pH 7.2 sterile PBS was added to the cellular sediment, which was then macerated with a bio-vortexer (Biospec Inc., USA) and centrifuged at 2000 g for ten seconds.

The DNA extraction from liver and kidney was performed using an illustra Tissue & Cells Genomic Prep Mini Spin Kit (GE Healthcare, USA), as per the manufacturer's recommendations and concentration was measured in a spectrophotometer (NanoVue, GE Healthcare, USA).

Molecular detection was carried out through PCR by using the primer pair: LEP1 (5′GGCGGCGCGTCTTAAACATG3′) and LEP2 (5′TTCCCCCCATTGAGCAAGATT3′), that amplified 331 bp for*Leptospira* spp. [18].

PCR reactions was performed in 0.2 mL microtubes with total volumes of 25 µL, containing PCR buffer solution (50 mM KCl, 10 mM of Tris-HCl pH 8.0), $MgCl_2$ (1.5 mM), dNTP solution (0.2 mM), Taq Platinum DNA (1.0 U) (Invitrogen, Brazil), 10 ρM of each primer, ultra-pure water (Life Technologies, USA) and DNA (10 ng).

Amplification was performed in a Mastercycler® EP Gradient Thermal Cycler (Eppendorf, Germany). Thermal cycling conditions were 94°C for three minutes, 30 cycles of 94°C for one minute, annealing at 63°C for one minute, and extension at 72°C for two minutes, with an additional ten minutes at 72°C at the end to complete extension of the amplified segments. Visualization of amplified products was accomplished by electrophoresis. For this 1.5% agarose gel was prepared with 1 µL/mL SYBR® Safe DNA gel stain (Life Technologies, USA). PCR product (10 µL) and 4 µL of 100 bp molecular ladder (Life Technologies, USA) were used. To all samples, 2 µL of a BlueJuice™ Gel Loading Buffer (Life Technologies, USA) was added. The gel was submitted to the electrophoresis run in an HE99 horizontal cube (GE Healthcare, USA) containing 1X TBE (0.1 M Tris, 0.09 M boracic acid, and 0.001 M EDTA) at 100 V for approximately one hour using an electrophoresis power supply (EPS 301, GE Healthcare, USA). The gel was visualized in a UV transilluminator and the image captured by a GelDoc-It® TS Imaging System (UVP, USA) and documented using VisionWorks® LS Image Acquisition and Analysis Software (UVP, USA). Controls were used for extraction and PCR technique. Contaminated liver and kidney suspensions were prepared with *L. interrogans* serovar Pyrogenes at 2.0×10^4leptospires/mL as the positive control, and ultrapure water (Life Technologies, USA) as the negative control.

Analytical sensitivity was tested using different known negative tissue samples (liver and kidney) by contaminating the samples with *L. interrogans* serovar Pyrogenes at concentrations of approximately 2.0×10^0; 2.0×10^1; 2.0×10^2; 2.0×10^3, and 2.0×10^4 microorganisms per milliliter of suspension from each organ sample [19].

RESULTS

From the 20 properties studied, 13 (65%) presented at least one seropositive animal. From the total 100 serum samples analyzed by MAT, 23 (23%) were reactive to one or more *Leptospira* spp. serovar.

Of the 29 *Leptospira* spp. serovars tested, only nine were reactive. Most animals were reactive to the Autumnalis serovar (n = 19) with titers varying from 100 to 1600. Other reactive serovars were Patoc (n = 3), Butembo (n = 2), Castellonis (n = 1), Djasiman (n = 1), Grippothyphosa (n = 1), Icterohaemorrhagiae (n = 1), Wolffi (n = 1) and Hardjo Prajitno (n = 1), whose titers varied from 100 to 200. The highest titer obtained was 1600 for Autumnalis serovar in a single animal (Table 1).

Table 1: Distribution of *Leptospira* spp. serovars and antibody titers from sheep herds in Sorocaba region, São Paulo state, southeast Brazil

Property	Animals analyzed/ positive	Serovars											
		Autumnalis			Butembo	Castellonis	Djasiman	Grippothyphosa	Icterohaemorrhagiae	Wollfi	Patoc		Hardjoprajitno
		100	200	1600	100	100	100	100	200	200	100	200	100
A	5/1	1	–	–	–	–	–	–	–	–	–	–	–
B	5/0	–	–	–	–	–	–	–	–	–	–	–	–
C	5/1	1	–	–	–	–	–	–	–	–	–	–	–
D	5/2	1	1	–	–	–	–	–	–	–	–	–	–
E	5/2	1	1	–	–	–	–	–	–	–	–	–	–

F	5/1	1	–	–	–	–	–	–	–	–	–	–	–
G	5/2	1	1	–	–	–	–	–	–	–	–	–	–
H	5/2	1	1	–	–	–	–	–	–	–	–	–	–
I	5/0	–	–	–	–	–	–	–	–	–	–	–	–
J	5/1	–	1	–	–	–	–	–	–	–	–	–	–
L	5/3[a]	1	2	–	1	–	–	–	–	–	–	–	–
M	5/3[b]	1	1	–	–	–	–	–	–	1	–	1	–
N	5/0	–	–	–	–	–	–	–	–	–	–	–	–
O	5/0	–	–	–	–	–	–	–	–	–	–	–	–
P	5/0	–	–	–	–	–	–	–	–	–	–	–	–
Q	5/1	–	–	–	–	–	1	–	–	–	–	–	–
R	5/1	–	1	–	–	–	–	–	–	–	–	–	–
S	5/0	–	–	–	–	–	–	–	–	–	–	–	–
T	5/0	–	–	–	–	–	–	–	–	–	–	–	–
U	5/3[C]	1	–	1	1	1	–	1	1	–	1	–	1
Total	100/23	10	9	1	2	1	1	1	1	1	1	1	1

[a]One animal reactive to two serovars, Autumnalis (200) and Butembo (100).

[b]One animal reactive to two serovars, Autumnalis (200) and Patoc (200).

[c]One animal reactive to two serovars, Autumnalis (100) and Castellonis (100) and another to five serovars, Autumnalis (1600), Butembo (100), Grippothyphosa (100), Icterohaemorrhagiae (200), and Patoc (100).

(–) non-reactive animals.

In the culture results, from the 20 properties studied, we found five (25%) positive from at least one animal. Of the liver and kidney samples from 100 animals submitted to culture in Fletcher medium, four liver samples (three with and one without antibiotic) and four kidney samples (three with and one without antibiotic) were positive for *Leptospira* spp., corresponding to seven animals. Only one animal presented simultaneous positivity in both organs. Microorganisms were observed in the culture after one month of incubation at 29°C, confirmed by visualization of spirochetes in a dark field microscope. No opalescence ring formation was seen (Dinger zone).

PCR results from the 20 properties studied revealed that eight (40%) were positive for *Leptospira* spp. in at least one animal. In liver and kidney samples from 100 animals submitted to PCR, seven liver and seven kidney samples were positive for *Leptospira* spp., corresponding to 12 animals. Two sheep were positive for both kidney and liver samples. The analytical sensitivity was 2.0×10^2 leptospires/mL.

Out of the 20 properties analyzed, 13 (65%) were reactive by at least one of the diagnostic tests used. Twenty-three animals were reactive by MAT, seven were positive in the Fletcher medium culture, and twelve were positive by PCR (Table 2).

Table 2: Results for microscopic agglutination test (MAT), culture and PCR of liver and kidney from sheep herds in Sorocaba region, São Paulo state, southeast Brazil

Culture		**MAT**	**PCR**		**Number of animals**
Liver	**Kidney**		**Liver**	**Kidney**	
–	–	–	–	–	75
–	–	+	–	–	13
–	–	+	–	+	3
–	+	+	–	+	1
–	+	–	–	+	1
–	+	+	+	+	1
+	+	+	+	+	1
+	–	–	+	–	1
–	–	+	+	–	2
+	–	+	+	–	2

+ positive; – negative.

DISCUSSION

Due to the paucity of data on the prevalence of leptospirosis in sheep flocks from different municipalities of the state of São Paulo, this study aimed to verify the occurrence of *Leptospira* spp. in different properties of the Sorocaba region, São Paulo state, using slaughterhouses as a strategic sample collection point. Thus, it was possible to establish the occurrence of leptospirosis in the flocks studied and highlight the most frequent serovars of *Leptospira* spp. from these regions.

According to serological results, 65% of the properties had positive animals, indicating that leptospirosis is present in the majority of sheep flocks in the Sorocaba region, thus demonstrating the importance of this disease in these animals.

The positive serology found in this study can be linked to previous contact with thc ctiological agcnt without disease development until the presence of ill carrier animals [20].

The most important probable infecting serovar was Autumnalis. This result corroborates the investigation by Viegas *et al.* [7] and Caldas *et al.* [8] in Bahia. This contrasts with Herrmann *et al.* [12], who reported Hardjo as the most prevalent serovar in sheep in Rio Grande do Sul state and Lilenbaum *et al.* [21], who observed that the most important serovars in Rio de Janeiro were Hardjo and Shermani.

Autumnalis is commonly isolated in wild animals, especially rodents, which could indicate them as possible leptospirosis transmitters in the sheep flocks studied [22]. This hypothesis is supported by the form of extensive farming observed in the present study.

Other probable infecting serovars were Djasiman, Hardjoprajitno, Wolffi, and Patoc, each reactive in only one animal. Wolffi and Hardjoprajitno are linked to the infection in bovines, Djasiman is found in wild animals, whereas Patoc is observed as a saprophytic serovar [23].

Some studies have demonstrated certain evidence that sheep are maintenance hosts for Hardjo, serving as a reservoir for bovines [24]. However, only one animal in this study demonstrated probable infection from this serovar.

Most reactive animals presented low antileptospirosis antibody titers, probably due to prior contact with the antigen. Only one animal presented a high titer of 1600 for Autumnalis with co-agglutination for other serovars, thus presenting serological reaction characteristic of acute infection [20].

Of the *Leptospira* spp. cultures from 100 renal and 100 hepatic samples cultured in Fletcher medium with and without antibiotic, eight were positive (four kidney and four liver) corresponding to five animals with positive serology (one was simultaneously positive in both kidney and liver) and two negatives. The isolation rate was 4% (8/200), better than values obtained by Azevedo *et al.* [2].

The low *Leptospira* spp. isolation rate could be dependent on various factors including type of medium used, serovar involved, sample processing time, type of material collected from the aseptic form, contamination, and selection of antibiotics used [25].

Failure to isolate the agent in the other 18 serologically positive animals could be explained by dealing with animals that had been in contact with a *Leptospira* without evolution of infection or disease or even by the factors cited by Thiermann *et al.* [25].

On the other hand, two serologically negative animals presented positive isolation, one for the kidney and the other for the liver. This exposes two probable scenarios: for the liver, the animal was in the initial infection phase without presenting MAT-detectable antibody titers; and in the kidney, the animal may have been infected by a different serovar than those tested in MAT without there being a cross-reaction.

Although this is a laborious, slow high-cost technique requiring months for results with little success in isolating the agent, identifying the serovar is highly important in epidemiological studies, as the isolated agent can be studied later to improve pathogen characterization and study its pathogenicity and other relevant analyses.

The presence of viable leptospires in the liver and kidneys of apparently healthy sheep at slaughter adds weight to the possibility of the disease being transmitted to the slaughterhouse and to meat packers who handle these materials. Furthermore, animal renal carriers could transmit the agent to rural workers from direct contact with urine or the contaminated environment.

The PCR of 100 renal and 100 kidney samples detected leptospires in 7% (14/200) samples (seven kidney and seven liver) corresponding to 12 positive animals (two animals were simultaneously positive for kidney and liver). Of the 23 serologically positive animals, leptospires were detected in ten while two did not present detectable antibodies by MAT.

Although PCR detected a higher positive sample rate than the culture technique, 13 serologically positive animals were negative. This can also be explained by what happened in culture, namely the absence of leptospire isolation in 18 seropositive sheep, probably because the animals had contact with the agent; but there was no progression of the disease.

The PCR technique was more practical and faster in detecting *Leptospira* spp. than culture in Fletcher medium and has the possibility of improving the sensitivity of diagnostic techniques in the early phase of infection and/or disease [19].

MAT is the worldwide reference test for leptospirosis diagnosis with high sensitivity and specificity. However, some difficulties with interpretation exist: there is a limitation in establishing whether serologically positive animals really are infected. Also, verification of a cross-reaction between different serovars can impede the establishment of the infecting serovar.

The presence of antileptospire antibodies often does not reflect the current situation of infection or the disease in animals, but rather only establishes host immunological response, which could be from prior contact without development of infection or the disease. This can be verified in the present study by the large number of serologically leptospire positive and negative animals from culture or PCR. This is reinforced by the weak concordance between serology and the agent's presence in studied tissue.

In comparing the techniques and their concordance proportion, results from culture and PCR techniques in both tissues (liver and kidney) presented a good concordance (Kappa of 0.97). But when the results are analyzed only by looking at positive samples, of the seven positive liver and kidney samples by PCR, three were negative in both tissues in culture, corresponding to 42.8% negativity; in other words culture detected 42.8 times less than PCR. In addition, the sensitivity results from the two techniques for detecting the agent, taking serologically positive animals as the basis, showed PCR to be more sensitive than culture. This has also been found in other comparison studies [18].

The results from the three diagnostic techniques shows the probable stages of infection in the sheep, in agreement with Levett [20]. Seventy-five animals were negative in all tests performed, indicating absence of infection; thirteen animals were positive only in serology, probably indicating prior contact with the etiological agent without disease development, or an animal after the convalescence phase that is no longer a renal carrier, but still presents detectable antibodies (immunological memory). Four animals were serologically positive with kidney culture and/or PCR positive, which probably indicates chronic infection and renal colonization stage (renal carrier) with detectable antibodies. Four serologically positive animals that had liver culture and/or PCR positive were probably found in the acute infection phase, in leptospiremia and with detectable antibodies, but still without renal colonization. Two positive animals by both liver and kidney culture and/or PCR were possibly in the end acute stage, still with leptospiremia, detectable antibodies, and renal colonization. One animal was serologically negative with kidney culture and/or PCR positive, which suggests an infection by a serovar other than those used in the battery of antigens in MAT, it did not present cross-reaction to the tested serovars, and was found in the convalescence and renal carrier phase. Another serologically negative animal with positive liver culture and/or PCR probably had a recent infection, with leptospiremia, but still without detectable antibodies or renal colonization.

According to the probable infection stage found in animals with positive hepatic culture and/or PCR, seven sheep (30.4%) from the 23 serologically positive animals presented acute phase infection, which could indicate that infection is persistent on these properties.

CONCLUSIONS

The occurrence of *Leptospira* spp. among sheep herds from Sorocaba region, state of São Paulo, Brazil, was 23% whereas the most important probable infecting serovar was Autumnalis, as determined by MAT. PCR was faster, more practical and sensitive than culture for detecting *Leptospira* spp. Our results reinforce the importance of sheep in the epidemiological context of leptospirosis in Brazil.

ACKNOWLEDGMENTS

The authors would like to thank the State of São Paulo Research Foundation (FAPESP) for the scholarship (2008/52537-0) and financial support (2008/53714-2) and the Regional Laboratory of Sorocaba – Adolfo Lutz Institute.

AUTHORS' CONTRIBUTIONS

PB participated in the design of the study, carried out the blood collection, performed the diagnostic tests, the analysis of the results and took part in the article writing. FHS and HL participated in the analysis of the results. VBRP participated in the analysis of the results and article writing. SBL participated in the design of the study, the analysis of the results and article writing. All authors read and approved the final manuscript.

REFERENCES

1. Corrêa WM, Corrêa CNM (Eds): Leptospiroses In *Enfermidades infecciosas dos mamíferos domésticos*. Rio de Janeiro: Medsi; 1992:219–231.
2. Azevedo SS, Alves CJ, Andrade JSL, Santos FA, Freitas TD, Batista CSA: Isolation of *Leptospira* spp. from kidneys of sheep at slaughter. *Arq Inst Biol São Paulo* 2004, 71(3):383–385.
3. Lilenbaum W, Varges R, Brandão FZ, Cortez A, de Souza SO, Brandão PE, Richtzenhain L, Vasconcellos SA: Detection of*Leptospira* spp. in semen and vaginal fluids of goats and sheep by polymerase chain reaction. *Theriogenology* 2008, 69(7):837–842. 10.1016/j.theriogenology.2007.10.027
4. Ellis WA, Bryson DG, Neill SD, McParland PJ, Malone FE: Possible involvement of leptospires in abortion, stillbirths and neonatal deaths in sheep. *Vet Rec* 1983, 112(13):291–293. 10.1136/vr.112.13.291
5. Ellis GR, Partington DL, Hindmarsh M, Barton MD: Seroprevalence to *Leptospira interrogans* serovar *hardjo* in merino stud rams in South Australia. *Aust Vet J* 1994, 71(7):203–206. 10.1111/j.1751-0813.1994.tb03402.x
6. Santa Rosa CA, Castro AFP: Presença de aglutininas anti-leptospira em soros de ovinos e caprinos no Estado de São Paulo. *Arq Inst Biol São Paulo* 1963, 30: 93–98.
7. Viegas EA, Viegas SARA, Caldas EM: Aglutininas anti-leptospira em hemo-soro de caprinos e ovinos no Estado da Bahia.*Arq Esc Med Vet Univ Fed Bahia* 1980, 5(1):20–34.
8. Caldas EM, Sampaio MB, Viegas EA, Viegas SARA, Dias EMM: Aglutininas antileptospira em ovinos e caprinos na região Nordeste do Estado da Bahia. *Arq Esc Med Vet Univ Fed Bahia* 1983, 8(1):88–98.
9. Langoni H, Marinho M, Baldini S, Silva AV, Cabral KG, Silva ED: Pesquisa de aglutininas anti-leptospiras em soros ovinos do Estado de São Paulo, Brasil, utilizando provas de macroaglutinação em placa e soroaglutinação microscópica. *Rev Bras Med Vet* 1995, 17(6):264–268.
10. Martins G, Lilenbaum W: The panorama of animal leptospirosis in Rio de Janeiro, Brazil, regarding the seroepidemiology of the infection in tropical regions. *BMC Vet Res* 2013, 9: 237. doi:10.1186/1746–6148–9-237. [http://www.biomedcentral.com/1746–6148/9/237] 10.1186/1746-6148-9-237
11. Carvalho SM, Mineiro AL, Castro V, Genovez ME, Azevedo SS, Costa FA: Leptospirosis seroprevalence and risk factors for sheep in Maranhão state, Brazil. *Trop Anim Health Prod* 2014, 46(2):491–494. 10.1007/s11250-013-0505-1
12. Herrmann GP, Lage AP, Moreira EC, Haddad JPA, Resende JR, Rodrigues RO, Leite RL: Soroprevalência de aglutininas anti- *Leptospira* spp. em ovinos nas Mesorregiões Sudeste e Sudoeste do Estado do Rio Grande do Sul, Brasil. *Ciênc Rural* 2004, 34(2):443–448.

13. Escócio CF, Genovez ME, Castro V, Paulin LMS, Piatti RM, Okuda LH, Gabriel FHL, Chiebao DP, Felicio PS, Almeida MCS: Perfil sanitário de rebanhos ovinos criados exclusivamente ou consorciados com bovinos na região de Sorocaba - São Paulo. In *35° Congresso Brasileiro De Medicina Veterinária: 19–22 Out 2008, Gramado, RS*. Gramado: Conbravet; 2008. [http://www.sovergs.com.br/conbravet2008/anais/cd/resumos/R0693–2.pdf]
14. Brasil. Ministério da Saúde. Secretaria de Vigilância em Saúde: *Guia Leptospirose: Diagnóstico e Manejo Clínico. Ministério da Saúde, Secretaria de Vigilância em Saúde, 2009. Em.* ftp://ftp.cve.saude.sp.gov.br/doc_tec/ZOO/LEPTO09_GUIA_MANEJO.pdf
15. World Health Organization: *Guidelines for the control of leptospires*. Geneva: WHO Offset Publication; 1982.
16. Passos EC, Vasconcellos SA, Ito FH, Yasuda PH, Nürmberger Junior R: Isolamento de leptospiras a partir do tecido renal de hamsters experimentalmente infectados com *Leptospira interrogans* sorotipo *pomona* . Emprego das técnicas da pipeta Pasteur e a das diluições seriadas em meios de cultura de Fletcher tratado com 5-fluoruracil ou o sulfato de neomicina. *Rev Fac Med Vet Zootec Univ São Paulo* 1988, 25(2):221–235. 10.11606/issn.2318-3659.v25i2p221-235
17. Heinemann MB, Garcia JF, Nunes CM, Gregori F, Higa ZM, Vasconcellos SA, Richtzenhain LJ: Detection and differentiation of *Leptospira* spp. serovars in bovine semen by polymerase chain reation and restriction fragment length polymorphism. *Vet Microbiol* 2000, 73(4):261–267. 10.1016/S0378-1135(00)00150-4
18. Mérien F, Amouriaux P, Perolat P, Baranton G, Saint-Girons I: Polymerase chain reaction for detection of *Leptospira* spp. in clinical samples. *J Clin Microbiol* 1992, 30(9):2219–2224.
19. Shimabukuro FH, Domingues PF, Langoni H, Silva AV, Pinheiro JP, Padovani CR: Pesquisa de suínos portadores renais de leptospiras pelo isolamento microbiano e reação em cadeia pela polimerase em amostras de rins de animais sorologicamente positivos e negativos para leptospirose. *Braz J Vet Res Anim Sci* 2003, 40(4):243–253.
20. Levett PN: Leptospirosis. *Clin Microbiol Rev* 2001, 14(2):296–326. 10.1128/CMR.14.2.296-326.2001
21. Lilenbaum W, Varges R, Ristow P, Cortez A, Souza SO, Richtzenhain LJ, Vasconcellos SA: Identification of *Leptospira* spp. carriers among seroreactive goats and sheep by polymerase chain reaction. *Res Vet Sci* 2009, 87(1):16–19. 10.1016/j.rvsc.2008.12.014
22. da Silva RC, Zetun CB, Gimenes Bosco SM, Bagagli E, Rosa PS, Langoni H: Toxoplasma gondii and *Leptospira* spp. infection in free-ranging armadillos. *Vet Parasitol* 2008, 157(3–4):291–293.
23. Salaberry SRS: Epidemiologia das principais doenças infecciosas de ovinos do município de Uberlândia, MG. *Thesis*2010. Faculdade de Medicina Veterinária, Universidade Federal de Uberlândia
24. Gerritsen MJ, Koopmans MJ, Peterse D, Olyhoek T: Sheep as maintenance host for *Leptospira interrogans* serovar *hardjo*subtype *hardjobovis* . *Am J Vet Res* 1994, 55(9):1232–1237.
25. Thiermann AB: Leptospirosis: current developments and trends. *J Am Vet Med Assoc* 1984, 184(6):722–725.

CHAPTER 14

LUNGWORM INFECTION IN SMALL RUMINANTS IN AND AROUND WOLAITA SODDO TOWN, SOUTHERN ETHIOPIA

Rahmeto Abebe[1], Mulugeta Melesse[2] and Solomon Mekuria[1]

[1]School of Veterinary Medicine, Hawassa University, Hawassa, Ethiopia

[2]Hadiya Zone Animal and Fisheries Resources Development Department, South Ethiopia, Hossana, Ethiopia

ABSTRACT

This study was conducted between November 2010 to April 2011 to estimate the prevalence of lungworm infection in small ruminants, determine the parasite species and identify the potential risk factors in and around Wolaita Soddo town, Southern Ethiopia. Faecal samples were collected from 360 randomly selected small ruminants (204 sheep and 156 goats) and processed with the modified Baerman technique for the extraction of first stage larvae. Overall, 45 (22.1%) sheep and 30 (19.2%) goats were found infected with lungworms. No significant difference was observed in the prevalence of lungworm infection between sheep and goats ($p>0.05$). Dictyocaulus filaria was the single lungworm species identified in both sheep and goats. The risk factors analyzed were sex, age, management system (zero-grazing or free-ranging), deworming history and body condition score (BCS). Management system, deworming history and BCS were significantly associated with the prevalence of D. filaria infection in sheep and goats (p0.05). In conclusion, the association of lungworm infections with the management system and deworming status of the animals in the present study are as expected. The association of infection with BCS requires further research to investigate if improving the nutritional status, thereby improving BCS, will result in lower prevalence of lungworm infection. Also, as the present sample size is thought to be small, further study with a larger sample size is required to determine the effect of age and host species difference in susceptibility to lungworm infection. One of the limitations of this study is that it is a one season survey and thus, a further year-round investigation is warranted to establish the association between seasonal variation and infection.

INTRODUCTION

Ethiopia is a country of huge livestock resources of which small stock is an integral part of the system. The country owns an estimated population of 24.2 million sheep and 22.6 million goats [1] which play an important role in the rural economy and enable the country to earn substantial amounts of foreign currency through export of skins and other byproducts. Despite the country has a huge potential of small ruminants, the country is unable to exploit these resources due to various reasons including endoparasitic infections.

Sheep and goats can be infected by many different kinds of endoparasites including lungworms. These lungworms are widely distributed throughout the world but are particularly common in countries with temperate climates, and in the

Citation: Rahmeto Abebe, Mulugeta Melesse and Solomon Mekuria, Lungworm Infection in Small Ruminants in and Around Wolaita Soddo Town, Southern Ethiopia, doi:10.4172/2157-7579.1000302.

highlands of tropical and sub-tropical countries [2]. The three economically important species of lungworms in sheep and goats are the nematode Dictyocaulus filaria , Muellerius capillaris and Protostrongylus rufescens . D. filaria is one of the most pathogenic lungworm of sheep and goats which lives in the lumen of the bronchial tree and commonly associated with chronic bronchitis and localized occlusion of the bronchial tree with atelectasis [3]. P. rufescens and M. capillaris are located in the lung parenchyma [3] and infections with these parasites are mainly associated with respiratory disturbances, development of focal pneumonia, and secondary bacterial infections of the lungs [4]. Infections with lung worms are either clinical or sub clinical [3].

In Ethiopia, the prevalence of lungworm infection in sheep and goats and the species of the parasite involved have been reported by many researchers such as Alemu et al., Regassa et al., Ibrahim and Godefa, Fentahun et al., Eyob and Matios, Terefe et al., Kebede et al. [5-11]. According to these studies, the prevalence of lungworm infection in Ethiopia ranges from 13.4–72.4% in sheep and 26.5–62.7% in goats. Nonetheless, much of the available data are from the northern and western parts of the country and information on the subject from the southern part of the country is scarce. Furthermore, as Ethiopia is a country with diverse ecological and climatic conditions, occurrence, species diversity and risk factors may vary from area to area and thus, it is found important to study the parasite in all parts of the country.

Therefore the objective of this study was to estimate the prevalence of lung worm infections, to investigate the lungworm species involved and to identify the associated risk factors in small ruminants in selected areas of southern Ethiopia [12,13].

MATERIALS AND METHODS

Study Area

The study was conducted between November 2010 to April 2011 in Wolaita Soddo town and its surroundings. Wolaita Soddo is a town and separate district in south-central Ethiopia located 385 km from Addis Ababa, the capital of Ethiopia. The town is the administrative center of the Wolaita Zone of the Southern Nations, Nationalities, and Peoples Region. Geographically, the town is situated at 6°54′N 37°45′E and has an elevation between 1600 and 2100 m above sea level.

Study Population

The study population consisted of 360 small ruminants (204 sheep and 156 goats) randomly selected from the sheep and goat populations in the study area. All the study animals were local breeds. Of the total sampled animals, 129 were female while 231 males. The age of the animals was determined based on the farmers' response and crosschecked by teeth inspection. Based on the response the animals were categorized in to three age groups: ≤ 1 yr, 1-3 year and >3 year old. The number of animals in each age category was 131, 197 and 32, respectively. Body condition scoring (BCS) was performed according to Ethiopia Sheep and Goat Productivity Improvement Program [14]. The assessment revealed that 178, 48 and 134 animals had good, moderate and poor BCS, respectively. With regard to the management system, 295 (81.9%) study animals were free-ranging on communal lands (extensively managed) whereas 65 (18.1%) kept under zerograzing system (intensively managed). As to their deworming status, 218 animals were known to be treated with a broad spectrum anthelminthic (i.e albendazole) within 3 months prior to the onset of the study while 142 animals did not receive any treatment.

Study Design and Sample Size Determination

A cross-sectional study design was employed to address the objective of the study. The sampling procedure used was a simple random sampling technique which means that all the animals in the study area had equal chance of being part of the sample. The sample size was determined according to Thrusfield [15] taking in to account an expected prevalence of 16% for sheep and 11.5% for goats, 5% absolute precision and 95% confidence level. Accordingly, the sample size required for the study was computed to be 204 for sheep and 156 for goats.

Sample collection and larval identification

Faecal samples were collected directly from the rectum of the selected animals in a universal bottle. While collecting the faecal samples, data about the species of animal, sex, age, body condition score (BCS), management system (zero-grazing vs free-ranging), and date of sampling were recorded on the format prepared for this purpose. The samples collected were transported to Sodo Regional Veterinary Laboratory within six hours of collection. In the laboratory, the Baermann technique was employed for the extraction of lungworm larvae from the faecal samples as described by Foreyt [16]. Identification of the species of lungworm encountered was carried out based on the characteristic morphological features described in literature by Taylor et al. and Bowman [3,4].

Statistical Analysis

Data obtained from questionnaire survey and faecal examination were entered into Microsoft excel spreadsheet after coding. All statistical analyses were performed on STATA 11.1 software (StataCorp 4905 Lakeway Drive, College Station, Texas 77845 USA). The prevalence of lung worm infection was calculated by dividing the number of animals affected by the total number of animals examined. The association between the prevalence of lung worm infection and the hypothesized risk factors (animal species, age, sex, deworming history, BCS and management system) was analyzed by univariable logistic regression test. A p value<0.05 was considered significant.

RESULTS

Prevalence of Lung Worm Infection

Out of 204 sheep and 156 goats examined, 45 sheep (22.1%) and 30 goats (19.2%) were found to be infected with lung worms. No significant difference was observed in the prevalence of infection between sheep and goats (p>0.05). D. filaria was the only species of lung worm identified in both sheep and goats (Table 1).

Table 1: Prevalence of D. filDriD infection in sheep and goats in and around Wolaita Soddo. CI: &onfidence Interval; OR: Odds Ratio

Host species	No. Animals examined	No. animals pos	Prevalence (%)	95% CI for prevalence	OR (95% CI)	p
Goats	156	30	19.2	13.5 - 26.4	1	
Sheep	204	45	22.1	16.7 - 28.5	1.2 (0.8 - 2.0)	0.513
Over all	360	75	20.8	16.8 - 25.4		

Hypothesized Risk Factor Analysis

In sheep, among the presumed risk factors, BCS and deworming history were found to be strongly associated with the prevalence of D. filaria infection ($p<0.001$) while sex and age of the animals didn't have significant effect ($p>0.05$). Furthermore, all the animals infected were extensively managed ones (Table 2).

Table 2: Logistic regression analysis of D. filaria infection in sheep with different risk factors. OR: Odds Ratio; CI: & confidence Interval; BCS: Body Condition Score; Ref: Reference Category

Variable	No. animals examined	No. animals pos.	Prevalence (%)	OR (95% CI)	p
Sex					
Male	89	17	19.1	Ref	
Female	115	28	24.4	1.4 (0.7-2.7)	0.371
Age					
≤ 1 Year	79	23	29.1	Ref	
1-3 Year	109	20	18.4	0.5 (0.3-1.1)	0.085
>3 Year	16	2	12.5	0.3 (0.1-1.7)	0.184
Management system					
Intensive	32	0	0		
Extensive	172	45	26.2		
BCS					
Good	102	9	8.8	Ref	
Moderate	28	11	39.3	6.7 (2.4-18.6)	0
Poor	74	25	33.8	5.3 (2.3-12.2)	0
Deworming history					
Dewormed	118	13	11	Ref	
Non dewormed	86	32	37.2	4.8 (2.3-9.9)	0

In goats, the prevalence of lungworm infection was significantly associated with management system, BCS and deworming history ($p<0.05$ for each factor). As in sheep, sex and age of the animals were not significantly associated with infection ($p>0.05$) (Table 3).

Table 3: Logistic regression analysis of D. filaria infection in goats with different risk factors. Note: OR: Odds Ratio; CI: & confidence Interval; BCS: Body Condition Score; Ref: Reference Category

Variable	No. animals examined	No. animals pos.	Prevalence (%)	OR (95% CI)	p
Sex					
Male	40	6	15	Ref	
Female	116	24	20.7	1.5 (0.6 -3.9)	0.433
Age					
≤1 Year	52	14	26.9	Ref	
1-3 Year	88	14	15.9	0.5 (0.2-1.2)	0.119
>3 Year	16	2	12.5	0.4 (0.1-1.9)	0.247
Management system					
Intensive	33	2	6.1	Ref	
Extensive	123	28	22.8	4.6 (1.0 -20.3)	0.046
BCS					
Good	76	5	6.6	Ref	
Moderate	20	7	35	7.6 (2.1-27.8)	0.002
Poor	60	18	30	6.1(2.1-17.6)	0.001
Deworming history					
Dewormed	100	9	9	Ref	
Non dewormed	56	21	37.5	6.1 (2.5-14.5)	0

DISCUSSION

In this study, lungworm larvae were observed in 22.1% of sheep and 19.2% goats examined. The prevalence recorded in both sheep and goats is lower than reports of the previous studies in Ethiopia (24.3% −72.4% for sheep; 26.5%–62.7% for goats) [5,6,8-11,15-17]. The lower prevalence in the current study could be attributed to better awareness of farmers to deworm their small ruminants against lungworms and other helminthic infection, apart from geographic variation. This was evidenced by the fact that more than 60% of the small ruminants included in this study were dewormed with broad spectrum anthelminthics.

D. filaria was the only species of lungworm identified in both sheep and goats in the present study. The small lungworms, P. rufescens and M. capillaris , were not detected. The absence of small lungworms in the present study area could be associated with their life cycle and the season of the study. Unlike D. filaria , which has a direct life cycle, P. rufescens and M. capillaris have an indirect life cycle requiring a molluscan intermediate host to complete their development [3]. As this study was conducted in a dry season, the climatic conditions in the study area might not be conducive for the survival and breeding of the intermediate hosts. In agreement with this finding, many of the previous studies [8,11,15,16,] also reported D. filaria as the predominant species circulating in Ethiopian sheep and goats managed under traditional husbandry system although mixed infections with the small lungworms was stated in low proportions. In contrast, other studies reported the preponderance of the small lungworms over D. filaria [5,6,11,12]. Apart from year and season of the studies, this difference might be ascribed to the variations in ecological conditions required for the breeding of the intermediate host between the current and previous study areas [18-20]. The aforementioned studies were conducted in the west and northeast part of Ethiopia while the present study was carried out in the southern part. Outside Ethiopia, surveys in Turkey, India and Iran [21-25] also reported D. filaria as the sole or predominant lungworm while in Morocco, Czech Republic, Norway and Bulgaria the most prevalent species identified was M. capillaris [26-28].

The current study revealed lack of significant difference in the prevalence of D. filaria infection between sheep and goats ($p>0.05$). Consistent with the present finding, most of the previous studies in which D. filaria was the predominant lungworm, reported absence of significant variation between the two hosts [9,13,17,19]. In contrast, in two studies dominated by the small lungworms [5,12], a significantly higher prevalence was noted in goats than in sheep. Our finding is also contrary to what is generally stated that goats appear to be more susceptible to infection than sheep and are thought to play a prominent role in the dissemination of the infection where both are grazed together [3]. The present and most of the previous studies in Ethiopia suggest that variations between sheep and goats in susceptibility to lungworm infections depend on the species of the parasite involved. That is, when D. filaria is the sole or predominant species encountered, no significant difference is observed in prevalence between the two hosts but in infections where small lungworms are the most prevalent goats are more susceptible than sheep. Nonetheless, this fact needs to be substantiated in the future by experimental studies involving the two hosts. The use of adequate sample size computed for sheep and goats separately should also be considered in future studies. In agreement with the present study, lack of significant variation between sheep and goats for D. filaria infection was also reported by a study in Iran [24].

In the present study, although D. filaria prevalence tended to decrease with age, the variation among the three age categories of animals was not significant in both sheep and goats ($p>0.05$). The prevalence in the younger animals (≤ 1 Year) was higher than in older animals (>3 Years) but the difference was not significant. This finding is consistent with some of the previous studies [5,9,15-17]. In contrast to the current findings, other authors [6,8,10,11] reported a significantly higher infection of D. filaria in young than adult animals. The absence of significant variation between young and old animals in the present study might be due to failure of the older animals to develop strong immunity to reinfection associated with the dry season feed shortage. It could also be attributed to sampling of small and disproportionate number of animals between the two age categories. Nevertheless, further investigation using large and proportional sample size is warranted in a season where adequate feed is available to determine the effect of age on lungworm infection.

The analysis of lungworm infection with the management system in goats showed that the prevalence was significantly higher in extensively than intensively managed animals ($p<0.05$) while all the sheep infected were extensively managed ones. The odds ratio (OR) of infection in extensively managed goats was 4.6 times higher than that in intensively kept. This is as expected and attributed to differences in feeding system between the two groups of animals. The intensively managed animals were zero-grazed and consequently, less likely to be infected with lungworm larvae. Of the intensively managed ones, only two animals had lungworms probably through some contamination of hay or bedding material. Similarly, the prevalence of lungworm infection was significantly higher in non-dewormed sheep and goats than dewormed ones ($p<0.001$) and this finding is also as expected. The odds of infection were 4.8 and 6.1 times higher respectively in non-dewormed sheep and goats than dewormed animals.

In both sheep and goats, the prevalence of D. filaria infection was significantly associated with BCS ($p<0.05$). It was observed that sheep with moderate or poor condition were 6.7 or 5.3 times more likely to shed D. filaria larvae than those in good condition. Similarly, the odds of infection in goats with moderate or poor BCS were 7.6 or 6.1 higher than those with good BCS. This, partly, may be attributed to the nutritional status of the animals. This study was conducted in the dry season where feed shortage is a serious problem for small ruminants kept under extensive management system in Ethiopia. Therefore, in the dry season free-ranging animals are not able to meet their maintenance requirements, and lose a substantial amount of weight. It is well known that poor nutrition lowers both the resistance (ability to resist the parasites) and resilience (ability to tolerate or ameliorate the effects of the parasite) of the animal thus enhancing the establishment of worms and increasing the prevalence in poorly conditioned animals [27]. In connection to lungworm, it is reported that poorly nourished animals appear to be less competent in getting rid-off lungworm infection although it is not unusual for well-fed animals to succumb to lungworm infection [28].

In conclusion, the overall prevalence of D. filaria infection in the current study was 22.1% in sheep and 19.2% in goats. As expected, management system (zerograzing or not) and deworming history in the last 3 months (yes/no) were significantly associated with presence of lungworm infection. BCS also was significantly associated with lungworm infection with animals with moderate or poor condition being at least 5.3 times more likely to be infected than animals in good condition. Further research is required to investigate if improving the nutritional status, thereby improving BCS, will result in lower prevalence of lungworm infection. Also, as the sample size in this study was thought to be small, a further study with a larger sample of sheep and goats is needed to determine the effect of age and host species difference in susceptibility to lungworm infection. Finally, one of the limitations of this study is that it is a one season observation and reflects the prevalence of the parasite only in the dry season. Thus, further year-round studies are warranted to establish the association between seasonal variation and lungworm infection.

ACKNOWLEDGEMENTS

The authors would like to thank Wolaita Soddo Regional Laboratory staff for their immense technical support during the laboratory work.

REFERENCES

1. Central Statistical Agency (2012) Federal Democratic Republic of Ethiopia Central Statistical Agency, Agricultural Sample Survey 2011/12. Report On Livestock and Livestock Characteristics.
2. Hansen J, Perry B (1994) The epidemiology, diagnosis and control of helminth parasites of ruminants. ILRAD, Nairobi, Kenya.
3. Taylor MA, Coop RL, Wall RL (2007) Veterinary Parasitology. (3rd Edn), Blackwell Publishing Ltd.
4. Panayotova-Pencheva MS, Alexandrov MT (2010) Some pathological features of lungs from domestic and wild ruminants with single and mixed protostrongylid infections. Vet Med Int 2010: 741062.
5. Alemu S, Leykun EG, Ayelet G, Zeleke A (2006) Study on small ruminant lungworms in northeastern Ethiopia. Vet Parasitol 142: 330-335.
6. Regassa A, Toyeb M, Abebe R, Megersa B, Mekbib B, et al. (2010) Lungworm infection in small ruminants: Prevalence and associated risk factors in Dessie and Kombolcha districts, Northeastern Ethiopia. Veterinary Parasitology 169: 144-148.
7. Ibrahim N, Godefa Y (2012) Prevalence of ovine lungworm infection in Mekelle town, North Ethiopia. The Internet Journal of Veterinary Medicine 9: 1-7.
8. Fentahun T, Seifu Y, Chanie M, Moges N (2012) Prevalence of lungworm infection in small ruminants in and around Jimma town, Southwest Ethiopia. Global Veterinaria 9: 580-585.
9. Eyob E, Matios L (2013) The prevalence and risk factors associated with ovine lungworm infestation in the Asella province, Central Ethiopia. Journal of Parasitology and Vector Biology 5: 116-121.
10. Terefe Y, Tafess K, Fekadie G, Kebede N (2013) Prevalence of lungworm infection in small ruminants in North Gondar zone, Amhara National Regional State, Ethiopia. Journal of Parasitology and Vector Biology 5: 40-45.
11. Kebede S, Menkir S, Desta M (2014) On farm and abattoir study of lungworm infection of small ruminants in selected areas of Dale district, Southern Ethiopia. Int J CurrMicrobiol App Sci 3: 1139-1152.
12. Ethiopian Sheep and Goats Productivity Improvement Project (ESGPIP) (2008) Technical Bulletin No. 8: Body condition scoring of sheep and goats.
13. Thrusfield M (2005) Veterinary Epidemiology (3rd Edn), Blackwell Science, UK.
14. Foreyt WJ (2001) Veterinary Parasitology Reference Manual. (5th Edn), Owa State University Press, Blackwell Publishing, USA.
15. Addis M, Fromsa A, Ebuy Y (2011) Study on the prevalence of lungworm infection in small ruminants in Gondar town, Ethiopia. Veterinary Research 4: 85-89.
16. Moges N, Bogale B, Chanie M (2011) Dictyocaulusfilaria and Muelleriuscapillaris are important lungworm parasites of sheep in Wogera district, Northern Ethiopia. International Journal of Animal and Veterinary Advance 3: 465-468.
17. Weldesenebet D, Mohamed A (2012) Prevalence of small ruminant lung worm infection in Jimma town. Global Veterinaria 8: 153-159.
18. Yildiz K1 (2006) Prevalence of lungworm infection in sheep and cattle in the Kirikkale province. TurkiyeParazitolDerg 30: 190-193.
19. Girisgin O, Senlik B, Girisgin AO, Akyol V (2008) Studies on sheep lungworms in Bursa province of Turkey: Determination of prevalence and relationships between larval output and parasite burden in the lungs. Pakistan J Zool 40: 365-369.
20. Dar LM, Darzi MM, Mir MS, Kamil SA, Rashid A, et al. (2012) Prevalence and Pathology of Lung Worm Infection in Sheep in Kashmir Valley, India. AnimSciAdv 2: 678-685.
21. Borji H, Azizzadeh M, Ebrahimi M, Asadpour M (2012) Study on small ruminant lungworms and associated risk factors in northeastern Iran. Asian Pac J Trop Med 5: 853-856.
22. Yagoob G, Hossein H, Ehsan A (2014) Prevalence of small ruminant lung-worm infestation in Tabriz city, Iran. Indian Journal of Fundamental and Applied Life Sciences 4: 320-323.
23. Berrag B, Urquhart GM (1996) Epidemiological aspects of lungworm infections of goats in Morocco. Vet Parasitol 61: 81-85.
24. Kudrnácová M, Kanková S, Langrová I, Jankovská I, Salaba O (2013) A study on lungworms occurrence in farm-bred sheep from north Bohemia (Czech Republic). ScientiaAgriculturaeBohemica 44: 6–9.

25. Domke AV, Chartier C, Gjerde B, Leine N, Vatn S, et al. (2013) Prevalence of gastrointestinal helminths, lungworms and liver fluke in sheep and goats in Norway. Vet Parasitol 194: 40-48.

26. Panayotova-Pencheva MS (2011) Species composition and morphology of protostrongylids (Nematoda: Protostrongylidae) in ruminants from Bulgaria. Parasitol Res 109: 1015-1020.

27. Walkden-Brown SW, Kahn LP (2002) Nutritional Modulation of Resistance and Resilience to Gastrointestinal Nematode Infection: A Review. Asian-Aust J AnimSci 15: 912-924.

28. Radostits OM, Gay CC, Hinchclift KW, Constable PD (2007) Veterinary Medicine: A textbook of the diseases of cattle, horses, sheep, pigs and goats. (10th Edn), Saunders Ltd, Elsevier.

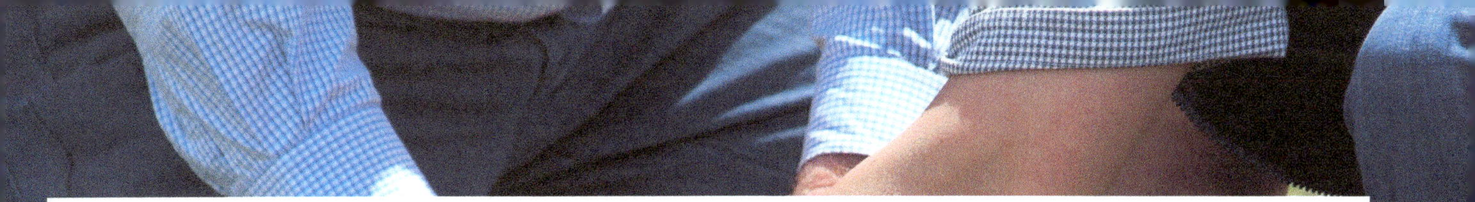

CHAPTER 15

CLINICAL MASTITIS IN EWES; BACTERIOLOGY, EPIDEMIOLOGY AND CLINICAL FEATURES

Tormod Mørk[1], Steinar Waage[2], Tore Tollersrud[1], Bjørg Kvitle[1] and Ståle Sviland[1]

[1]Department of Animal Health, National Veterinary Institute, Dep, N-0033 Oslo, Norway

[2]Department of Production Animal Clinical Sciences, Norwegian School of Veterinary Science, Dep, N-0033 Oslo, Norway

ABSTRACT

Background

Clinical mastitis is an important disease in sheep. The objective of this work was to identify causal bacteria and study certain epidemiological and clinical features of clinical mastitis in ewes kept for meat and wool production.

Methods

The study included 509 ewes with clinical mastitis from 353 flocks located in 14 of the 19 counties in Norway. Clinical examination and collection of udder secretions were carried out by veterinarians. Pulsed-field gel electrophoresis (PFGE) was performed on 92 *Staphylococcus aureus* isolates from 64 ewes.

Results and Conclusion

***S. aureus* was recovered from 65.3% of 547 clinically affected mammary glands, coagulase-negative staphylococci from 2.9%, enterobacteria, mainly *Escherichia coli*, from 7.3%, *Streptococcus* spp. from 4.6%,*Mannheimia haemolytica* from 1.8% and various other bacteria from 4.9%, while no bacteria were cultured from 13.2% of the samples. Forty percent of the ewes with unilateral clinical *S. aureus* mastitis also had a subclinical *S. aureus* infection in the other mammary gland. Twenty-four of 28 (86%) pairs of *S. aureus* isolates obtained from clinically and subclinically affected mammary glands of the same ewe were indistinguishable by PFGE. The number of identical pairs was significantly greater than expected, based on the distribution of different *S. aureus* types within the flocks. One-third of the cases occurred during the first week after lambing, while a second peak was observed in the third week of lactation. Gangrene was present in 8.8% of the clinically affected glands; *S. aureus* was recovered from 72.9%, *Clostridium perfringens* from 6.3% and *E. coli* from 6.3% of the secretions from such glands. This study shows that *S. aureus* predominates as a cause of clinical ovine mastitis in Norway, also in very severe cases. Results also indicate that *S. aureus* is frequently spread between udder halves of infected ewes.**

Citation: Tormod Mørk, Steinar Waage, Tore Tollersrud, Bjørg Kvitle and Ståle Sviland, DOI: 10.1186/1751-0147-49-23.

BACKGROUND

Mastitis is an important disease in sheep. Clinical cases are often severe; systemic signs are present and the condition is obviously painful. Clinically affected glands frequently suffer partial or complete damage and do not resume normal function. Reduced milk yield leads to decreased growth of the lambs [1, 2, 3]. Additional losses associated with clinical mastitis are costs of treatment and culling of ewes due to permanent udder damage [3, 4, 5, 6, 7]. In very severe cases, gangrene may develop in the mammary gland and the ewe may die. Thus, mastitis has a major impact on both economy and animal welfare in sheep production.

Although a wide range of microorganisms may cause ovine mastitis, most cases are reported to be due to staphylococci [8]. Several reports indicate that coagulase-negative staphylococci (CNS) are the most common cause of subclinical mastitis in dairy ewes [9, 10, 11, 12, 13, 14], while both CNS and *Staphylococcus aureus* are frequent causes in meat sheep [5, 15, 16]. With regard to organisms associated with clinical mastitis, there are fewer reports published. *S. aureus* has been reported to be the most common causal organism in both meat [5, 15, 17, 18, 19] and dairy ewes [13, 20, 21]. *Mannheimia haemolytica* [5, 18, 19, 22], *Escherichia coli* [13, 18,19] and various streptococci [15, 18, 19] are other important causative organisms.

Differences in climate, production forms and management practices may give rise to differences both in the epidemiology, bacteriology and clinical manifestations of mastitis. In Norway, sheep are kept exclusively for meat and wool production. They are housed during the winter and early spring, including the lambing season.

The objective of this study was to identify bacteria associated with clinical ovine mastitis in Norway. In addition, certain epidemiological and clinical features of the disease were studied.

METHODS

Animals and Clinical Data

Udder secretions were collected and clinical data recorded from 509 ewes with clinical mastitis. The ewes belonged to 353 flocks located in 14 counties in Norway (Figure 1). The geographical distribution of the cases is shown in Table 1. Clinical mastitis was present in one gland in 471 ewes and in both glands in 38 ewes. The study was carried out in 2002, 2003 and 2004. Only cases that occurred between 1 week prepartum and 8 weeks postpartum were included. In Norway, lambing generally takes place in April and May.

Table 1: Distribution by region and county of 547 milk samples obtained from ovine mammary glands with clinical mastitis, and of the 509[a] ewes and 353 flocks from which the samples originated

Region	County	No. of flocks	No. of ewes	No. of glands
East	Akershus	13	27	31
	Hedmark	68	121	128
	Oppland	60	85	86
	Buskerud	4	5	6
South	Aust-Agder	34	56	57
	Vest-Agder	4	6	7
	Rogaland	40	48	53
West	Hordaland	22	26	28
	Sogn og Fjordane	25	25	29
	Møre og Romsdal	32	39	40
North	Sør-Trøndelag	33	46	50
	Nord-Trøndelag	6	10	13
	Nordland	3	3	4
	Troms	9	12	15

[a] Four hundred and seventy-one ewes with unilateral and 38 with bilateral intramammary infection.

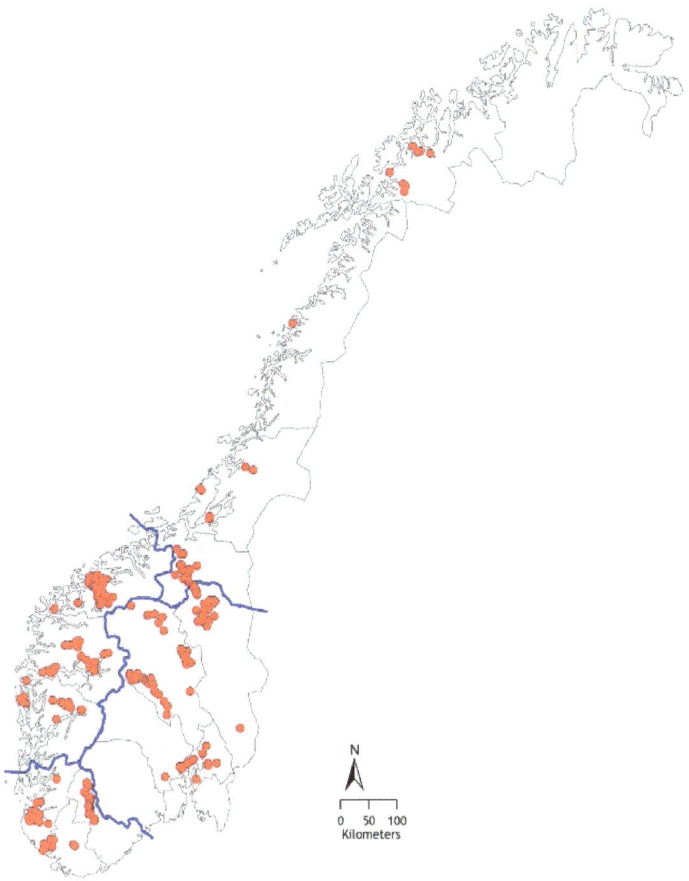

Figure 1: Map of Norway showing the location of the sheep flocks from which cases of clinical mastitis were obtained. Thin lines show county boundaries and thick lines region boundaries.

Data and Sample Collection

Thirty-two veterinary practitioners contributed to the study. When called to a case of clinical mastitis, the veterinarian was to examine the ewe, collect udder secretions and record information regarding the identity, age, date of parturition, the number of lambs and the clinical condition of the ewe on a standardized form. Clinical data included the rectal temperature, an assessment of the severity of systemic signs (graded as none, weak, moderate or severe) and local clinical signs of the affected gland, including whether or not gangrene was present (i.e., cold and blue udder and teat skin).

Prior to treatment, samples were collected aseptically from the clinically affected glands in 10-ml sterile plastic vials by the veterinary practitioner according to the International Dairy Federation's standards [23]. Additionally, samples were taken from the clinically unaffected gland of 252 of the ewes with unilateral clinical mastitis. The samples were sent by mail to the laboratory as soon as possible after sampling, or frozen and stored at -20°C until submission.

If a ewe experienced more than one episode of mastitis during the observation period, only the first episode was included in the study.

Microbiological Methods

The samples were examined at the National Veterinary Institute or at the TINE Mastitis Laboratory in Molde, Norway, and bacteria were identified according to the recommendations of the International Dairy Federation [23] with additions. The National Veterinary Institute and the TINE Mastitis Laboratory are both quality assured in accordance with NS-EN ISO/IEC 17025. Briefly, the secretions were brought to room temperature, assessed visually and characterized by appearance before they were mechanically shaken and 10 µl plated on Bacto Blood Agar Base No 2 (Difco Laboratories, Detroit, MI, USA) containing 5% washed bovine erythrocytes and incubated for 48 hours in a 5% CO_2 atmosphere at 37°C. Cultures were read at 24 and 48 hours. If growth was not detected after incubation for 24 hours, the original sample was incubated for 4 hours at 37°C and 50 µl aliquots plated and incubated for 24 hours under aerobic (5% CO_2 atmosphere) and anaerobic conditions.

Bacterial species were identified tentatively by their gross colony morphology and by Gram staining, and further confirmatory tests were used as necessary. All suspected staphylococcal colonies were tested using the tube coagulase test (Becton Dickinson Microbiology Systems, Bedford,

MA, USA). Coagulase-positive staphylococci were streaked on peptone agar (p-agar) (Difco, Sparks, MD) supplemented with 7 mg/l of acriflavin (Sigma-Aldrich Chemie, Steinheim, Germany) [24], and incubated at 37°C for 24 hours. Bacterial growth in the full length of the streak on p-agar was considered confirmative of *S. aureus*. Isolates identified as *S. aureus* were stored at -70°C in Bacto Heart Infusion Broth (Difco) with 15% glycerol. *E. coli* was identified by the lactose and indole tests, and other enterobacteria were identified to the species or genus level by using a microtube identification system (API 20 E®; bioMérieux S.A., Marcy-l›Etoile, France). *Streptococcus uberis,Streptococcus dysgalactiae, Streptococcus agalactiae, Streptococcus* spp. and *Enterococcus* spp. were distinguished by the CAMP reaction, the aesculin and inulin tests and by culture on the bromthymolblue lactose-sucrose agar. Bacteria within the family *Pasteurellaceae* were identified to the species level by the CAMP reaction, the indole, mannitol, sorbitol, trehalose, dulcitol, oxidase and beta-galactosidase tests and the haemolysis patterns. *Clostridium perfringens* was differentiated from other *Clostridium* spp. by colony morphology, immobility and the presence of a zone of partial haemolysis and a zone of complete haemolysis. *Arcanobacterium pyogenes* was identified by Gram staining and the presence of pinpoint colonies surrounded by a narrow zone of clear haemolysis at 48 hours. None of the samples were from ewes with arthritis, conjunctivitis or pneumonia; therefore, the mammary secretions were not checked for the presence of mycoplasms.

Total DNA was prepared and pulsed-field gel electrophoresis (PFGE) performed as described previously [25] on 92 *S. aureus* isolates from 21 flocks in which at least one ewe had bilateral *S. aureus* intramammary infection (IMI) and where at least two ewes experienced clinical *S. aureus* mastitis. The band patterns were compared visually. Isolates with indistinguishable patterns were considered identical PFGE types while those with at least one band difference were considered to be different types.

Statistical Methods

The chi-square test was used to compare the frequencies of cases within different time intervals in relation to parturition and the relative proportions of clinical *S. aureus* cases and gangrenous mastitis cases in ewes of different parity and with different number of lambs. The distribution of pairs of *S. aureus* PFGE types within flocks (equal vs. unequal) in ewes with bilateral IMI was compared with the corresponding distribution that would be expected if all *S. aureus* isolates found within each flock were paired randomly. All isolates from the flocks that supplied two or more cases of clinical *S. aureus* mastitis, of which at least one ewe had bilateral IMI, were included, and Fisher›s exact test was used to test the probability of identical distributions of the observed and expected pairs.

$P < 0.05$ was considered statistically significant.

RESULTS

Bacteriological and Epidemiological Findings

The distribution of bacteria cultured from secretions from the glands with clinical mastitis is shown in Table 2.*S. aureus* was the predominant pathogen and was found in 65.3% of the samples from affected glands. In the samples from the southern, eastern, western and northern regions, *S. aureus* was found in 76.0%, 59.0%, 63.9% and 69.5%, respectively.

Table 2: Results of culture of secretions recovered from 547 mammary glands with clinical mastitis

Bacteriological finding	n	%
Staphylococcus aureus	357	65.3
Coagulase-negative staphylococci	16	2.9
Streptococcus uberis	9	1.6
Streptococcus dysgalactiae [a]	8	1.5
Streptococcus spp. [b]	8	1.5
Enterococcus spp.	4	0.7
Escherichia coli	35	6.4
Klebsiella pneumoniae	2	0.4
Enterobacter spp.	3	0.5
Mannheimia haemolytica	10	1.8
Arcanobacterium pyogenes	4	0.7
Clostridium perfringens	7	1.3
Pasteurella spp. [c]	4	0.7
No growth	72	13.2
Contaminated samples [d]	8	1.5

[a] Subsp. *dysgalactiae*.

[b] Other than *Str. dysgalactiae* and *Str. uberis*.

[c] *Pasteurella mairii* (2 samples), *Pasteurella multocida* (2 samples).

[d] If blood agar plates contained more than two different types of colonies.

Information about the date of parturition was received from 318 of the 471 cases of unilateral clinical mastitis. The distribution of the observed clinical mastitis cases in relation to the time of parturition is shown in Figure2. The relative proportion of cases was greatest during the first week after lambing. Sixty-four (20.1%) of the 318 ewes for which the times of lambing and treatment were recorded, were treated for clinical mastitis during the first two days after parturition. The proportion of cases was significantly greater in the first ($P < 0.005$) and the third ($P < 0.05$) week postpartum as compared with the second week postpartum.

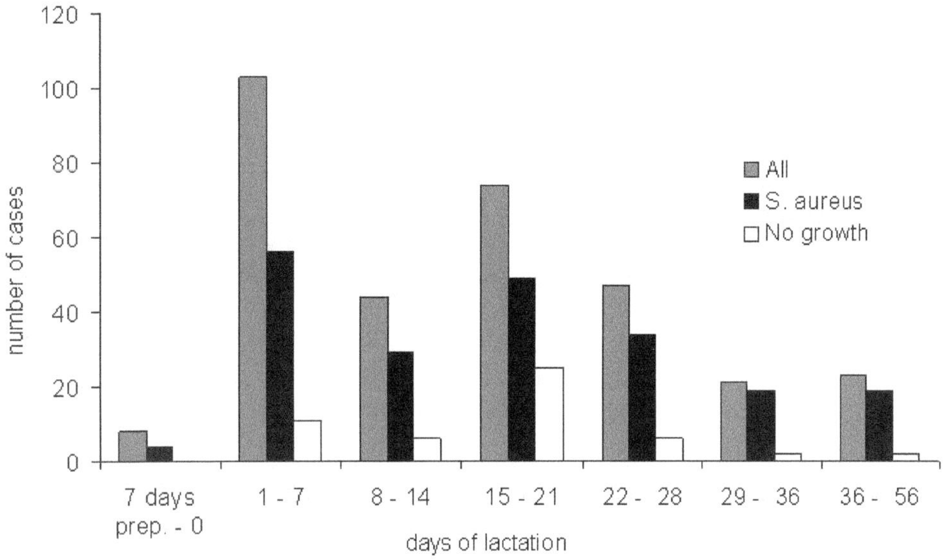

Figure 2: Distribution of 318 cases of clinical mastitis in relation to weeks of lactation.

The proportion of the clinical *S. aureus* cases among all the clinical cases did not differ significantly between weeks of lactation, between ewes of different parities or between ewes with different number of lambs (data not shown).

In 180 ewes with unilateral clinical *S. aureus* mastitis, from which samples from both mammary glands were examined, *S. aureus* was found in secretions from 72 (40.0%) of the glands without clinical signs. In 72 ewes with unilateral clinical mastitis not caused by *S. aureus*, a subclinical *S. aureus* infection was found to be present in 10 (13.9%) of the glands without clinical signs.

S. aureus PFGE Types in ewes with Bilateral IMI

A total of 22 different PFGE types were found among 92 *S. aureus* isolates from 21 farms. Comparisons of *S. aureus* pairs revealed that 24 (86.0%) of 28 pairs had indistinguishable band patterns (Table 3). Given the PFGE types of all *S. aureus* isolates within each flock, expected flock-specific distributions of PFGE type pairs based on all possible random pairwise combinations of isolates were arranged. The number of pairs with identical types observed in the flocks was significantly greater than that expected, when assuming a random distribution of isolates ($P < 0.0001$).

Table 3: Distribution within flocks of 22 different PFGE types of 92 *S. aureus* isolates from ewes with intramammary infection (IMI). Only flocks in which at least one ewe experienced bilateral *S. aureus* IMI and two ewes experienced clinical mastitis are included. The observed pairs of PFGE types from the ewes with bilateral *S. aureus* IMI are shown. Also shown is the expected distribution of pairs with equal and unequal PFGE type combinations when assuming random pairwise distribution of the observed isolates within each flock.

				Expected pairs (n)	
Flock	Ewes with IMI (n)	*S. auerus* types (n) present in flock	Bilateral PFGE type combinations	Equal	Unequal
F1	6	K, P, Q (4), R	QQ	6	15
F2	9	I, J, L (7), M	LL	21	24
F3	2	R (3)	RR	3	0
F4	3	R (4)	RR	6	0
F5	2	H (2), O (2)	HH, OO	2	4
F6	2	D (2), H	DD	1	2

F7	2	H, I, U	IU	0	3
F8	2	H (3), X	HH, HX	3	3
F9	2	D, H (3)	DH, HH	3	3
F10	2	I, M, V	IV	0	3
F11	6	H (5), I, W	HH	10	11
F12	3	H, I (3)	II	3	3
F13	3	H (4), I (2)	HH, HH, II	7	8
F14	3	F, J (3)	JJ	3	3
F15	2	H, S (2)	SS	1	2
F16	2	D (3)	DD	3	0
F17	4	H (2), I (2), N, G (2)	HH, II, GG	3	18
F18	2	C (2), E	CC	1	2
F19	2	C (2), G	CC	1	2
F20	3	I (2), R, T	II	1	5
F21	2	A (2), B	AA	1	2

Clinical Signs

Of the 471 cases of unilateral clinical mastitis systemic signs were recorded in 325 (Table 4) and the rectal temperature was measured in 342. Moderate or severe systemic signs were present in 159 (48.9%) ewes and 193 (56.4%) ewes had a rectal temperature above 40.0°C. Thirty-seven (11.8%) out of 313 ewes showed no systemic signs and had a rectal temperature below 40.1°C.

Table 4: Distribution of 325 of the 471 ewes with unilateral clinical mastitis by causal organism and the systemic signs[a]

Pathogen	**1**	**2**	**3**	**4**	**Total**
	No. (%)	**No. (%)**	**No. (%)**	**No. (%)**	
All	51 (15.7)	115 (35.4)	119 (36.6)	40 (12.3)	325
S. aureus	30 (13.5)	77 (34.5)	89 (39.9)	27 (12.1)	223
Enterobacteria	2 (7.7)	9 (34.6)	11 (42.3)	4 (15.4)	26
No growth	11 (34.4)	12 (37.5)	4 (12.5)	5 (15.6)	32

[a] 1 = no systemic signs, 2 = weak systemic signs, 3 = moderate systemic signs, 4 = severe systemic signs.

Gangrene was present in 48 (8.8%) of 547 clinically affected udder halves and *S. aureus* was found in 35 (72.9%), *C. perfringens* in 3 (6.3%), *E. coli* in 3 (6.3%) and *A. pyogenes* in 1 (2.1%). Bacteria were not found in 4 (8.3%) samples from such cases and two samples were contaminated. The degree of systemic influence was recorded in 33 ewes with gangrenous mastitis. Thirty (90.9%) of these cases exhibited moderate or severe signs. The proportion of the gangrenous mastitis cases among all the clinical cases did not differ significantly between weeks of lactation, between ewes of different parities or between ewes with different number of lambs (data not shown).

DISCUSSION

A random and representative selection of sheep flocks was not deemed feasible for this type of study. However, in order to have a reasonably representative geographical spread of the mastitis cases ewes from 14 of the 19 counties in Norway were included. Thus, the present flocks were housed and pastured under various conditions, and the variations in climatic conditions, flock size and management routines of Norwegian sheep production were reasonably well represented. During the lambing season and subsequent weeks the ewes are paid close attention. Later, most flocks are moved to pastures in the forests or mountains. For this reason, the study was restricted to cases that occurred between 1 week prepartum and 8 weeks postpartum in order to obtain clinical cases of recent origin.

S. aureus was found in 65% of the samples from clinically affected glands. The dominance of *S. aureus* as a cause of clinical ovine mastitis has also been shown in regional studies in Norway, where *S. aureus* was isolated from udder secretions of between 64 and 87% of the ewes [26, 27]. In the present study, the largest proportion of *S. aureus* was found in the southern region (76%). A similar proportion of such cases (75%) was previously observed in a study including cases from one of the municipalities of this region [28]. Studies of clinical mastitis in meat sheep in other countries have found varying, though mostly relatively great, proportions of *S. aureus* infections (20–60%) [5, 17, 18, 19, 20, 22]. In a study of dairy sheep in Jordan, Lafi et al. [13] found that 22% of the clinical mastitis cases were caused by *S. aureus*.

The main *S. aureus* reservoirs in sheep are suggested

to be infected mammary glands and teat lesions [29]. However, *S. aureus* can also be cultured from intact teat skin and other body sites [10, 30, 31]. In dairy flocks, transfer during milking is considered an important mechanism for the spread of this organism [29]. In flocks of meat sheep, transmission of *S. aureus* between ewes could be a result of the herdsman transmitting *S. aureus* between ewes during manual udder control, or the udder being exposed to bedding material contaminated from infected ewes [6, 7]. Some lambs occasionally suck other ewes than their dam, which might be a mechanism for the spread of *S. aureus* [32]. In Norway, routine examination of teats and udders are performed after weaning, and ewes with palpable abnormalities or which have experienced clinical mastitis are usually slaughtered before the breeding season. This contributes to decreasing the reservoir of *S. aureus*, but it obviously does not eliminate it.

Studies in other countries have reported prevalences of subclinical *S. aureus* IMI to be between 1 and 6% [12,13, 15, 33]. This indicates that subclinically infected glands are an important reservoir of *S. aureus* that can only be detected through bacteriological examination. In this study, 14% of the ewes with unilateral clinical mastitis caused by other pathogens than *S. aureus* had a subclinical *S. aureus* infection in the other mammary gland, while 40% of the ewes with clinical *S. aureus* infection in one gland had a subclinical *S. aureus* infection in the other. PFGE typing showed that 86% of the pairs of isolates from ewes with bilateral *S. aureus* IMI were indistinguishable. This percentage was much higher than what would be expected if the isolates from each of the flocks were paired at random, thus demonstrating a considerably greater tendency for spread of *S. aureus*between the udder halves of a ewe than between ewes within a flock.

The very low percentage of *M. haemolytica* in the clinically affected glands in this study (1.8%) contrasts results of clinical mastitis surveys in meat sheep in the UK and Ireland, where the proportions of cases caused by this organism were found to be approximately 50% and 21%, respectively [5, 18]. Enterobacteria, mainly *E. coli*, were obtained from 7.3% of the clinically affected udder halves, which is similar to the proportions found in other studies on meat sheep [5, 18, 22]. However, the number of clinical cases caused by Gram negative bacteria and *A. pyogenes* may be underestimated because the samples were frozen before bacteriological analysis [34, 35].

It is noteworthy that nearly 85% of the ewes exhibited systemic signs and that gangrene was present in as much as 9% of the clinically affected udder halves, clearly showing that ovine clinical mastitis must be considered a serious animal welfare problem. However, mild cases of clinical mastitis are most likely underrepresented in this study. According to Norwegian legislation, antibiotic treatment of animals must be initiated by a veterinarian and, for economical reasons, farmers might be reluctant to call for a veterinary surgeon to treat mild clinical cases.

Most mastitis cases occurred close to lambing. One-third of the ewes developed clinical mastitis during the first week after lambing, and a second peak, although somewhat smaller, was observed in the third week postpartum. This is in accordance with data from the Norwegian Sheep Recording System [36]. Likewise, studies in the UK and Ireland found that cases of acute clinical mastitis occurred most frequently during the first week of lactation, while a second peak occurred between the third and fourth week [5] or the fourth and seventh week [18] after lambing. Clinical cases around parturition might be newly acquired IMI or aggravations of existing subclinical infections [37]. The proportion of very severe cases, in which gangrene had developed, was not greater among cases occurring close to lambing as compared with those occurring later. The second peak could be explained by increased milk demand from the lambs and the eruption of incisors, which increases the risk of teat lesions. It has been reported that teat lesions frequently are present in ewes with clinical mastitis three to four weeks after lambing [38].

CONCLUSION

This study shows that *S. aureus* is the most common cause of clinical mastitis in sheep in Norway and that this organism is frequently spread between glands in infected ewes. Further studies identifying predisposing factors, including reservoirs, transmission routes and factors facilitating *S. aureus* infection of the ovine mammary gland, are needed in order to improve strategies to reduce the occurrence of mastitis in sheep.

ACKNOWLEDGEMENTS

Of the veterinary surgeons who kindly contributed to the study, the authors would particularly like to thank Gunvald Mosdøl, Olav Koltveit, Grethe Steihaug, Dag Aasland, Jan I. Holøymoen, Anne Aaby, Anders Avdem, Berit C. Brændvang, Aud Solberg, Odd S. Skregelid and Knut I. Dragset.

AUTHORS' CONTRIBUTIONS

TM, SW, TT and SS have been involved in the design of the study and the protocols. TM has been responsible for the field project. BK, TM and SS have performed most of the microbiological work in the laboratory. BK has performed the PFGE. SW and SS have been responsible for data analysis in cooperation with TM and TT. TM drafted the manuscript, but all the authors have contributed substantially to the final manuscript. All authors have read and approved the final manuscript.

REFERENCES

1. Fthenakis GC, Jones JET: The effect of experimentally induced subclinical mastitis on milk yield of ewes and on the growth of lambs. Br Vet J. 1990, 146: 43-49.
2. Johnston WS, Maclachlan GK, Murray IS: A survey of sheep losses and their causes on commercial farms in the north of Scotland. Vet Rec. 1980, 106: 238-240.
3. Larsgard AG, Vaabenoe A: Genetic and environmental causes of variation in mastitis in sheep. Small Rumin Res. 1993, 12: 339-347. 10.1016/0921-4488(93)90069-T.
4. Gibson IR, Hendy PG: Mastitis in dry ewes. Vet Rec. 1976, 98: 511-512.
5. Jones JET: Mastitis in sheep. Breeding for Disease Resistance in Farm Animals. Edited by: Owen JB, Axfor RFE. 1991, Bangor: Tucson, AZ, CAB International, 412-423.
6. Kirk JH, Glenn JS: Mastitis in ewes. Compend Cont Educ Pract Vet. 1996, 18: 582-591.

7. Watson DJ, Buswell JF: Modern aspects of sheep mastitis. Br Vet J. 1984, 140: 529-534.
8. Bergonier D, Berthelot X: New advances in epizootiology and control of ewe mastitis. Livest Prod Sci. 2003, 79: 1-16. 10.1016/S0301-6226(02)00145-8.
9. Ariznabarreta A, Gonzalo C, San Primitivo F: Microbiological quality and somatic cell count of ewe milk with special reference to staphylococci. J Dairy Sci. 2002, 85: 1370-1375.
10. Burriel AR: Dynamics of intramammary infection in the sheep caused by coagulase-negative staphylococci and its influence on udder tissue and milk composition. Vet Rec. 1997, 140: 419-423.
11. Fthenakis GC: Prevalence and aetiology of subclinical mastitis in ewes of Southern Greece. Small Rumin Res. 1994, 13: 293-300. 10.1016/0921-4488(94)90078-7.
12. Gonzalo C, Ariznabarreta A, Carriedo JA, San Primitivo F: Mammary pathogens and their relationship to somatic cell count and milk yield losses in dairy ewes. J Dairy Sci. 2002, 85: 1460-1467.
13. Lafi SQ, Al-Majali AM, Rousan MD, Alawneh JM: Epidemiological studies of clinical and subclinical ovine mastitis in Awassi sheep in northern Jordan. Prev Vet Med. 1998, 33: 171-181. 10.1016/S0167-5877(97)00048-2.
14. Pengov A: The role of coagulase-negative *Staphylococcus* spp. and associated somatic cell counts in the ovine mammary gland. J Dairy Sci. 2001, 84: 572-574.
15. Watson DL, Franklin NA, Davies HI, Kettlewell P, Frost AJ: Survey of intramammary infections in ewes on the New England Tableland of New South Wales. Aust Vet J. 1990, 67: 6-8.
16. Hariharan H, Donachie W, Macaldowie C, Keefe G: Bacteriology and somatic cell counts in milk samples from ewes on a Scottish farm. Can J Vet Res. 2004, 68: 188-192.
17. Kryzanowski J, Wawron W, Malinowski V, Gluszak J, Orlik S: Bacterial flora isolated from the secretion of mastitic udders of ewes and their sensitivity to antibiotics. Med Vet. 1983, 39: 462-464.
18. Onnasch H, Healy AM, Brophy PO, Kinsella A, Doherty ML: A study of mastitis in sheep. Res Vet Sci. 2002, 72: 42-10.1016/S0034-5288(02)90120-7.
19. Quinlivan TD: Survey observations on ovine mastitis in New Zealand stud Romney flocks. 2. The bacteriology of ovine mastitis. N Z Vet J. 1968, 16: 153-160.
20. Al-Samarrae SAG, Sharma VK, Yousif AA: Mastitis in sheep in Iraq. Vet Rec. 1985, 116: 323-
21. Kirk JH, Glenn JS, Maas JP: Mastitis in a flock of milking sheep. Small Rumin Res. 1996, 22: 187-191. 10.1016/S0921-4488(96)00881-4.
22. Bocklisch H, Wetzstein D: Clinical, diagnostic laboratory and therapeutic studies of mastitis in a large sheep breeding flock (article in German). Tierärztl Prax. 1994, 22 (6): 524-528.
23. International Dairy Federation: Laboratory methods for use in mastitis work. 1981, Brussels: IDF, Document 132
24. Capurro A, Concha C, Nilsson L, Östensson K: Identification of coagulase-positive staphylococci isolated from bovine milk. Acta Vet Scand. 1999, 40: 315-321.
25. Mørk T, Tollersrud T, Kvitle B, Jørgensen HJ, Waage S: Genetic diversity of *Staphylococcus aureus* isolated from ovine intramammary infections in Norway. Vet Microbiol. 2005, 106: 265-273. 10.1016/j.vetmic.2004.12.020.
26. Kvitrud A, Lysne I: Examinations of mastitis in sheep (article in Norwegian). Nord Vet Med. 1959, 11: 129-140.
27. Sæter EA, Eieland E: Ovine mastitis in mountain districts in Norway (article in Norwegian). Nord Vet Med. 1961, 13: 32-44.
28. Indrebø A, Mosdøl G: Mastitis in the ewe. Microbiological findings and sensitivity to antibiotics (article in Norwegian). Nor Vet Tidsskr. 1991, 103: 107-113.
29. Vautor E, Abadie G, Guibert JM, Huard C, Pepin M: Genotyping of *Staphylococcus aureus* isolated from various sites on farms with dairy sheep using pulsed-field gel electrophoresis. Vet Microbiol. 2003, 96: 69-79. 10.1016/S0378-1135(03)00207-4.
30. Scott MJ, Jones JET: The carriage of *Pasteurella haemolytica* in sheep and its transfer between ewes and lambs in relation to mastitis. J Comp Pathol. 1998, 118: 359-363. 10.1016/S0021-9975(07)80011-9.
31. Vautor E, Abadie G, Guibert JM, Chevalier N, Pepin M: Nasal carriage of *Staphylococcus aureus* in dairy sheep. Vet Microbiol. 2005, 106: 235-239. 10.1016/j.vetmic.2004.11.019.
32. Bergonier D, de Cremoux R, Rupp R, Lagriffoul G, Berthelot X: Mastitis of dairy small ruminants. Vet Res. 2003, 34: 689-716. 10.1051/vetres:2003030.
33. Deutz A, Pernthaner A, Schlerka G, Baumgartner W: Investigations on cell count of milk and distribution of bacterial mastitis in Lower Austrian sheep and goat flocks (article in German). Wien Tierärztl Mschr. 1990, 77: 70-77.
34. Sanchez A, Contreras A, Jimenez J, Luengo C, Corrales JC, Fernandez C: Effect of freezing goat milk samples on recovery of intramammary bacterial pathogens. Vet Microbiol. 2003, 94: 71-77. 10.1016/S0378-1135(03)00066-X.
35. Schukken YH, Grommers FJ, Smit JA, Vandegeer D, Brand A: Effect of freezing on bacteriologic culturing of mastitis milk samples. J Dairy Sci. 1989, 72: 1900-1906.
36. Vatn S: Epidemiology of mastitis in Norwegian sheep. Proceedings of the 6th International Sheep Veterinary Congress:17–21 June 2005; Hersonissos. Edited by: Fthenakis GC, McKaller FA. 2005, 6th International Sheep Veterinary Congress, 318-319.
37. Watkins GH, Burriel AR, Jones JET: A field investigation of subclinical mastitis in sheep in southern England. Br Vet J. 1991, 147: 413-420.
38. Indrebø A: Mastitis and teat injuries in the ewe in relation to age, partus and number of lambs (article in Norwegian). Nor Vet Tidsskr. 1991, 103: 197-204.

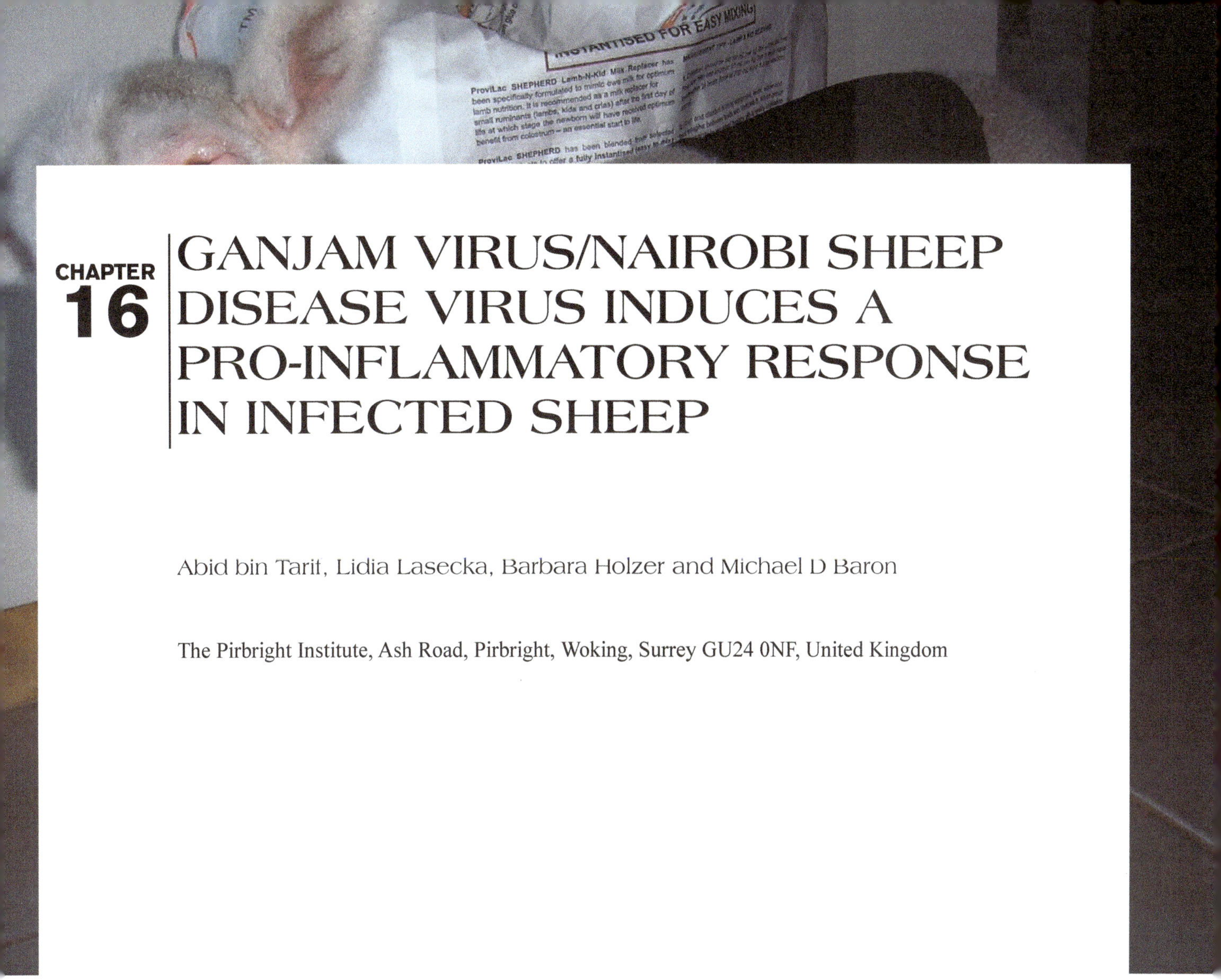

CHAPTER 16

GANJAM VIRUS/NAIROBI SHEEP DISEASE VIRUS INDUCES A PRO-INFLAMMATORY RESPONSE IN INFECTED SHEEP

Abid bin Tarit, Lidia Lasecka, Barbara Holzer and Michael D Baron

The Pirbright Institute, Ash Road, Pirbright, Woking, Surrey GU24 0NF, United Kingdom

ABSTRACT

Partly due to climate change, and partly due to changes of human habitat occupation, the impact of tick-borne viruses is increasing. Nairobi sheep disease virus (NSDV) and Ganjam virus (GV) are two names for the same virus, which causes disease in sheep and goats and is currently known to be circulating in India and East Africa. The virus is transmitted by ixodid ticks and causes a severe hemorrhagic disease. We have developed a real-time PCR assay for the virus genome and validated it in a pilot study of the pathogenicity induced by two different isolates of NSDV/GV. One isolate was highly adapted to tissue culture, grew in most cell lines tested, and was essentially apathogenic in sheep. The second isolate appeared to be poorly adapted to cell culture and retained pathogenicity in sheep. The real-time PCR assay for virus easily detected 4 copies or less of the viral genome, and allowed a quantitative measure of the virus in whole blood. Measurement of the changes in cytokine mRNAs showed similar changes to those observed in humans infected by the closely related virus Crimean Congo hemorrhagic fever virus.

INTRODUCTION

Nairobi sheep disease (NSD) was first identified at the beginning of the 20th century by Montgomery as a disease affecting sheep and goats in parts of Kenya [1]. It has since been identified in several places in East Africa. A similar disease has also been reported in north east India, where it was called Ganjam [2]. The recent application of molecular sequencing techniques to the viruses that cause these diseases (NSDV and GV, respectively) revealed that they are the same virus [3, 4], with different strains existing on the two continents. Whether the virus has existed for an historically long time in both places, or is a relatively recent import from one part of the world to another has yet to be determined. It is possible that the virus was imported to Africa from India as a consequence of the same kind of livestock movement that introduced rinderpest virus to Africa in the 1880 s [5].

Citation: Abid bin Tarif, Lidia Lasecka, Barbara Holzer and Michael D Baron, Ganjam virus/Nairobi sheep disease virus induces a pro-inflammatory response in infected sheep, DOI: 10.1186/1297-9716-43-71.

The virus is spread by hard (Ixodid) ticks, and appears to be dependent on the tick vector for dissemination, with no direct transmission between animals. This obligate vector step may explain why the virus is not seen as a major economic threat, since young animals in endemic areas tend to be protected by maternal antibodies through the period where they are first exposed to the virus via a bite from an infected tick, after which they have their own immune protection. The disease tends to be only noticed on introduction of naive livestock into an endemic area, e.g. for the purposes of improving local breeds by crossing. The disease that ensues is regarded as one of the most pathogenic in small ruminants, with mortality rates as high as 90%; animals die from acute haemorrhagic fever [1, 6]. Disease is only seen in sheep and goats, with no disease seen or viraemia detected when cattle, buffalo, equids or other mammals are infected [1, 7], although the limitations of early virus detection methods (pathogenesis in neonatal mouse brains) have to be borne in mind. NSDV was originally seen as a disease with a relatively restricted distribution, a distribution largely dependent on that of the *Rhipicephalus appendiculatus* tick [1, 8]; in contrast, GV has been reported predominantly in *Haemaphysalis* species in India [7, 9]. Recent studies, especially using molecular detection techniques, have found the virus in tick samples from a much wider geographical area, and it now appears that it is distributed over most of the Indian sub-continent as well as much wider in East Africa than the restricted area in Kenya originally reported [9].

NSDV/GV is a bunyavirus of the genus *Nairovirus*; other members of the genus include *Dugbe virus* and *Kupe virus*, both isolated from cattle ticks in East Africa, and the human pathogen *Crimean Congo hemorrhagic fever virus* (CCHFV). CCHFV is another tick-borne virus which appears to be spreading, with increasing outbreaks in Russia, Turkey, India and Pakistan and recent detection of the virus in tick samples from Spain [10]. The spread of CCHFV, or at least outbreaks of disease, seems to be a consequence of a combination of changes in land use and climate, leading to increased contact between people and ticks, and possibly changes in the range of the tick vectors as well as their competence to propagate the virus [11]. The range of NSDV/GV may likewise be spreading, and its impact will also increase as we push more and more for breed improvement and maximising land use to manage the increasing global demands for food. For this reason, and because it has promise as a good model system to study the nairoviruses (while work on CCHFV is restricted to BSL4 laboratories, and lacks an in vivo system to study disease), we have initiated work on NSDV/GV with a view to characterising the virus and its pathology.

Early studies described the clinical signs of the disease in detail, as well as establishing the dependence on the tick vector. We have recently shown that the virus can block the actions of both type 1 (interferon α/β) and type 2 (interferon γ) interferons, as well as inhibit the induction of interferon β in infected cells [12]. We report here the results of an initial study of the replication of the virus in sheep and the major cytokine responses in infected animals. We found a fundamentally pro-inflammatory response, with specific differences between responses to a pathogenic and a non-pathogenic virus. As part of the project, we have developed a sensitive, NSDV/GV-specific, real-time PCR assay for detecting viral RNA which may be useful in other labs for screening diagnostic samples where nairovirus infection is suspected.

MATERIALS AND METHODS

Viruses and Cells

Except where indicated, media and cells were obtained from the Central Sterilisation Unit, this institute. MDBK (Madin-Darby bovine kidney) cells and Vero-SLAM (African green monkey kidney, expressing human SLAM) cells (the gift of Dr Rick De Swart, Department of Virology, Erasmus MC, The Netherlands) were grown in Dulbecco's modified Eagle's medium (DMEM) supplemented with 5% foetal calf serum (FCS). Although SLAM was not required for growth of NSDV, Vero-SLAM cells were the Vero cells in general use in our laboratory and it was known that the virus can infect these cells. BHK21/clone 13 (baby hamster kidney) cells were obtained from ATCC (LGC Standards, Teddington, UK) and cultured in Glasgow modified Eagle's Medium (GMEM) containing 10% FCS. PO (sheep, kidney) cells (from the Collection of Cell Lines in Veterinary Medicine (CCLV), Friedrich Loeffler Institute, Riems, Germany) and BSR-T7 (a BHK-derived cell line constitutively expressing T7 RNA polymerase) cells (a gift from Prof K. K. Conzelman) were grown in DMEM medium enriched with 10% FCS. SSF (primary sheep skin fibroblast) cells and BSF (primary bovine skin fibroblast) cells were prepared previously as described by Childerstone et al. [13]. These cells were maintained in Iscove's modified Dulbecco's medium (IMDM) (Life Technologies, Paisley, UK) containing 10% FCS. BFA (bovine foetal aortic endothelium) cells were obtained from the European Cell Culture Collection) and grown on Nutrient Mixture F-12 Ham medium (Sigma, Dorset, UK) containing 20% FCS. Primary ovine endothelial cells were either obtained from Dr H-H Takamatsu (The Pirbright Institute) and maintained in IMDM containing 10% FCS or prepared from ovine pulmonary artery and aorta essentially as described [14] and maintained in medium M131 supplemented with microvascular growth supplement (MVGS) (Life Technologies).

The Nairobi sheep disease virus (NSDV) isolate (ND66-PC9) was obtained from Dr Piet van Rijn, Central Veterinary Institute of Wageningen, Netherlands. The Ganjam virus (GV) isolate (IG619, TVPII 236) was obtained from World Reference Center for Emerging Viruses and Arboviruses at the Galveston National Laboratory, and was the kind gift of Prof Robert B Tesh, University of Texas Medical Branch, Galveston, Texas, USA. Virus stocks were grown in BHK21/clone 13 cells using GMEM containing 2% FCS, penicillin (100 U/mL), streptomycin sulphate (100 μg/mL), 2 mM L-glutamine and 5% tryptose phosphate broth solution. The virus titre was determined as the 50% tissue culture infectious dose ($TCID_{50}$) in BHK21 cells. Both strains grew to similar final titres (~10^6/mL) and were used after two additional passages in BHK cells. Multiplicity of infection (MOI) was calculated as $TCID_{50}$ per plated cell.

Multi-Step Growth Curves of Virus

Cells were plated in 6-well dishes 6-9 h before use, apart from primary endothelial cells, which were plated 18 h before infection to ensure good attachment. Cells were infected with

NSDV or GV at a MOI of 0.01; after 1 h incubation at 37°C, 5% CO2, the inoculum was removed, the cells were washed once with growth medium and incubated in fresh medium at 37°C, 5% CO2. At 0, 12, 24, 36, 48 and 72 hours post infection (hpi) samples were frozen at -80°C. Each virus time course was carried out at least in duplicate. When all samples had been collected, they were thawed and centrifuged at 2500 rpm, 4°C for 10 min to remove cell debris. The supernatants were stored at -80°C. The amount of viruses in each sample was determined by titration on BSR-T7 cells (for NSDV) or BHK21 (for GV). CPE (cytopathic effect) was scored at 3-5 days post infection (dpi) and virus titre was calculated as $TCID_{50}$/mL by the Spearman-Kärber method [15].

Animal Study

The animal study described in this paper was subject to full ethical review and licensing under the Animals (Scientific Procedures) Act 1986 of the United Kingdom, and was approved by the competent authority with Project Licence number 70/7014. Six outbred sheep (female Dorset breed animals at 7-8 months of age) were obtained from commercial suppliers. Three animals were infected subcutaneously with 10^4 $TCID_{50}$ units of either the NSDV or GV isolate at the first passage in BHK 21/clone 13 cells from receipt of samples. The rectal temperature of the animals was measured before the experiment began and each day during the experiment. Blood samples were taken prior to infection and on the indicated days post infection into vacutainers for serum (coagulated blood) and leucocytes (EDTA as anti-coagulant) as well as into Tempus® vacutainers (Life Technologies) for stabilisation of total RNA. Serum samples were separated and stored at -20°C. White cell counts were determined from duplicate samples on the day of sampling, using a Cellometer Auto T4 (Nexcelcom, Lawrence, MA, USA). Red cells were pelleted by centrifugation and the supernatant (essentially plasma plus buffy coat cells) stored at -80°C until used for virus isolation or RNA extraction.

RT-qPCR of Viral RNA and Ovine Cytokines

RNA was prepared from the whole blood samples in Tempus tubes using the Tempus® Spin RNA Isolation kit (Life Technologies). RNA was extracted from white cell samples using RNeasy mini kits (Qiagen, West Sussex, UK). All oligonucleotide primers were from Sigma. Reverse transcription was carried out as instructed by the manufacturer using Superscript II (Life Technologies) with either genome-specific primer (0.1 pmol/µL final concentration) or Oligo(dT)-Anch ($(T)_{16}VN$) (5 pmol/µL final concentration). cDNA was diluted 4-fold (3-fold if RNA concentration was low) in water and heated at 75°C for 15 min before use in PCR. PCR was performed in 10 µL (initial gradient PCRs) or 20 µL (real-time PCR) reactions using Applied Biosystems SYBR® Green PCR Master Mix (Life Technologies). Real-time PCR reactions were carried out on a Rotorgene 2000 (Qiagen) and analysed using Rotor-Gene software v6; the threshold for determining the Ct was set at normalised fluorescence=0.01. The PCR program used consisted of a 10 min activation step at 95°C followed by 40 cycles of 15 s at 95°C, 30 s at the appropriate annealing temperature (Table 1) and 30 s at 72°C. Final primer concentrations for each real-time PCR assay were as listed in Table 1. Each reaction contained 15 ng (whole blood) or 3 ng (white cells) of RNA as cDNA.

Table 1: PCR primer pairs and reaction conditions used in the work described in this paper

Target	Primer sequences	Ta[1]	[Primer][2]	Reference
NSDV/GV (F1/R1A)	TGACCATGCAGAACCAGATYG	62	300nM	this paper
	GAAACAAGCCTCATGCTAACCT			
NSDV/GV (F2/R2)	GGAGAATGGCAAAGAGGTTGT	64	300nM	this paper
	GTAAATCCGATTGGCAGTGAAG			
NSDV/GV F3b (RT primer)	GTCTTTGAACTYTGACCA	n/a	n/a	this paper
IL-1β	CCTTGGGTATCAGGGACAA	60	300nM	[16]
	TGCGTATGGCTTTCTTTAGG			
IL-4	ACCTGTTCTGTGAATGAAGCCAA	60	300nM	[17]
	CCCTCATAATAGTCTTTAGCCTTTCC			
IL-6	TCCAGAACGAGTTTGAGG	60	400nM	[16]
	CATCCGAATAGCTCTCAG			
IL-8	ATGAGTACAGAACTTCGA	57	300nM	[16]
	TCATGGATCTTGCTTCTC			
IL-10	TGCTGTTGACCCAGTCTCTG	60	200nM	this paper
	AGGGCAGAAAACGATGACAG			
IL-12A	TGGGCATTGTCTGTCTTCTG	60	200nM	this paper
	TTCTTCCAGGGAGGGTTTCT			

IL-12B	GCTGGGAGTACCCTGACACG	61	500nM	[17]
	GTGACTTTGGCTGAGGTTTGGTC			
IL-18	ACTGTTCAGATAATGCACCCCAG	60	300nM	[17]
	TTCTTACACTGCACAGAGATGGTTAC			
Interferon β	CCAGATGGTTCTCCTGCTGTGT	63	300nM	this paper
	GACCAATACGGCATCTTCCTTC			
TNFα	GAATACCTGGACTATGCCGA	60	200nM	[16]
	CCTCACTTCCCTACATCCCT			
TGFβ	GTGGACATCAACGGGTTCAG	60	300nM	this paper
	TGTCCAGGCTCCAGATGTAG			
Interferon γ	CTCCGGCCTAACTCTCTCCT	60	300nM	this paper
	AGGCCCACCCTTAGCTACAT			
GAPDH	GGTGATGCTGGTGCTGAGTA	60	300nM	[16]
	TCATAAGTCCCTCCACGATG			
SDHA	ACCTGATGCTTTGTGCTCTGC	60	200nM	[16]
	CCTGGACGGGCTTGGAGTAA			
G6PDH	CGAGGCTGTGTACACCAAGA	60	300nM	this paper
	ATGTGGTGGAGCAGTGGAGT			

1: Ta: annealing temperature.

2: [Primer]: primer concentration.

Statistical Analysis

Real-time PCR data from the animal experiment was analysed using the General Linear Model form of ANOVA as implemented in Minitab 16 with a model in which the virus used and the days post infection were fixed factors. Due to the loss of some animals at day 7, analysis was restricted to the data from days 0, 2, 4 and 7. The two virus isolates were compared using the ANOVA of the linear model, and the significance of any increase or decrease of transcription on day 2, 4 and 7, compared to the value at day zero, was determined using Dunnett's correction for multiple comparisons.

RESULTS

Characteristics of Virus Isolates in Cell Culture

Two isolates of NSDV/GV were available to us, one of NSDV Entebbe strain (ND66-PC9) originally prepared by Terpstra from samples taken in Uganda in 1956 [18] and passed 75 times in tissue culture, the other of GV (IG619), originally isolated in India, but with no recorded passage history. Both isolates were found to grow to good titres (10^6 $TCID_{50}$/mL) on BHK21/clone13 cells, as previously reported for NSDV [6] (data not shown). We assessed their ability to grow in a variety of other cultured cells, both continuous lines and primary cells (Figure 1). The NSDV isolate grew well, to titres of 10^6 $TCID_{50}$/mL, in all the cell lines tested with the exception of MDBK cells, an established bovine kidney line, where the peak titre was only 10^4 $TCID_{50}$/mL. This was not due to a species-specific restriction, since the virus grew equally well in bovine and ovine skin fibroblasts, and in bovine and ovine endothelial cells (Figure 1). This isolate grew well also in another hamster kidney-derived cell line (BSR-T7). Cytopathic effect (CPE) was observed in most of the cell types, though it appeared more slowly in the primary skin fibroblasts. In contrast, the GV isolate grew well only in BHK21/clone13 cells, Vero cells or the bovine foetal endothelial cell line, and showed strong CPE only in the BHK cells, which were therefore used for titration of GV stocks. This virus grew poorly in ovine or bovine kidney cell lines, or in primary goat or sheep endothelial cells, and essentially did not grow in the primary ovine or bovine skin fibroblasts (Figure 1). In general NSDV growth peaked at earlier time points (at 36 and 48 h post infection), whereas the GV displayed a slower growth rate, and the virus titre did not peak by the end of the time course. These data suggested that the extended passage of the NSDV isolate in BHK cells has adapted it to cell culture in general; other studies in our laboratory have shown this isolate replicates well in human cells as well (A549 cells). The GV isolate appeared to be significantly more restricted in the cell lines it will enter and replicate in. However, there seems to be no species specific restriction since each virus isolate grew equally well in hamster, monkey and human-derived cell lines as well as in bovine and ovine cells. An interesting observation was that this isolate grew significantly worse in BSR-T7 cells (max titre 10^4) compared to BHK21/clone13 cells, despite the fact that they are both subclones of BHK cells, and it grew better in Veros than in BSR-T7 cells, despite the observation that both cells are defective in production of type 1 interferon [19, 20].

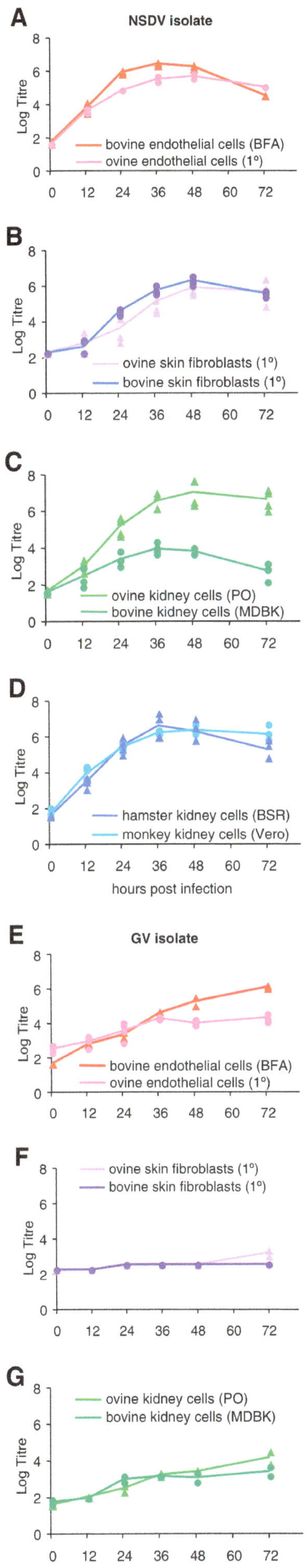

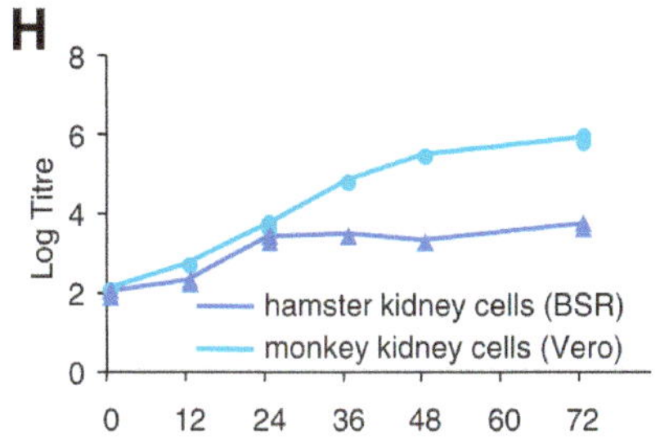

Figure 1: Growth of NSDV/GV isolates in cultured cells. The NSDV isolate (A-D) or the GV isolate (E-H) were used to infect different primary (1°) or permanent cell lines as described in "Materials and methods". At the indicated times post infection the cells were frozen and the titre ($TCID_{50}$/mL) of virus in the cell-free supernatant determined. Each experiment was carried out 2-4 times; symbols representing individual experiments may overlap.

Development of Real-Time Assay for NSDV/GV Genome

In order to be able to track and quantitate the growth and spread of the virus isolates in samples taken during animal studies, we developed a real-time PCR based assay for viral RNA. We selected primers based on the available sequences of the S segments of NSDV, GV, CCHFV, Dugbe virus and Kupe virus. The S segment was chosen because there is more extensive sequence data for that segment than the M or L segments, and primers were selected for the reverse transcription (RT) step and for a Sybr Green-based real-time PCR. We used a genome-specific primer (F3b) for the reverse transcription (RT) step as the assay was to be used for quantitation; random hexanucleotide primers, while possibly more sensitive, are not compatible with RNA quantitation [21]. Preliminary tests showed that lower background and higher sensitivity was achieved using a single primer external to the PCR target than by using the same primers for the RT and PCR steps. We sought to find primer sets that were conserved in NSDV/GV but not in any of the other nairoviruses, so that the assay could also be used as a diagnostic for NSDV/GV should the need arise in the future. The location of the primers in the overall alignment are shown in Figure 2, and the sequence of the primers used are listed in Table 1, along with the reaction conditions (annealing temperature and primer concentration). All primer pairs were optimised for annealing temperature by gradient PCR, and the optimal primer concentration determined (e.g. Figure 3B). Primer pairs F1-R1a and F2-R2 both worked well with similar sensitivity (Figure 3C-F), detecting fewer than 10 copies of target. We tested whether the primers would react with Dugbe virus, since this virus is also found associated with livestock. No reaction was seen with a clone of Dugbe virus S segment (Figure 3G-H). No reaction product was seen in samples without template (NTC controls), and this assay was used to measure viral genome RNA in the subsequent animal experiment.

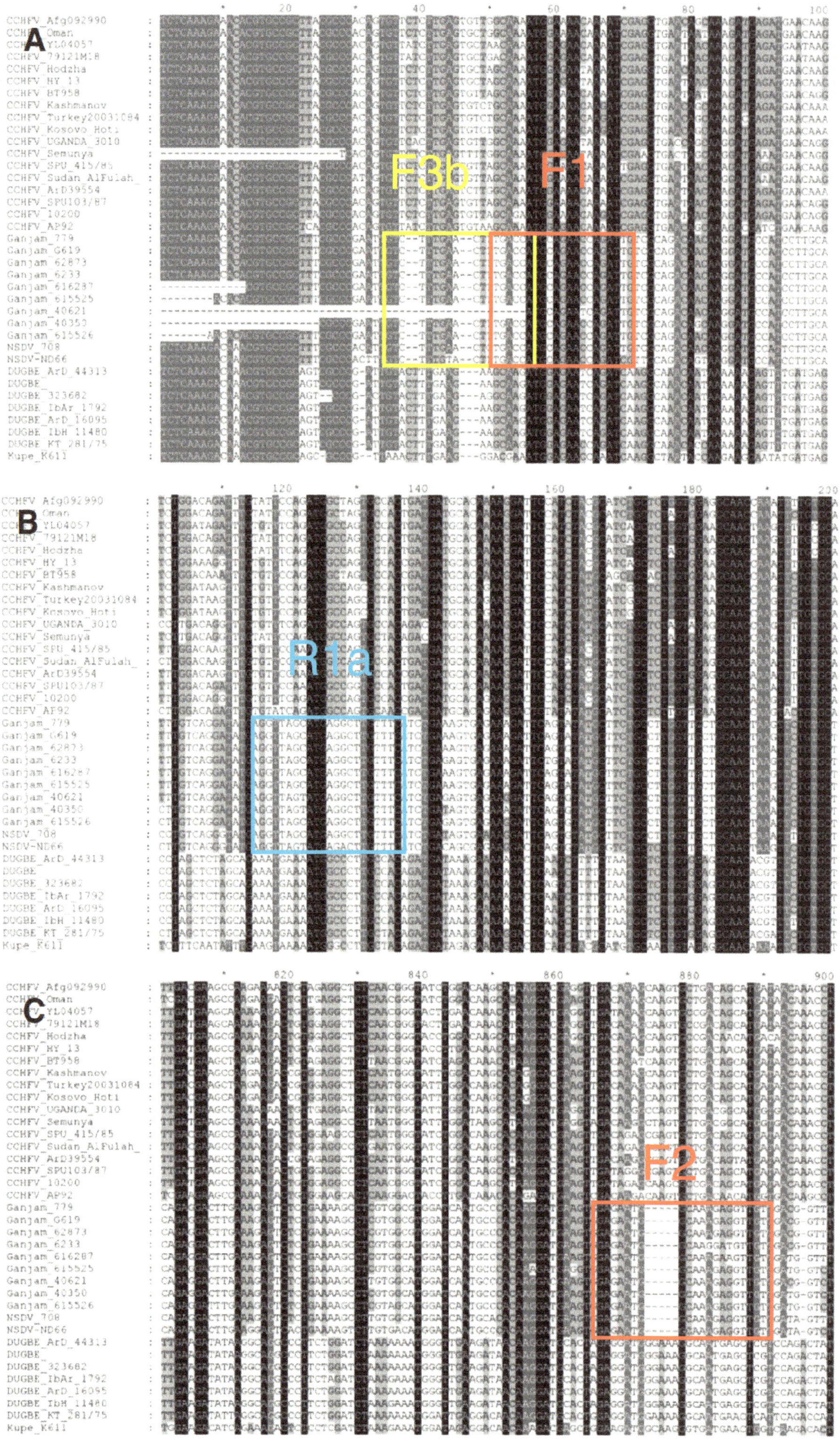
A
F3b
F1
B
R1a
C
F2
CCHFV_Afg092990
CCHFV_Oman
CCHFV_YL04057
CCHFV_79121M18
CCHFV_Hodzha
CCHFV_HY_13
CCHFV_BT958
CCHFV_Kashmanov
CCHFV_Turkey20031084
CCHFV_Kosovo_Hoti
CCHFV_UGANDA_3010
CCHFV_Semunya
CCHFV_SPU_415/85
CCHFV_Sudan_AlFulah_
CCHFV_ArD39554
CCHFV_SPU103/87
CCHFV_10200
CCHFV_AP92
Ganjam_779
Ganjam_G619
Ganjam_62873
Ganjam_6233
Ganjam_616287
Ganjam_615525
Ganjam_40621
Ganjam_40350
Ganjam_615526
NSDV_708
NSDV-ND66
DUGBE_ArD_44313
DUGBE_
DUGBE_323682
DUGBE_IbAr_1792
DUGBE_ArD_16095
DUGBE_IbH_11480
DUGBE_KT_281/75
Kupe_K611

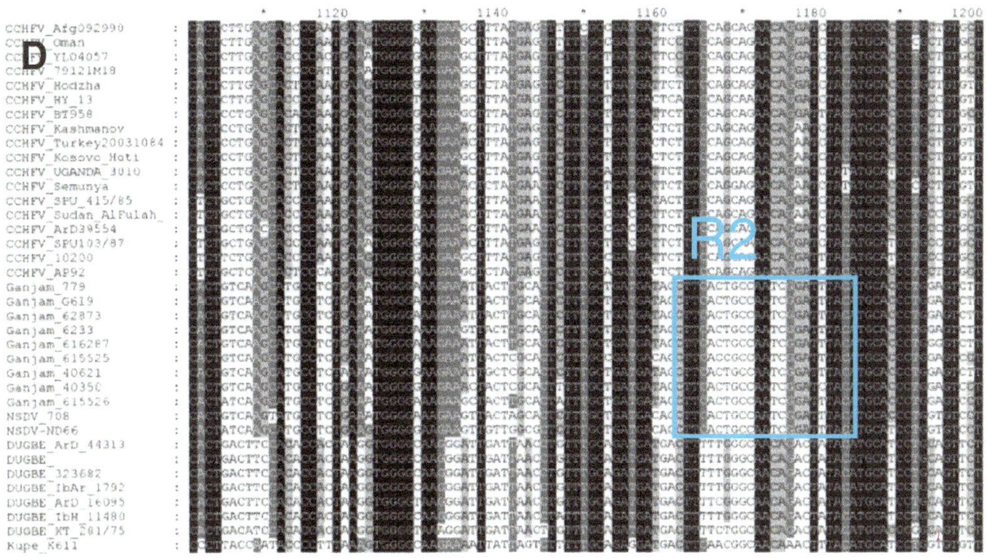

Figure 2: Identification of specific primers for NSDV/GV PCR. An alignment of all available S segments for nairoviruses (CCHFV, NSDV, GV, Dugbe virus and Kupe virus) was made and extracted blocks from this alignment are shown to illustrate the differences between NSDV/GV and other nairoviruses at the points selected for use as RT and PCR primers.

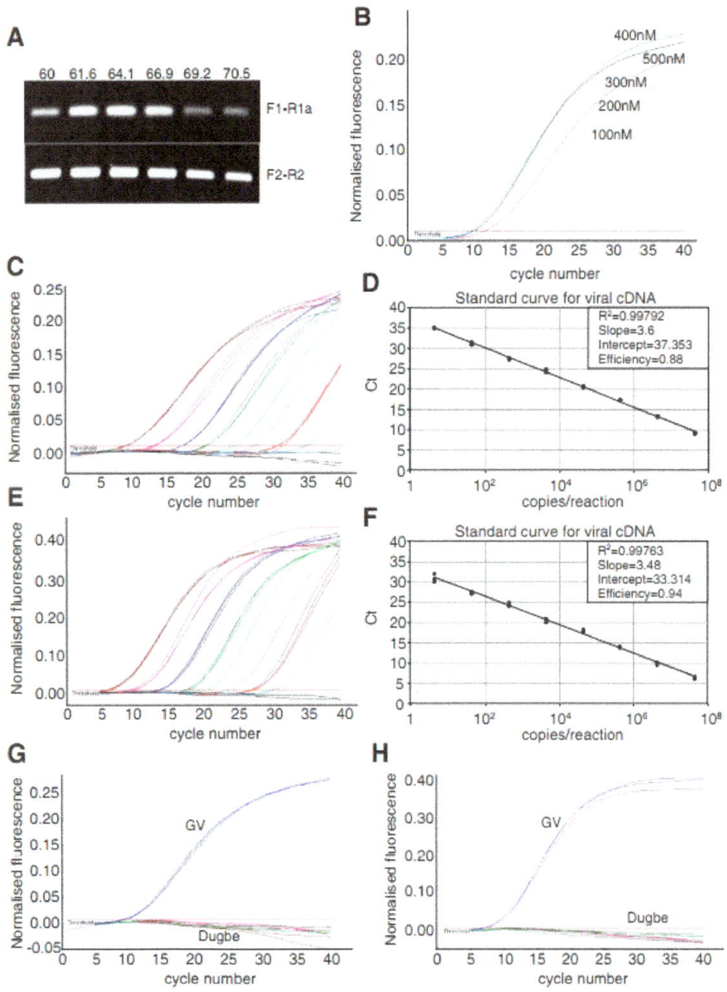

Figure 3: Optimisation and validation of PCR primers for NSDV/GV detection and quantitation. A) Example gradient PCRs of F1/R1a and F2/R2 primer pairs. B) Example real-time PCR with 100-500nM primer concentration for F1/R1a primer pair. C) Sensitivity determination for real-time PCR with F1-R1a primer pair; serial dilutions were made of GV S segment DNA template from 4 to 4×10^7 copies per reaction and the real-time PCR carried out with F1/R1a. D) Plot of data from (C). E), F) Similar sensitivity determination and standard curve for primer pair F2/R2. G) Real-time PCR results for F1/R1a primer pair with 4×10^7 copies of GV (blue) or Dugbe virus (brown) S segment; purple and green lines are negative controls. H) As (G), but with F2/R2 primer pair.

Real-Time PCR Measurement of Cytokine mRNA Levels

A set of primers specific for a range of ovine cytokines was prepared, either using published primer pairs or designed from ovine mRNA sequences taken from the data base. The reaction conditions for each primer pair were optimised as described for the viral RNA assay, using an anchored oligo(dT) oligonucleotide ($(T)_{16}VN$) to prime the RT reactions. Some published primer pairs for specific ovine cytokines were found to have low reaction efficiency, and new primers were designed for those assays. A complete listing of the primers used and reaction conditions for the relevant assays is given in Table 1.

Pathogenicity and Virus Growth in Animals

Each virus isolate was passaged a further two times in BHK21/clone13 cells to prepare stock, and 10^4 $TCID_{50}$units of virus were injected subcutaneously into 3 sheep per isolate. The animals infected with GV isolate IG619 showed higher and more prolonged pyrexia as well as profound leucopoenia (Figure 4). One of this group became extremely weak and apathetic by 7 dpi, developing clear hyperaemia in the coronary band (Figure 4), with gum lesions and bloody diarrhoea; this animal was euthanised at this point for post-mortem. A second animal with less severe clinical signs from the same group, and one animal from the group infected with the tissue culture-adapted NSDV isolate were sacrificed and post-mortem examination carried out at the same time. The animal with severe clinical signs had an enlarged spleen and multiple internal haemorrhages on blood vessels and the lining of the lower gut (Figure 4), while the other animal from the same group showed less in the way of pathology. The animals infected with NSDV-Entebbe showed only a transient pyrexia and leucopoenia, and the animal killed at 7 dpi showed no pathology at post mortem. The remaining animals were kept for a further four days, by which time temperatures had returned to normal.

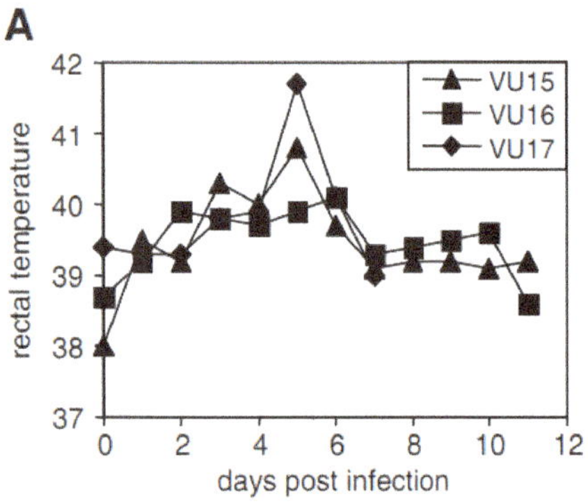

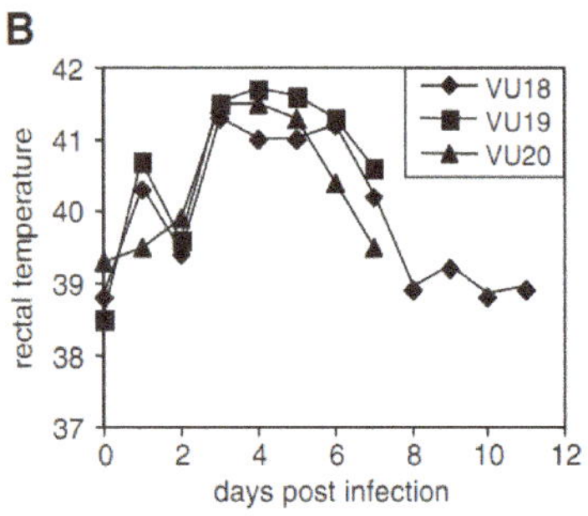

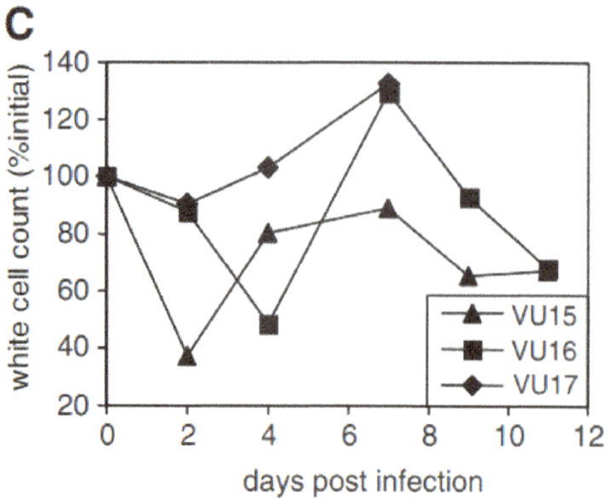

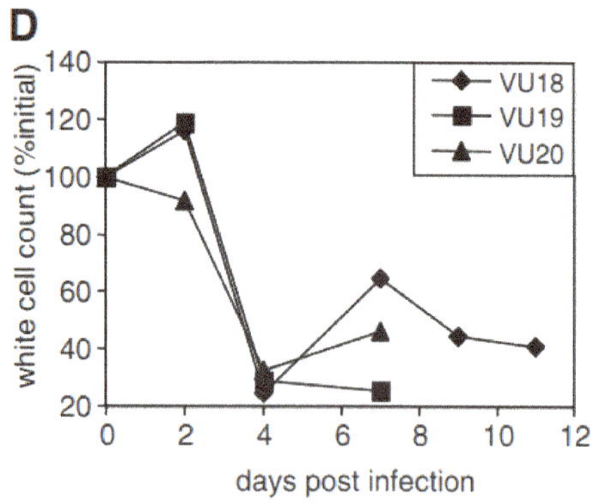

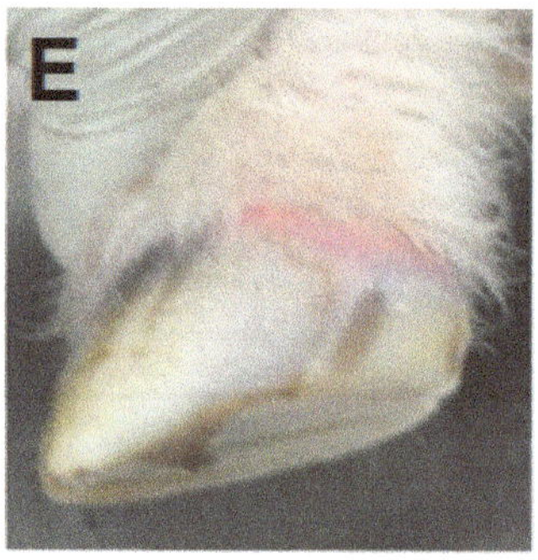

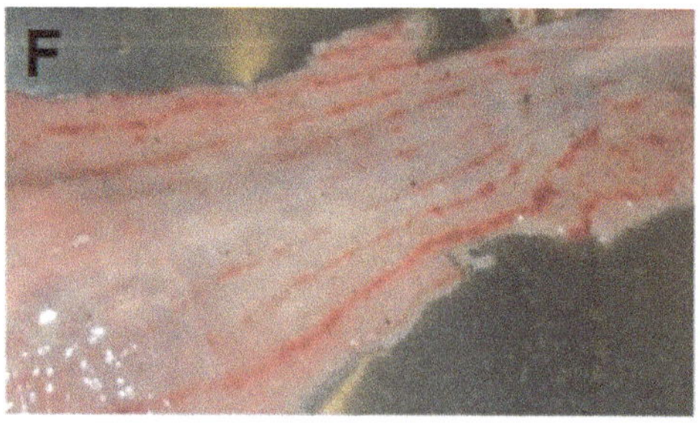

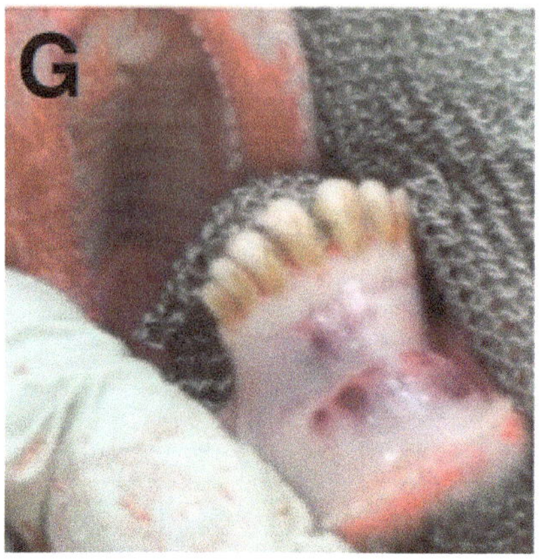

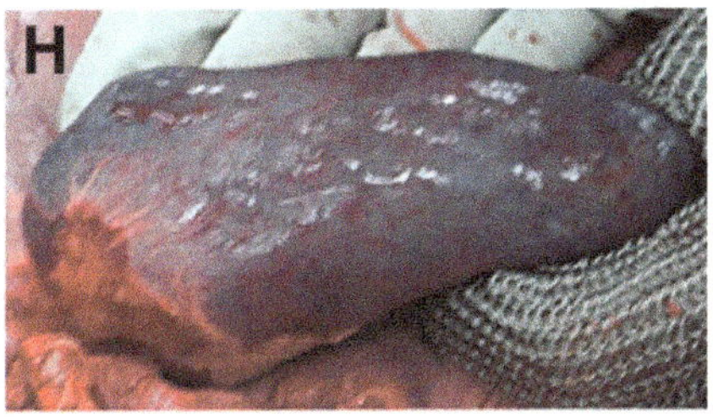

Figure 4: Effects of NSDV and GV isolates on sheep. Three animals (VU15-17) were infected with the NSDV isolate and three (VU18-20) were infected with the GV isolate. Animals VU17, VU19 and VU20 were sacrificed at 7 days post infection, when VU19 showed extreme clinical signs. A, B) rectal temperatures for the animals over the course of the experiment. C, D) white cell counts on the indicated days post infection, calculated for each animal as % white cell count on day 0. E-H show examples of pathology from VU19: E) Inflamed coronary band on hoof. F) zebra striping of caecum. G) haemmorrhage of gums. H) swollen spleen.

RNA was prepared from whole blood samples taken directly into RNA stabilising solution (Ambion "Tempus" vacutainers) and the relative level of viral genome RNA in each sample determined. Due to the small sample numbers and the wide variation in virus load observed in different animals, not all days in which virus genome was detected appeared statistically different from zero, but the pattern of responses was nevertheless clear. Viral RNA levels were higher in the GV IG619-infected animals, peaking at around 4 dpi and falling rapidly after 7 dpi (Figure 5A). Similar results were obtained from RNA isolated from a crude white cell preparation (Figure5B) consisting of blood from which red cells were removed (buffy coat & plasma). Virus isolation from this preparation was successful for GV at days of peak viral RNA, but the NSDV isolate could not be recovered. Several white cell samples from NSDV and GV-infected animals were found to be extremely toxic to cell cultures.

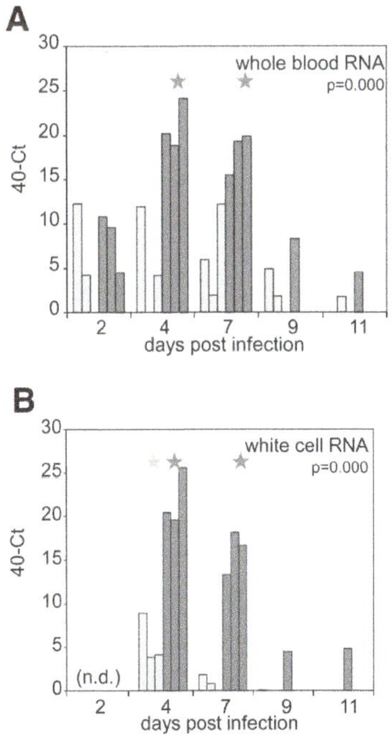

Figure 5: Real-time PCR assay of viral genome RNA. Viral genome was quantitated in (A) whole blood and (B) white cells isolated on different days post infection, for animals infected with NSDV isolate (light bars) or GV isolate (dark bars). Values are expressed as 40-Ct so that an increase in value corresponds to an increase in viral RNA. n.d. = not determined (samples lost before assay). The probability (p) value shown is that for the contrast of the two virus isolates and indicates the probability that the differences arose by chance. A star above a group of bars for a particular combination of virus and dpi indicate a significant difference from 0 at a threshold of $p = 0.05$.

The RNA prepared from whole blood which had been stabilised with complete cell lysis immediately on isolation was used to study cytokine mRNA levels during the course of infection (Figure 6). Infection with either isolate led to rapid increases in levels of IL-1β, IL-8 and IL-12 mRNA, with a later increase in IFN-γ mRNA levels as the infection was resolving. The pathogenic virus isolate caused a noticeably higher level of transcription of IL-6, IL-10 and TNFα mRNAs, and a clear if transient suppression of transcription of IL-4 and TGFβ. No consistent effect was seen in the levels of IL-18 or IFNβ mRNA in the animals of either group. A set of three housekeeping genes (glyceraldehyde phosphate dehydrogenase (GAPDH), glucose-6-phosphate dehydrogenase (G6PDH) and succinate dehydrogenase (SDHA)) showed no variation between samples (not shown), indicating that RNA recovery and the RT reactions had not introduced any significant bias into the results.

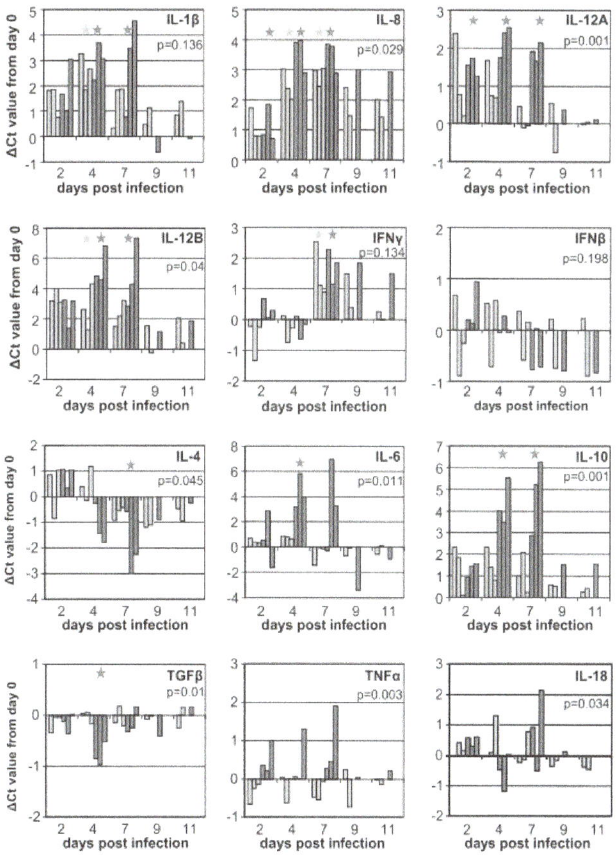

Figure 6: Effects of infection on transcription of cytokine mRNAs. Cytokine mRNA levels were determined in total blood RNA from animals infected with the NSDV isolate (light bars) or the GV isolate (dark bars). Due to the variable initial Cts seen in samples from different animals, values for day N are expressed as Ct(day 0)-Ct(day N), so that an increase in specific mRNA appears as an increase in the plotted value. The probability (*p*) value shown is that for the contrast of the two virus isolates and indicates the probability that the differences

arose by chance. A star above a group of bars for a particular combination of virus and dpi indicate a significant difference from 0 at a threshold of $p=0.05$.

DISCUSSION

It is clear from the studies in tissue culture that the NSDV isolate has adapted in some way to allow it to grow well in most of the cell lines tested. At the same time, this isolate has essentially lost virulence in sheep. These findings are in accord with those of Terpstra [6], who found that NSDV of the 55th to 71st tissue culture passage had greatly reduced virulence, while generating a protective immune response in some animals. The nature of the attenuation remains to be determined. The attenuated virus clearly still grows in animals, though less than the pathogenic virus. This is not due to a defect in the replication machinery or assembly of the attenuated virus, as it is clear from the tissue culture studies that this virus replicates well; direct comparisons in which the two isolates are used to infect a compatible cell line (Vero cells) have shown that the NSDV isolate appeared to produce new viral protein and progeny virions slightly faster than the pathogenic isolate. Other studies in our laboratory have shown that both isolates block the actions of type 1 and type 2 interferons and the induction of type 1 interferon [12] equally well, suggesting that the decreased pathogenicity of the NSDV isolate is not associated with any loss of function in this area. One possible difference between the two isolates is a change in one or both surface glycoproteins of the virus to allow the adapted isolate to enter the cell lines tested more easily, but which has reduced the effectiveness of the virus at growing in the natural target cells in the animal. Further studies to identify the native receptor NSDV/GV are required before we can examine the receptor preference of these two isolates.

There have been no detailed studies on the nature of the pathogenesis in GV/NSDV infections; GV has only recently been identified as a widespread infection in India [3, 9], and it is likely that the virus has been, in the past, frequently ignored or confused with diseases having similar signs in sheep/goats (e.g. peste des petits ruminants, Rift Valley fever), on either continent. The pyrexia seen here with the pathogenic isolate is similar to that reported previously [1, 6]; the profound leucopoenia has not previously been reported for NSDV infections, although it is a common clinical sign of viral hemorraghic fever, and may be caused by the same large scale apoptosis of leukocytes seen in CCHFV-infected mice [22] or Ebola virus haemorrhagic fever [23]. Loss of white cells has been reported in CCHFV-infected humans [24].

The cytokine responses observed in this study suggest a similar pattern to that seen in CCHFV infections in humans (reviewed in [25]) and in some other haemorrhagic fevers. The pathogenesis of CCHFV is poorly understood, not least because most cases occur in areas with limited clinical pathology facilities, and work on the disease requires specialized buildings and equipment (BSL4 containment). Nevertheless, serology on CCHF patients has shown increases in IL-6 and IL-10 and increased TNFα in clinically severe (hospitalised) cases [26,27], and monocyte-derived dendritic cells infected with CCHFV release IL-6, IL-10 and TNFα [28], while we showed that pathogenic NSDV/GV was associated with increases in these cytokines as well as of IL-12, and a decrease in IL-4, all concordant with a Th1, proinflammatory response, which has been proposed for CCHFV [26, 29]. One study found reduced levels of IL-12 in CCHF patients [30], but this may be a matter of timing, since the levels of IL-12 in NSDV/GV infection declined rapidly after 7 days. The observed cytokine responses would be expected to give rise to lymphohistocytosis (often associated with CCHF [29]), while both IL-6 and TNFα are associated with the increase in endothelial permeability that is common in viral hemorrhagic fevers [31, 32]. Elevated TNFα is found in a number of other hemorrhagic fevers, including infection with Hantaan virus [33], Ebola virus [34] or Puumala virus [35]. It does need to be pointed out that most of those studies have measured serum cytokine proteins, while in this instance we have looked only at the levels of specific mRNAs, since specific assays for ovine cytokines have not yet been developed. This means that we will have missed some changes due to cytokines secreted by other organs (e.g. IL-6 produced by the liver); on the other hand, the real-time PCRs are very sensitive, and the serial samples allow us to pick up quite small changes in transcription patterns.

The real-time PCR detection of viral genome was much more sensitive than virus isolation, as has been seen with other viruses. Interestingly, white cell RNA was almost as sensitive as whole blood RNA for detecting virus, especially the more wild-type, pathogenic isolate, despite the fact that low yields of RNA from the white cell preparation meant that it was necessary to use less of this RNA in the RT-PCR than whole blood RNA, suggesting that the viral RNA in the blood is mostly associated with white cells, and that EDTA blood or other anticoagulated blood will be a suitable sample for laboratory testing/diagnosis.

ACKNOWLEDGEMENTS

This work was supported by grants BB/F00740X/1 and BB/F006764/1 from the United Kingdom Biotechnology and Biological Sciences Research Council. We would like to thank Prof R B Tesh and Dr P. van Rijn for the gift of the GV and NSDV isolates, Dr R Waters for carrying out the post mortem examination of the infected sheep, Drs H-H Takamatsu and K Darpel for helpful discussions about preparing endothelial cells and the ovine cytokine responses, and Drs S. Gubbins and D Schley for advice on statistical analysis.

AUTHORS' CONTRIBUTIONS

AbT processed all the samples from the animal study and carried out all the real-time PCR studies. LL prepared endothelial cells and carried out all the studies on virus growth in cell culture. BH characterised and sequenced the virus isolates. MDB conceived of, designed and directed the study, carried out the animal work and prepared the manuscript. All authors read and approved the final manuscript.

REFERENCES

1. Montgomery E: On a tick-borne gastro-enteritis of sheep and goats occuring in British East Africa. J Comp Pathol. 1917, 30: 28-57.
2. Dandawate CN, Shah KV: Ganjam virus: a new arbovirus isolated from ticks Haemaphysalis intermedia Warburton and Nuttall, 1909 in Orissa, India. Indian J

Med Res. 1969, 57: 799-804.

3. Yadav PD, Vincent MJ, Khristova M, Kale C, Nichol ST, Mishra AC, Mourya DT: Genomic analysis reveals Nairobi sheep disease virus to be highly diverse and present in both Africa, and in India in the form of the Ganjam virus variant. Infect Genet Evol. 2011, 11: 1111-1120. 10.1016/j.meegid.2011.04.001.
4. Marczinke BI, Nichol ST: Nairobi sheep disease virus, an important tick-borne pathogen of sheep and goats in Africa, is also present in Asia. Virology. 2002, 303: 146-151. 10.1006/viro.2002.1514.
5. Spinage CA: Cattle Plague: A History. 2003, New York, Boston, Dordrecht: Kluwer Academic/Plenum
6. Terpstra C: Nairobi Sheep Disease. 1969, Utrecht: University of Utrecht
7. Dandawate CN: Studies on Ganjam virus with reference to viremia in vertebrate hosts & development of antibodies. Indian J Exp Biol. 1977, 15: 1058-1059.
8. Davies FG: Nairobi sheep disease in Kenya. The isolation of virus from sheep and goats, ticks and possible maintenance hosts. J Hyg (Lond). 1978, 81: 259-265. 10.1017/S0022172400025092.
9. Sudeep AB, Jadi RS, Mishra AC: Ganjam virus. Indian J Med Res. 2009, 130: 514-519.
10. Estrada-Pena A, Palomar AM, Santibanez P, Sanchez N, Habela MA, Portillo A, Romero L, Oteo JA: Crimean-Congo hemorrhagic fever virus in ticks, Southwestern Europe, 2010. Emerg Infect Dis. 2012, 18: 179-180. 10.3201/eid1801.111040.
11. Estrada-Pena A, Jameson L, Medlock J, Vatansever Z, Tishkova F: Unraveling the ecological complexities of tick-associated crimean-congo hemorrhagic Fever Virus transmission: a gap analysis for the Western palearctic. Vector Borne Zoonotic Dis. 2012, 12: 743-752. 10.1089/vbz.2011.0767.
12. Holzer B, Bakshi S, Bridgen A, Baron MD: Inhibition of interferon induction and action by the nairovirus Nairobi sheep disease virus/Ganjam virus. PLoS One. 2011, 6: e28594-10.1371/journal.pone.0028594.
13. Childerstone AJ, Cedillo-Baron L, Foster-Cuevas M, Parkhouse RM: Demonstration of bovine CD8+ T-cell responses to foot-and-mouth disease virus. J Gen Virol. 1999, 80: 663-669.
14. Ryan US: Isolation and culture of pulmonary endothelial cells. Environ Health Perspect. 1984, 56: 103-114.
15. Finney DJ: Statistical Method in Biological Assay. 1964, London: Charles Griffen & Co Ltd, 2
16. Smeed JA, Watkins CA, Rhind SM, Hopkins J: Differential cytokine gene expression profiles in the three pathological forms of sheep paratuberculosis. BMC Vet Res. 2007, 3: 18-10.1186/1746-6148-3-18.
17. Li H, Cunha CW, Davies CJ, Gailbreath KL, Knowles DP, Oaks JL, Taus NS: Ovine herpesvirus 2 replicates initially in the lung of experimentally infected sheep. J Gen Virol. 2008, 89: 1699-1708. 10.1099/vir.0.2008/000554-0.
18. Terpstra C: Physical and biological properties of Nairobi sheep disease virus. Vet Microbiol. 1983, 8: 531-541. 10.1016/0378-1135(83)90002-0.
19. Conzelmann KK: Reverse genetics of Mononegavirales. Biology of negative strand RNA viruses: The power of reverse genetics. Edited by: Kawaoka Y. 2004, Berlin Heidleberg New York: Springer, 1-42.
20. Mosca JD, Pitha PM: Transcriptional and posttranscriptional regulation of exogenous human beta interferon gene in simian cells defective in interferon synthesis. Mol Cell Biol. 1986, 6: 2279-2283.
21. Lekanne Deprez RH, Fijnvandraat AC, Ruijter JM, Moorman AF: Sensitivity and accuracy of quantitative real-time polymerase chain reaction using SYBR green I depends on cDNA synthesis conditions. Anal Biochem. 2002, 307: 63-69. 10.1016/S0003-2697(02)00021-0.
22. Bente DA, Alimonti JB, Shieh WJ, Camus G, Stroher U, Zaki S, Jones SM: Pathogenesis and immune response of Crimean-Congo hemorrhagic fever virus in a STAT-1 knockout mouse model. J Virol. 2010, 84: 11089-11100. 10.1128/JVI.01383-10.
23. Geisbert TW, Hensley LE, Gibb TR, Steele KE, Jaax NK, Jahrling PB: Apoptosis induced in vitro and in vivo during infection by Ebola and Marburg viruses. Lab Invest. 2000, 80: 171-186. 10.1038/labinvest.3780021.
24. Ergonul O, Celikbas A, Baykam N, Eren S, Dokuzoguz B: Analysis of risk-factors among patients with Crimean-Congo haemorrhagic fever virus infection: severity criteria revisited. Clin Microbiol Infect. 2006, 12: 551-554. 10.1111/j.1469-0691.2006.01445.x.
25. Weber F, Mirazimi A: Interferon and cytokine responses to Crimean Congo hemorrhagic fever virus; an emerging and neglected viral zonoosis. Cytokine Growth Factor Rev. 2008, 19: 395-404. 10.1016/j.cytogfr.2008.11.001.
26. Ergonul O, Tuncbilek S, Baykam N, Celikbas A, Dokuzoguz B: Evaluation of serum levels of interleukin (IL)-6, IL-10, and tumor necrosis factor-alpha in patients with Crimean-Congo hemorrhagic fever. J Infect Dis. 2006, 193: 941-944. 10.1086/500836.
27. Papa A, Bino S, Velo E, Harxhi A, Kota M, Antoniadis A: Cytokine levels in Crimean-Congo hemorrhagic fever. J Clin Virol. 2006, 36: 272-276. 10.1016/j.jcv.2006.04.007.
28. Connolly-Andersen AM, Douagi I, Kraus AA, Mirazimi A: Crimean Congo hemorrhagic fever virus infects human monocyte-derived dendritic cells. Virology. 2009, 390: 157-162. 10.1016/j.virol.2009.06.010.
29. Karti SS, Odabasi Z, Korten V, Yilmaz M, Sonmez M, Caylan R, Akdogan E, Eren N, Koksal I, Ovali E, Erickson BR, Vincent MJ, Nichol ST, Comer JA, Rollin PE, Ksiazek TG: Crimean-Congo hemorrhagic fever in Turkey. Emerg Infect Dis. 2004, 10: 1379-1384. 10.3201/eid1008.030928.
30. Saksida A, Duh D, Wraber B, Dedushaj I, Ahmeti S, Avsic-Zupanc T: Interacting roles of immune mechanisms and viral load in the pathogenesis of crimean-congo hemorrhagic fever. Clin Vaccine Immunol. 2010, 17: 1086-1093. 10.1128/CVI.00530-09.
31. Ferro T, Neumann P, Gertzberg N, Clements R, Johnson A: Protein kinase C-alpha mediates endothelial barrier dysfunction induced by TNF-alpha. Am J Physiol Lung Cell Mol Physiol. 2000, 278: L1107-L1117.

32. Desai TR, Leeper NJ, Hynes KL, Gewertz BL: Interleukin-6 causes endothelial barrier dysfunction via the protein kinase C pathway. J Surg Res. 2002, 104: 118-123. 10.1006/jsre.2002.6415.

33. Linderholm M, Ahlm C, Settergren B, Waage A, Tarnvik A: Elevated plasma levels of tumor necrosis factor (TNF)-alpha, soluble TNF receptors, interleukin (IL)-6, and IL-10 in patients with hemorrhagic fever with renal syndrome. J Infect Dis. 1996, 173: 38-43. 10.1093/infdis/173.1.38.

34. Hensley LE, Young HA, Jahrling PB, Geisbert TW: Proinflammatory response during Ebola virus infection of primate models: possible involvement of the tumor necrosis factor receptor superfamily. Immunol Lett. 2002, 80: 169-179. 10.1016/S0165-2478(01)00327-3.

35. Kanerva M, Vaheri A, Mustonen J, Partanen J: High-producer allele of tumour necrosis factor-alpha is part of the susceptibility MHC haplotype in severe puumala virus-induced nephropathia epidemica. Scand J Infect Dis. 1998, 30: 532-534. 10.1080/00365549850161629.

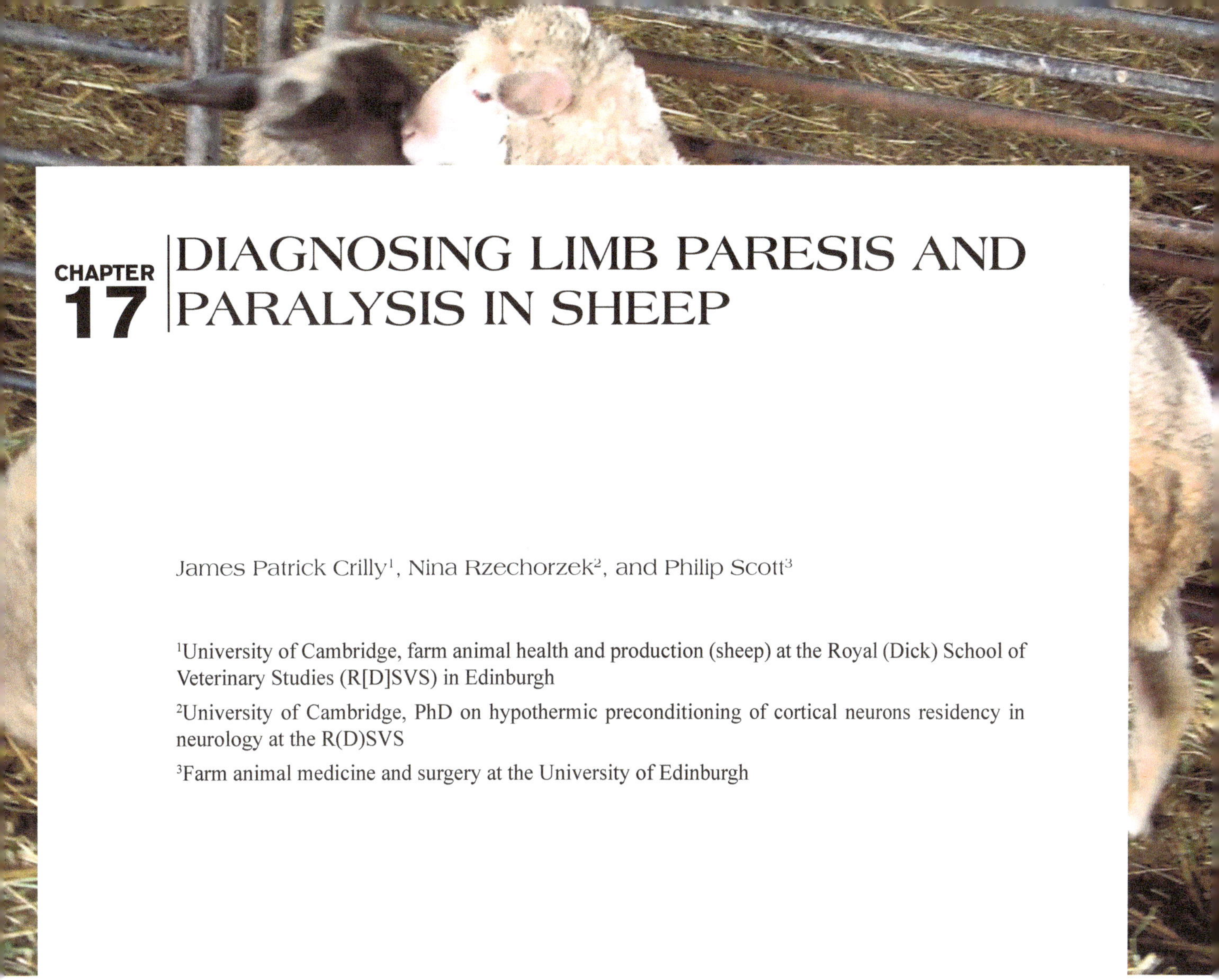

CHAPTER 17 DIAGNOSING LIMB PARESIS AND PARALYSIS IN SHEEP

James Patrick Crilly[1], Nina Rzechorzek[2], and Philip Scott[3]

[1]University of Cambridge, farm animal health and production (sheep) at the Royal (Dick) School of Veterinary Studies (R[D]SVS) in Edinburgh

[2]University of Cambridge, PhD on hypothermic preconditioning of cortical neurons residency in neurology at the R(D)SVS

[3]Farm animal medicine and surgery at the University of Edinburgh

ABSTRACT

Paresis and paralysis are uncommon problems in sheep but are likely to prompt farmers to seek veterinary advice. A thorough and logical approach can aid in determining the cause of the problem and highlighting the benefit of veterinary involvement. While this may not necessarily alter the prognosis for an individual animal, it can help in formulating preventive measures and avoid the costs – both in economic and in welfare terms – of misdirected treatment. Distinguishing between central and peripheral lesions is most important, as the relative prognoses are markedly different, and this can often be achieved with minimal equipment. This article describes an approach to performing a neurological examination of the ovine trunk and limbs, the ancillary tests available and the common and important causes of paresis and paralysis in sheep.

PARESIS may be defined as 'a deficiency in the generation of the gait or in the ability to support weight' and implies that a degree of voluntary movement is still present. Paralysis (plegia) is the complete loss of voluntary movement. Muscle weakness is associated with both conditions but may also be due to other causes.

HISTORY TAKING

With reference to the chief complaint, it is important to ask the farmer about onset, duration, evolution (static, progressive, waxing and waning, episodic) and lateralisation of clinical signs (unilateral, bilateral, more marked on the right or left). Ascertaining which animals and how many are affected is also important, as are any relevant husbandry factors. Examples include:

- What are the sheep currently being fed? Has the diet changed recently?
- Are there known/suspected mineral/trace element deficiencies on the farm?
- Has the affected animal/group/flock received any treatments recently?
- Is the flock open or closed?
- What is the origin of the affected animals?

Citation: James Patrick Crilly, Nina Rzechorzek and Philip Scott, Diagnosing limb paresis and paralysis in sheep, doi:10.1136/inp.h5547.

Neurological Examination

The core objectives of a neurological examination, together with the history, are to determine:

- Whether the condition is neurological;
- What part of the nervous system is affected;
- A list of differential diagnoses for the clinical signs observed;
- An appreciation of the severity of the disease (in order to give a prognosis).

A neurological examination should always be accompanied by a full clinical examination to avoid missing non-neurological causes of the presenting complaint (eg, orthopaedic), as well as those that manifest in neurological signs secondary to generalised metabolic, infectious, toxic or nutritional disturbances (Box 1).

Initial Assessment

An initial assessment should be made from a distance. The demeanour, stance and posture of the animal should be observed. If it is recumbent, is there opisthotonos (marked dorsal extension of the head and neck)? Do the limbs appear flaccid or rigidly extended? Does it display the Schiff–Sherrington phenomenon (Table 3)? If it is able, the animal should be encouraged to stand, walk and turn, and the following assessed:

- What stance does the animal adopt? Is it wide based or narrow based?
- What is the posture? Is there kyphosis (dorsal curvature of the spine), lordosis (ventral curvature of the spine), scoliosis (lateral deviation of the spine), torticollis (twisting of the neck) or an abnormal head carriage? Are the elbows, hocks or fetlocks dropped?
- Is the face symmetrical? If not, which areas are affected and how do they differ?
- Is the gait normal?
- Is there any ataxia (poor coordination when moving) and which limbs are affected? n Is the protraction–retraction of each limb normal, hypometric or hypermetric?
- Is the gait stiff or stilted?
- Is there any paresis or plegia? (Note, toe dragging indicates paresis; this is sometimes more easily heard than seen but hoof scuffing may give clues);
- Does the problem affect one limb, a pair of limbs or all four limbs?
- If the animal circles, are the circles tight or wide and in which direction?

Animals should be observed for involuntary movements such as tremor (involuntary oscillating contraction of antagonistic muscle groups) or myoclonus (sudden contraction followed by immediate relaxation of a specific muscle group).

Box 1: Common causes of recumbency in sheep

It is important to determine whether a recumbent sheep is down due to a primary nervous system lesion or is affected by a different problem that may be unrelated to the nervous system or that may affect it indirectly. Examples of commonly encountered causes of recumbency include:

Primary neurological disorders

- Listeriosis (infection of the trigeminal nerve and associated brainstem nuclei by *Listeria monocytogenes*);
- Spinal cord trauma.

Systemic disturbances that affect the nervous system (secondary neurological disorders)

- Hypocalcaemia (see Video 1);
- Hypomagnesaemia;
- Polioencephalomalacia (cerebrocortical necrosis), eg, thiamine deficiency.

Non-neurological problems

- Multiple limb lameness;
- Severe debility and emaciation*;
- Septicaemic and toxaemic states (eg, acute mastitis, metritis, clostridial disease)*;
- Severe pneumonia;
- Acute fasciolosis.

* These conditions may present with secondary neurological disorders

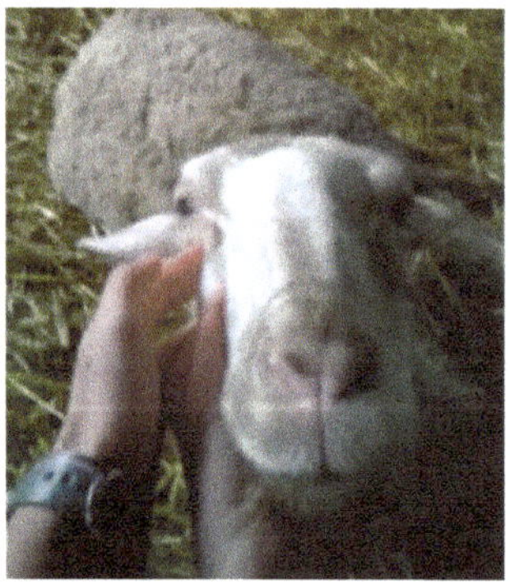

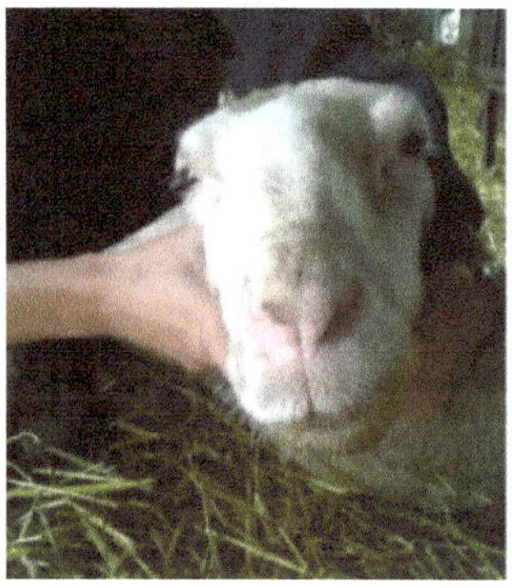

This ewe is recumbent due to listeriosis but the changes to facial symmetry are subtle (minor changes in the shape of the ocular and nasal aperture and set of the lip and ear) and the animal may be misdiagnosed if the cranial nerve function were not assessed

The assessment should then be followed by a general clinical examination and a specific neurological examination. Particular attention should focus on eliminating other causes if a neurological problem is suspected. For example, muscle wasting of a limb may be the result of prolonged disuse due to an orthopaedic cause of lameness, and cardiovascular or respiratory embarrassment may be responsible for episodes of collapse. Important differential diagnoses for recumbency (other than those covered in this article) are given in Box 1.

Table 1: Tests of cranial nerve function

Test/observation	Cranial nerve involved
Facial symmetry	VII
Ear position	VII
Ocular aperture	VII
Eye position	III, IV, VI
Auditory response (eg, to a hand clap)	VIII
Menace response	II, VII
Palpebral reflex	V, VII
Corneal reflex	V, VII, VI
Pupillary light reflex	II, III
Facial sensation	V
Jaw tone	V
Tongue tone and position	XII
Vestibulo-ocular reflex	VIII, III, VI, IV

Localising the Lesion

A neuroanatomical diagnosis is required before listing differential diagnoses of any neurological problem. Certain problems/pathologies are more common at particular sites than others. A systematic approach using only very basic tools can yield accurate information about a lesion's location and distribution (whether it is focal, multifocal or diffuse, and symmetrical or asymmetrical). The priority is to identify a single site that explains all of the neurological signs observed, since multifocal lesions are less common.

The stages of the close-up neurological examination can be performed in any order but should be methodical and consistent to avoid missing important information. The authors find it easiest to start at the head with assessment of mentation and behaviour, abnormal head carriage, head tremor, head turn or head tilt, facial symmetry and more specific testing of the cranial nerves (Table 1). When assessing the indicators of cranial nerve function, it must be remembered that non-neurological causes of abnormalities are also possible (eg, facial symmetry disrupted by swelling and tongue position, and movement disrupted by injury). The gag reflex is difficult to assess in sheep due to the narrow oral aperture and long buccal cavity. Facial and trigeminal nerve dysfunction is often accompanied by food packing into the cheeks, and the corneal reflex is a reliable test of cranial nerve VI function only if the eyelids are held open to observe the retraction of the globe.

The range of motion of the neck or a pain response elicited on manipulation or palpation of the neck, back, muscles or joints may identify a region for further investigation. Subsequently, if the animal is standing, tests of proprioception, such as a modified 'paper-slide test', should be performed (Box 2).

The animal can then be laid on its side and the spinal reflexes of the uppermost limbs tested, after which the animal should be turned over and the tests repeated on the contralateral limbs. Other spinal reflexes can be tested while the animal is standing or recumbent and are described in Box 2.

The animal can then be laid on its side and the spinal reflexes of the uppermost limbs tested, after which the animal should be turned over and the tests repeated on the contralateral limbs. Other spinal reflexes can be tested while the animal is standing or recumbent and are described in Box 2.

Box 2: Testing postural reactions and spinal reflexes

Proprioceptive positioning
It is more difficult to test postural reactions in sheep than in small animals or horses because they are less tolerant of their limbs being handled. The authors find the easiest method is to place a foot on a robust piece of plastic (eg, an old feed sack) and, ensuring the animal is weight bearing on that limb, drawing the plastic laterally to assess how rapidly the animal detects the displacement of the limb and how accurately it returns the limb to the accustomed position. Hopping tests, wheelbarrow tests, hemiwalking, and visual and tactile placing tests as performed in small animals can be performed with lambs and small adult sheep.

Cutaneous trunci (panniculus) reflex
This reflex has a segmental input and a unitary output at the level of C8-T1 running to the cutaneous trunci muscle of the flank. In response to a light stimulus (eg, a fly landing on the animal's side), the cutaneous trunci contracts several times. It is best stimulated by gently pinching the skin in the region of the sublumbar fossa and the corresponding area of the thoracic flank (it can frequently be elicited by touching the tip of a ballpoint pen on the skin). Sequential stimulation of the flank from the caudal to cranial aspect can help locate a spinal lesion, ie, the cutaneous trunci reflex cannot be stimulated below the lesion but is intact above it. Due to the overlap of dermatomes, precise localisation (ie, to a single nerve root segment) is often not possible.

Perineal reflex
To assess the perineal reflex, the skin of the perineal region is pinched firmly. A normal response entails contraction of the anal sphincter and ventroflexion of the tail, and should occur irrespective of which side of the perineum is pinched. A reduced response indicates damage to the sacral spinal cord segments or damage to the pudendal and caudal rectal nerves (Constable 2004).

Myotatic reflexes
Tests for myotatic reflexes involve an afferent (sensory) arm and an efferent (motor) arm that often involve the same nerve trunk; both arms communicate in the same spinal segment. Decreased reflexes are due to muscular disorders, peripheral neuropathies or damage to the spinal segment where the nerve(s) involved originate. An exaggerated reflex is most frequently due to a lack of descending inhibition resulting from a spinal lesion cranial to the spinal segment of nerve origin, but it may also be exaggerated if the antagonistic muscle tone is reduced. Clonus indicates a lack of descending inhibition. The most commonly used tests involve the following:

- Patellar reflex. This reflex tests the integrity of spinal cord segments L4-L6 and the femoral nerve. The stifle is flexed to tense the patellar tendon and the crus rested on an open palm (to avoid restricting its movement). The patellar tendon is struck with a narrow, hard object (eg, the handle of a pair of scissors). The intact reflex produces a rapid contraction of the quadriceps and extension of the stifle. When performing this test, it may help to displace the skin of the limb laterally to ensure that woolless skin overlies the tendon. Striking the muscle body or the bones will produce misleading results;
- Extensor carpi radialis (ECR) reflex. This reflex tests the integrity of spinal cord segments C7-T2. The carpus is flexed and the metacarpus rested on the open palm. The front of the carpus is palpated and the tendon of the ECR located. This is again lightly and sharply struck, and contraction of the ECR results in an extension of the carpus;
- Tendons of gastrocnemius (testing L7-S1 and the tibial nerve), biceps brachii (testing C6-C8), triceps brachii (testing C6-C8) and the muscle belly of the cranial tibial muscle (testing L6-S1 and the peroneal nerve) may be struck, but the authors find the response difficult to reliably produce in neurologically normal animals.

Withdrawal reflexes
A painful stimulus to the distal limb (eg, pinching between the toes with artery forceps) will produce a withdrawal of the limb and should elicit flexion at all joints of that limb. This involves multiple motor units and therefore tests the integrity of a single sensory input but multiple motor outputs. A neurologically normal animal should be conscious of the stimulus as well but as sheep are stoic animals this may be hard to judge.

Once the ability to withdraw the limb has been established, stimulation of different parts of the limb (eg, using a pen or forceps) can be used to assess the integrity of the sensory innervation to different parts of the limb. The crossed extensor reflex (extension of the contralateral limb when the withdrawal reflex is stimulated) is normal in neonates but indicates an upper motor neuron lesion if seen in an adult.

Neural control of the limb musculature can be divided into local reflex arcs (Fig 1) and a descending modulation of these, which largely reduces the responsiveness of the reflex arc. Disruption of the efferent arm of a local reflex arc (a lower motor neuron [LMN] lesion) results in hyporeflexia, flaccid paralysis and rapid loss of muscle mass. Such lesions affect (from the peripheral to central aspects) the neuromuscular junction, the nerve trunk itself, the plexi where these nerves form from segmental spinal nerves, the ventral nerve roots of the segmental nerves or the spinal cord where the nerves originate. Disruption of the descending neurons (an upper motor neuron [UMN] lesion) removes inhibition from the reflex arc resulting in hyper-reflexia, spastic paralysis and a slower loss of muscle mass (Fig 2). Such a lesion occurs in the spinal cord cranial to the segment where the nerve roots give rise to the nerves involved in the reflex arc. It is accompanied by loss of conscious sensation and proprioception caudal to the lesion. An LMN lesion may have only motor deficits (damage to peripheral nerve trunks will result in sensory deficits distal to the lesion) and may occur in the spinal cord or involve only the peripheral nervous system; UMN lesions are always central (Fig 3). This distinction is important because the peripheral nervous system has a greater regenerative capacity than the central nervous system (CNS).

At the end of the neurological examination it should be possible to locate the lesion within one of the following functionally anatomical groups:

- Forebrain
- Cerebellum
- Vestibular system
- Brainstem
- C1-C5
- C6-T2
- T3-L3
- L4-S3
- Peripheral nerve/muscle/neuromuscular junction.

Peripheral Nerve Lesions

Peripheral lesions may affect either a single nerve trunk or multiple nerves within the same limb. Generalised peripheral neuropathies do occur (botulism, for example) but are rare in sheep. The number of nerves affected and the degree of nerve disruption affect the clinical signs seen.

The large myelinated A fibres convey motor signals to the muscle fibres and also carry proprioceptive information and are the most vulnerable to injury (eg, hypoxia). C fibres are the smallest fibres and have the lowest conduction speed but are the more refractory to injury. They convey temperature, itch and deep pain sensation.

A mild insult may result in neuropraxia – a temporary dysfunction of the axon. Spontaneous recovery is relatively rapid, within a matter of days. If the insult is more severe, resulting in transection of the axons, then recovery is possible but this relies on the myelin sheath and connective tissue surrounding the nerve remaining intact. The axon can re-extend within this framework but this is a slow process. This type of injury is known as axonotmesis. If the nerve structure (i.e., axons and myelin sheaths) is highly disrupted (neurotmesis), then this axonal regeneration may well not reach its intended target, leading to a permanent loss of function. Whether reinnervation occurs depends on the size of the gap between the proximal and distal nerve segments. Neuroma (a swelling resulting from haphazard regrowth of the axons and often a cause of discomfort) is one potential outcome of failed regeneration. Functional deficits may also arise due to 'reorganisation', in which suboptimal repair results in the axon terminating in an 'off-target' site.

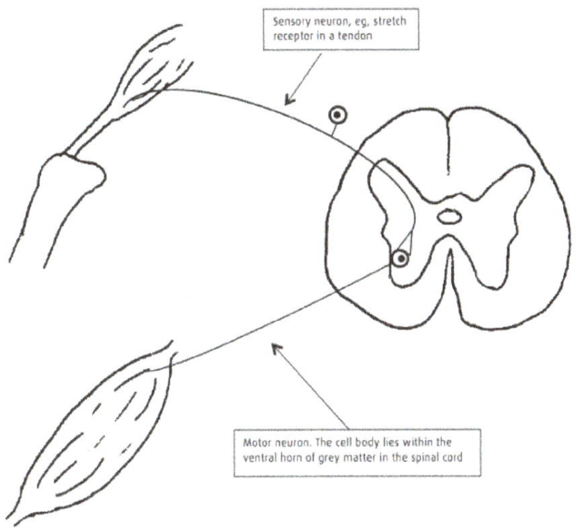

Figure 1: Simple reflex arc. The reflex arc provides the basis for neurological examination of the limbs and trunk. At its most simple, it involves just two neurons – the afferent (sensory) neuron and the efferent (motor) neuron. For example, increased tension in a tendon is detected by stretch receptors resulting in activation of the afferent neuron, which, through a direct synapse to a motor neuron, increases motor neuron activity and, thus, muscular contraction.

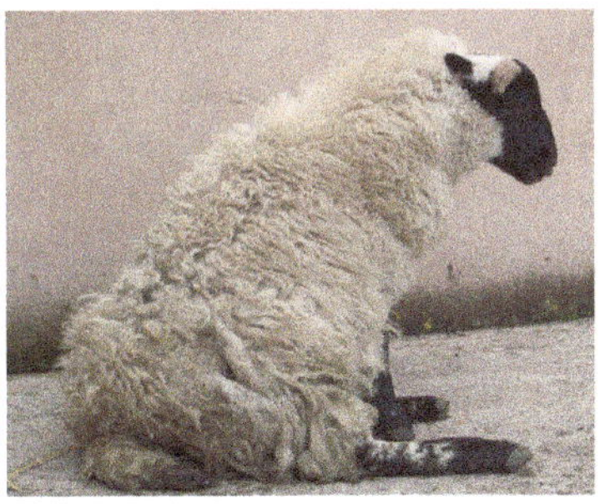

Figure 2: Scottish Blackface lamb with a compressive thoracolumbar lesion. Spinal lesions in the thoracolumbar region often result in animals adopting a dog-sitting position. The hindlimb myotatic reflexes (e.g., patellar reflex) are usually exaggerated in such cases.

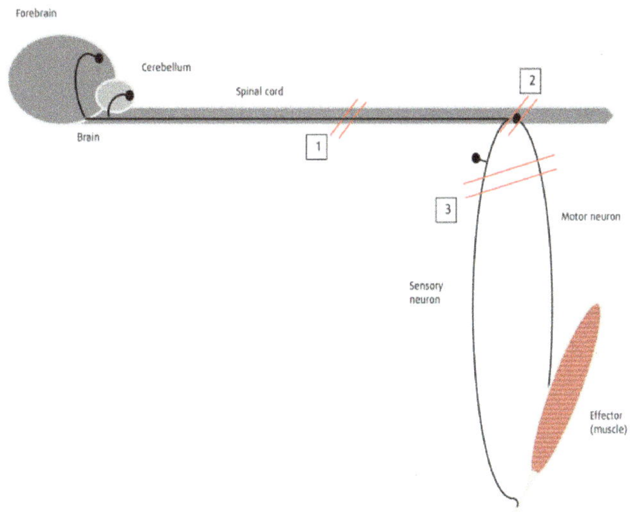

Figure 3: Schematic diagram showing upper motor neuron (UMN) and lower motor neuron (LMN) lesions relative to the spinal cord. UMN lesions (1) may occur anywhere cranial to the nerve roots that give rise to the nerves involved in the reflex/limb/muscle group in question. They disrupt the descending (inhibitory) axons that originate in the brain and also disrupt ascending pathways conveying sensation and proprioceptive information. LMN lesions may be central (2) or peripheral (3). Lesions in these locations may affect just motor neuron function or may affect both motor neurons and sensory neurons, leading to a loss of sensation as well as paresis/paralysis.

Presenting signs and common causes of some peripheral nerve lesions are listed in Table 2.

As spontaneous recovery is possible, and as long as any rectifiable problem has been attended to (eg, a foreign body removed, an abscess drained), then supportive care and minimising the accidental self-trauma that accompanies limb flaccidity can yield satisfactory results. For example, where fetlock 'knuckling' occurs, splinting of the distal limb to prevent trauma to the dorsum of the foot is indicated. Spontaneous recovery may take many weeks and clients must be prepared for a long wait without a guarantee of recovery.

Spinal Lesions

Spinal lesions have a poorer prognosis than peripheral nerve lesions due to the difference in response to injury. Unlike the nerve regeneration witnessed peripherally, axonal regeneration is poor in the central nervous system due to the physical barrier presented by the glial scar and the local factors produced by CNS glia and myelin debris that are non-permissive for growth (Kotter and others 2006).

The clinical signs associated with lesions of each of the major spinal cord segments are listed in Table 3 and will depend on the severity of disruption of the spinal cord and the precise location of the lesion. Reflexes and sensation may be reduced or completely absent and a degree of difference may occur between the left and right sides if the lesion is lateral to the spinal cord (eg, a perivertebral abscess extending into the spinal canal from the left may cause more severe deficits on the left side than the right side). Cervical lesions often produce more obvious gait deficits in the hindlimbs than the forelimbs.

Table 2: Presenting signs and potential causes of peripheral nerve lesions

Problem	Presenting signs	Potential causes
Brachial plexus avulsion	Dropped elbow, passively flexed fetlock and carpus, generalised decreased limb tone (unable to bear weight), easily abducted limb, decreased limb sensation, decreased extensor carpi radialis (ECR) reflex, possible disruption of the panniculus reflex, possible Horner's syndrome	Forelimb stuck in fence/gate, ill-fitting harness in rams
Radial nerve damage	Knuckling of the fetlock and carpus but the animal can bear weight, decreased sensation of antebrachium, metacarpus and foot, possible flexed elbow if the damage is higher up, decreased ECR reflex	Prolonged lateral recumbency, trauma to the lateral aspect of the forelimb
Sciatic nerve damage	Decreased sensation of the whole limb except the medial aspect, decreased tone except in the quadriceps and psoas musculature, decreased withdrawal reflex, intact or exaggerated patellar reflex	Iatrogenic damage due to injection into the hamstrings or caudal gluteal areas
Femoral nerve damage	Animal is unable to bear weight (if bilateral, the animal exhibits a frog-legged position), inability to extend the stifle, decreased patellar reflex, decreased skin sensation over the craniomedial crus	Hindlimb stuck over a gate/fence, trauma to the cranial aspect of the thigh, hyperextension of the hip
Distal limb nerve damage	Variable, depending on precisely which nerves are involved and the degree of damage	Trauma to a distal limb (eg, entrapped in wire)

Obturator nerve paralysis, which presents as weakness of the adductor and gracilis muscles leading to an inability to adduct the hindlimbs, is a known sequela to dystocia in cattle but is rare in sheep

Particular lesions are more commonly seen in certain spinal locations and further diagnostic evidence can be gathered from the history, signalment and diagnostic tests (see below). Common spinal lesions in sheep are listed in Table 4.

Scrapie

Scrapie is a transmissible encephalopathy of sheep and goats. Paresis and ataxia, especially of the hindlimbs, are common clinical signs (Healy and others 2003, Jeffrey and Gonzalez 2007); quadriplegia and recumbency are seen at a later date. Other clinical signs include separation from the rest of the flock, depression, anxiety or hyperexcitability, head tremor, low head carriage, pruritus (including a 'nibble' response to stimulation of the back), weight loss, bruxism, cud-dropping and an absent menace response (Healy and others 2003, Konold and Phelan 2014). Most of the sheep that are affected are more than two years of age (Jeffrey and Gonzalez 2007).

Definitive diagnosis is by detection of the proteaseresistant prion protein (PrPsc) in the brain on postmortem examination. Infection can be detected by the isolation of PrPsc from lymphoid tissue biopsies (eg, tonsillar tissue or rectal mucosa).

If scrapie is suspected in the UK, then the local APHA office must be notified.

Maedi-Visna

Maedi-visna is caused by maedi-visna virus (MVV), a small ruminant lentivirus. A variety of clinical syndromes follow infection, including progressive weight loss accompanied by dyspnoea and tachypnoea due to a lymphoid infiltrate of the interalveolar septa (maedi), indurative mastitis and, more rarely, arthritis and a neurological form (visna) (Pritchard and McConnell 2007).

Visna is most commonly seen in heavily infected flocks with widespread maedi, but there is some suggestion of different strains of MVV having different degrees of neurotropism (Payne and others 2004, Benavides and others 2006). Early clinical signs include unilateral paresis of a hindlimb (Fig 4) progressing to ataxia, hindlimb paralysis, recumbency and death. Other signs include fine head tremor, circling, progressive head tilt, visual impairment and separation from the rest of the flock (Pritchard and McConnell 2007). Affected animals are usually four to five years old but rapidly progressive disease has been reported in lambs as young as four months of age (Benavides and others 2007). Visna is more rapidly progressive than maedi, with affected animals dying or being euthanased within weeks of the onset of clinical signs. As visna is usually seen in flocks in which maedi is already present, suspicion may be high on clinical signs alone.

Table 3: Clinical signs associated with lesions of the spinal cord

Lesion location	Forelimb intrinsic reflexes	Forelimb conscious sensation and proprioception	Hindlimb intrinsic reflexes	Hindlimb conscious sensation and proprioception	Notes
C1-C5	Increased	Decreased	Increased	Decreased	
C6-T2	Decreased	Decreased	Increased	Decreased	Disruption of the spinal cord at the level of T1-T3 could theoretically abolish the origin of the sympathetic supply to the head leading to Horner's syndrome
T3-L3	Normal	Normal	Increased	Decreased	Schiff-Sherrington phenomenon may occur with severe acute lesions and involves an increased thoracic limb extensor tone with retention of voluntary movements and normal proprioceptive placing in these limbs, accompanied by hindlimb paresis/paralysis
L4-S2	Normal	Normal	Decreased	Decreased	
S2 onwards	Normal	Normal	Normal	Normal	Cauda equina syndrome seen: decreased tail tone, altered perineal sensation, disrupted perineal reflex, passive bladder distension

Table 4: Common causes of neurological signs that indicate a spinal cord lesion

Lesion	Location	Common signalment	Clinical signs	Treatment	Cause
Atlanto-occipital joint infection	Atlanto-occipital joint	Usually in young lambs (within the first two weeks of life)	Low head carriage, ataxia (hindlimb more noticeable), tetraparesis, neck pain (see Video 2)	Single injection of dexamethasone and seven days of procaine penicillin	Effectively a form of neonatal septic polyarthritis (joint ill), which is frequently caused by *Streptococcus dysgalactiae*
Compressive cervical myeloencephalopathy (wobbler syndrome)	Cervical	Texel and Beltex rams	Ataxia of all four limbs (see Video 3), paresis, may progress to tetraplegia	None	Fatty nodules on the floor of the spinal canal. There appears to be a hereditary component, so affected animals should not be bred from
Traumatic injury	Anywhere, frequently cervical	Often in rams that have been fighting	Clinical signs consistent with location, greater severity in cases of fracture	Mild cases frequently recover within a few days. Treatment should involve isolation, confinement and anti-inflammatory medication. Cases with unstable or displaced fractures should be euthanased	Often due to fighting among rams or other trauma (eg, being hit by car)
Vertebral body osteomyelitis	Frequently thoracolumbar but may be anywhere along the spinal cord	May be seen in any age of sheep but many cases involve lambs aged four to 12 weeks. It is usually a sporadic problem affecting individual animals	Dependant on location, onset usually sudden. If thoracolumbar, the animal will be bright, alert and responsive but with paresis or paralysis of the hindlimbs. It will often sit like a dog and move by pulling itself along using its forelimbs (see Videos 5 and 6)	Euthanasia	Thought to be due to bacterial infection of the vertebral body following bacteraemia but this is unproven
Delayed swayback	Clinical signs indicate a cranially progressive problem	Most commonly in lambs aged four to 12 weeks. It is usually a flock problem	Ascending paresis/ paralysis and ataxia, gradual onset (see Video 7)	If mildly affected, an animal may make slaughter weight. If severely affected, the animal should be euthanased	Copper deficiency during pregnancy
Sarcocystosis	Clinical signs frequently consistent with a thoracolumbar lesion	Usually lambs about one year of age. Multiple animals are usually affected	Hindlimb paresis/ paralysis, may be tetraparetic (see Video 8)	Mild cases may recover with nursing care but severe cases should be euthanased	Ingestion of sarcocyst oocysts (shed in dog faeces) by naïve animals

Affected animals are seropositive. Histopathology findings at postmortem examination include nonsuppurative encephalitis affecting the cerebellum. MVV can be demonstrated immunohistopathologically or by PCR in the cerebellum at postmortem examination.

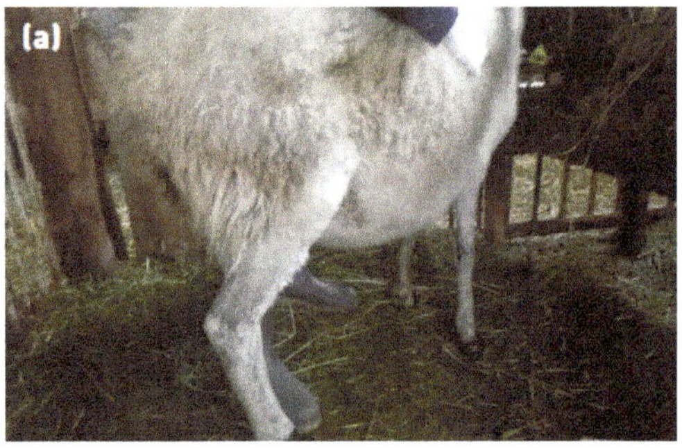

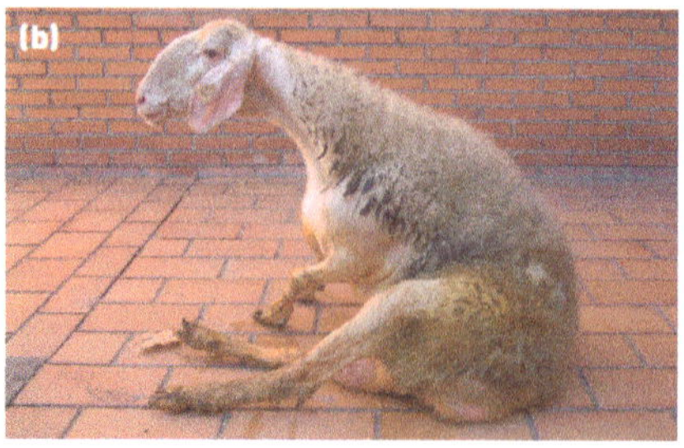

Figure 4: Limb paralysis due to infection with maedi-visna virus (MVV). Early in the disease course animals often show unilateral hindlimb paresis (a). The disease then progresses to ataxia, hindlimb paralysis (b), recumbency and death. Animals affected with visna are usually a small subsection of those infected with MVV in a flock (Picture b: Valentín Pérez and Julio Benavides).

Box 3: Technique for sampling cerebrospinal fluid

- Place the sheep in sternal recumbency with an assistant kneeling in front and grasping the animal's hocks. Positioning may be assisted by sedation of the animal
- Pull the hocks forward to extend the leg, flex the hip and flex the caudal spine; this widens the lumbosacral space. The landmarks that can be seen are the two wings of the ilium and the dorsal spinous processes
- With the thumb and ring finger on the wings of the ilium and the index finger lying along the dorsal spinous processes, feel the lumbosacral space as a depression just caudal to a line drawn between the two iliac crests, as shown in the photograph on the right
- Prepare this area surgically and place a small bleb of local anaesthetic beneath the skin
- Advance a needle slowly, perpendicular to the skin. A decrease in resistance will be felt as the point passes through the interarcuate ligament. The needle should be cautiously advanced until cerebrospinal fluid wells up in the hub
- Collect the fluid as it drips from the needle hub or attach a 5 ml syringe and apply gentle suction. No more than 2 ml should be aspirated
- Place the fluid in an EDTA tube immediately (Scott 1993)

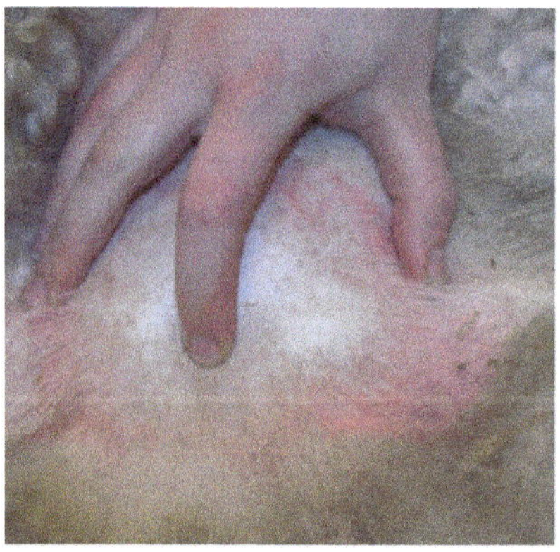

The lumbosacral space can be felt as a depression just caudal to a line drawn between the two iliac crests

Ancillary Diagnostic Techniques

Additional diagnostic techniques can help to confirm a diagnosis; however, those that are within the remit of specialist referral centres, such as computed tomography (CT) and magnetic resonance imaging (MRI), will not be considered here.

Cerebrospinal Fluid Sampling

Cerebrospinal fluid bathes the CNS and protects it from mechanical damage. It is produced at the choroid plexi within the ventricles of the brain. Under normal circumstances it is a clear, colourless fluid with a very low cell count, consisting mainly of macrophages. It can be sampled from two sites – the cisterna magna, which lies deep to the foramen magnum of the skull, and the lumbosacral space. Sampling from the cisterna magna requires deep sedation or general anaesthesia and carries with it the risk of iatrogenic brain damage. Sampling from the lumbosacral space is much easier, can be performed on the conscious animal and carries a lower risk of iatrogenic damage. Box 3 describes the sampling method. As there is rarely a significant difference between the samples obtained from either site, lumbosacral sampling is preferred in the majority of cases.

Changes to the CSF that are relevant include:

- *Blood Staining* – this is due to very recent haemorrhage or artefactual due to iatrogenic damage of vessels within the spinal canal. Sedimentation over several hours or centrifugation will clear the colour;

- *Xanthochromic Appearance* – yellow/orange discolouration is indicative of past haemorrhage; centrifugation will not clear the colour. Haemosiderophages may be seen among the cells present
- *Frothy Appearance*, which forms a stable foam when shaken – this indicates that the protein content is increased
- *Turbidity* – the cell count is much higher than normal (eg, in bacterial meningitis; in this case the fraction of neutrophils is also increased).

If there are no gross changes, the fluid should be submitted for laboratory analysis of the protein concentration because disruption of the flow of CSF (as occurs with a space-occupying lesion compressing the spinal cord) results in an increase in the protein concentration of the CSF caudal to the lesion – a phenomenon known as Froin's syndrome (Scott and Will 1991). This increase is too small to be detected using a refractometer. Analysis of the cell types present within the CSF can also aid in diagnosis and can be performed at a low cost using sedimentation with standard Diff-Quik staining of the sediment and simple light microscopy (see Lowrie and Anderson [2011] for a full description of this technique). Sarcocystis merozoites have also been identified in CSF samples from sheep with neurological signs (Formisano and others 2013).

Radiography

Radiography of the spine can detect gross distortions of the bones of the vertebral column or the limbs. The clarity of images of sheep is often limited by the fleece, which adds artefacts and prevents placement of the plate as close to the area in question as is possible in other species. Nonetheless, it can be helpful in the detection of fractures or gross changes associated with osteomyelitis or perivertebral infections (Fig 5).

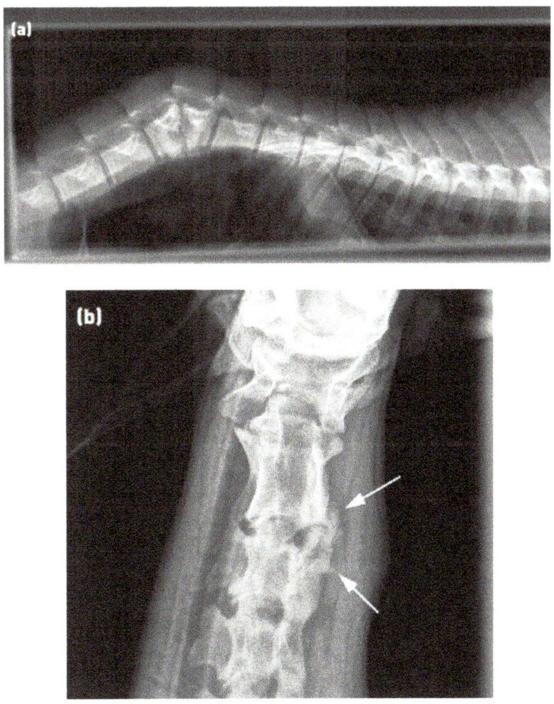

Figure 5: Radiograph showing (a) vertebral body destruction and disruption of the normal spinal architecture due to vertebral body osteomyelitis affecting the lumbar vertebrae. (b) New bone formation and loss of normal architecture (arrows) around the C2-C3 articulation on the right-hand side caused by a perivertebral abscess.

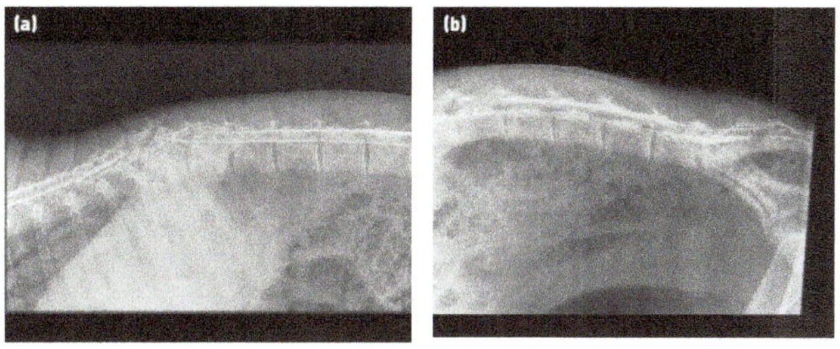

Figure 6: Myelograph showing (a) narrowing and dorsal deviation of both the dorsal and ventral columns of contrast material at the level of T11-T12. This lamb had vertebral body osteomyelitis resulting in erosion of vertebral bodies of T11 and T12. (b) Pooling of contrast material at the injection site (the lumbosacral junction). This myelograph has been taken too soon after administration of the contrast material as the dorsal contrast column is well established only as far as L3. The lesion in this case was at T10.

Ultrasonography

Ultrasonography can be used to detect perivertebral abscesses in the cervical area, for example, those derived from intramuscular injection in the neck using dirty needles or irritant substances (see Video 4). It may also be used to assess the degree of urinary bladder distension (Scott and Sargison 2010) that may occur as a result of damage to the pelvic nerves (eg, in cauda equina syndrome).

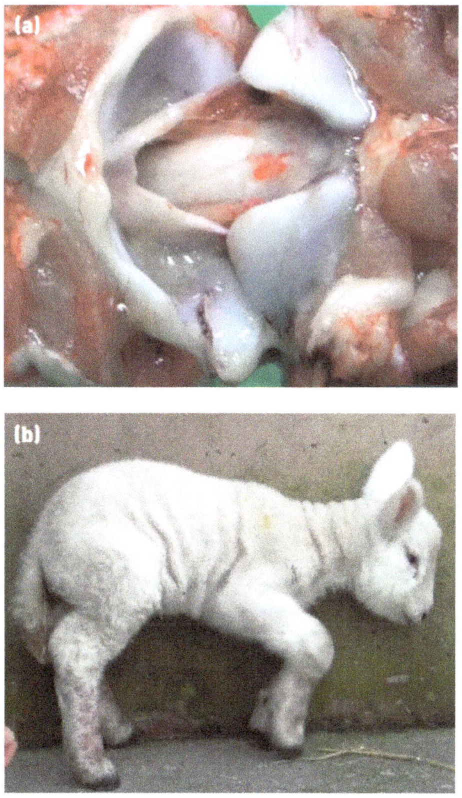

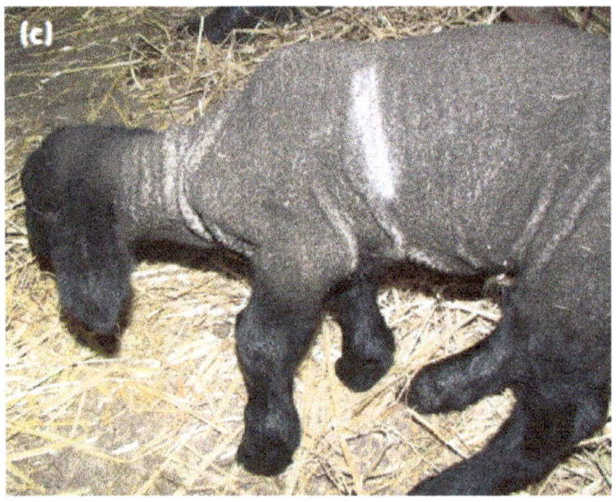

Figure 7: Atlanto-occipital joint infection. (a) Sepsis of the atlanto-occipital joint appears to be part of the same septic polyarthritis complex as the more frequently seen septic arthritides of limb joints (eg, carpus and tarsus). (b) and (c) Affected lambs show neck pain, low head carriage, ataxia and tetraparesis, which manifests frequently as flexion of the forelimbs.

Myelography

The injection of contrast material into the epidural space can be performed at the same lumbosacral site as for CSF sampling (Fig 6). Approximately 5 ml injected into a two- to three-month-old lamb (15 to 20 kg) will allow imaging of the thoracolumbar spine. Elevating the hindquarters after injection aids cranial spread of the contrast material. The dorsal and or ventral columns on the lateral view will appear narrowed if the spinal cord is compressed. Dorsoventral projections are often very hard to interpret in sheep.

While this technique can aid the detection of spinal cord compression that is not accompanied by bony changes, it may not add any further information on localisation and is probably too costly for all but the most valuable animals.

Flock Implications

The diagnosis of certain causes of paresis or paralysis may have implications for the flock as a whole. The response may be governed by law, as with suspected scrapie, or will have to be worked out between the vet and the flock owner.

Table 5: Common causes of paresis and paralysis, and examples of flock control measures

Problem	Examples of control measures at flock level
Atlanto-occipital joint infection	Improve colostrum intake, navel dipping and lambing shed hygiene. Tick control may be appropriate if the involvement of tick-borne fever or tick pyaemia is suspected
Swayback	Increase dietary provision of copper for pregnant ewes (beware overcompensation and subsequent copper toxicity)
Vertebral body osteomyelitis	Aetiology not fully elucidated but any risk factors for bacteraemia or immunosuppression should be identified and controlled
Sarcocystosis	Identify the at-risk pasture/feedstuff and remove young animals from it. Prevent dog access to sheep carcases and ensure feedstuffs cannot become contaminated by dog faeces
Abnormal localisation of *Taenia multiceps* lesions	This is a rare presentation; classical gid is also likely to be seen. Control is as for sarcocystosis and includes regular worming of farm dogs with praziquantel
Compressive cervical myeloencephalopathy ('wobbler syndrome')	Do not breed from affected rams (and ewes), identify and outcross or remove at-risk family lines
Traumatic injury	Identify and remove the causes (eg, take care when mixing rams, ensure any trailers used to transport animals are fit for purpose)
Perivertebral abscessation	Identify the causes and, where abscesses are thought to result from iatrogenic injury, review the injection site, technique, equipment and product
Maedi-visna	Test the flock serologically to establish prevalence levels – test and cull policies have been successful in eliminating disease. Complete depopulation followed by repopulation from accredited disease-free sources is also possible. If neither option is practical, mitigate the spread and effects of the disease by ensuring a relatively young age profile to the flock, avoid or limit the period of housing and keep good records to identify and remove offspring or ewes identified as being clinical cases of maedi–visna
Brachial plexus damage	Identify and remove the inciting causes, for example, poorly fitted raddle harnesses on rams, poor injection site choice, poorly designed pens or fences that allow entrapment of limbs, and unsympathetic handling causing panicking sheep to become entrapped or trampled
Damage to individual nerve trunks	Control is as for brachial plexus damage

Some sporadic problems, such as neuropathies due to injury or occasional cases of vertebral body osteomyelitis, may not require any changes to flock management if they occur in singly; however, larger numbers of these problems should prompt careful investigation to identify the risk factors. For example, if many cases of atlanto-occipital joint infection (Fig 7) are seen in a flock, then colostrum intake, lambing shed hygiene and tick challenge, as well as the incidence of related problems such as infectious polyarthritis, should be evaluated.

Other problems, such as swayback (which rarely occurs singly and has a management-related cause [insufficient copper available in the diet of the pregnant ewe]), should automatically prompt discussion of the cause of the disease and control of risk factors pertaining to it.

Causes of paresis and paralysis with flock implications and examples of control measures are summarised in Table 5.

SUMMARY

A logical approach incorporating a basic neurological examination can allow localisation of lesions causing paresis or paralysis. This, alongside history and signalment, will often allow a presumptive diagnosis that is sufficient to provide a prognosis and decide on treatment. Further diagnostic tests will allow confirmation of diagnoses made on clinical grounds. The individual prognosis and flock implications of the various causes of limb paresis/paralysis in sheep are widely variable and an accurate diagnosis is vital in ensuring the welfare of individuals and the health of the flock.

ACKNOWLEDGEMENT

Nina Rzechorzek is funded by a Wellcome Trust Integrated Training Fellowship for Veterinarians (096409/Z/11/Z). Funding sources did not have any involvement in the writing of this article or the decision to submit it for publication.

REFERENCES

1. BENAVIDES J., GARCÍA-PARIENTE C., FERRERAS M. C., FUERTES M., GARCÍA-MARÍN J. F., PEREZ V. (2007) Diagnosis of clinical cases of the nervous form of maedi–visna in 4- and 6-month old lambs. Veterinary Journal 174, 655–658
2. BENAVIDES J., GÓMEZ N., GELMETTI D., FERRERAS M. C., GARCÍA-PARIENTE C., FUERTES M., OTHERS (2006) Diagnosis of the nervous form of maedi–visna infection with a high frequency in sheep in Castilla y Leon, Spain. Veterinary Record 158, 230–235
3. CONSTABLE P. D. (2004) Clinical examination of the ruminant nervous system. Veterinary Clinics of North America: Food Animal Practice 20, 185–214
4. FORMISANO P., ALDRIDGE B., ALONY Y., BEEKHUIS L., DAVIES E., DEL POZO J., DUN K., ENGLISH K., OTHERS (2013) Identification of Sarcocystis capracanis in cerebrospinal fluid from sheep with neurological disease. Veterinary Parasitology 193, 252–255
5. HEALY A. M., WEAVERS E., MCELROY M., GOMEZ-PARADA M., COLLINS J. D., O'DOHERTY E., SWEENEY T., DOHERTY M. L. (2003) The clinical neurology of scrapie in Irish sheep. Journal of Veterinary Internal Medicine 17, 908–916
6. JEFFREY M., GONZALEZ L. (2007) Scrapie. In Diseases of Sheep. 4th edn. Ed Aitken I. D. Blackwell Publishing. pp 241–249 Google Scholar
7. KONOLD T., PHELAN L. (2014) Clinical examination protocol to detect atypical and classical scrapie in sheep. Journal of Visualized Experiments 83, e51101
8. KOTTER M. R., LI W-W., ZHAO C., FRANKLIN R. J. M. (2006) Myelin impairs CNS remyelination by inhibiting oligodendrocyte precursor cell differentiation. Journal of Neuroscience 26, 328–332
9. LOWRIE M., ANDERSON J. (2011) Cerebrospinal fluid: analysis and interpretation in small animals. In Practice 33, 78–85
10. PAYNE J. H., BAINBRIDGE T., PEPPER W. J., PRITCHARD G. C., WELCHMAN D. DE B., SCHOLES S. F. E. (2004) Emergence of an apparently neurotropic maedi-visna virus infection in Britain. Veterinary Record 154, 94
11. PRITCHARD G. C., MCCONNELL I. (2007) Maedi-visna. In Diseases of Sheep. 4th edn. Ed Aitken I. D. Blackwell Publishing. pp 217–223
12. SCOTT P. R. (1993) Collection and interpretation of cerebrospinal fluid in ruminants. In Practice 15, 298–300
13. SCOTT P. R. (2012) Clinical, ultrasonographic and pathological description of bladder distension with consequent hydroureters, severe hydronephrosis and perirenal fluid accumulation in two rams putatively ascribed to pelvic nerve dysfunction. Small Ruminant Research 107, 45–48
14. SCOTT P. R., SARGISON N. D. (2010) Ultrasound as an adjunct to clinical examination in sheep. Small Ruminant Research 92, 108–119
15. SCOTT P. R., WILL R. G. (1991) A report of Froin's syndrome in five ovine thoracolumbar epidural abscess cases. British Veterinary Journal 147, 582–584

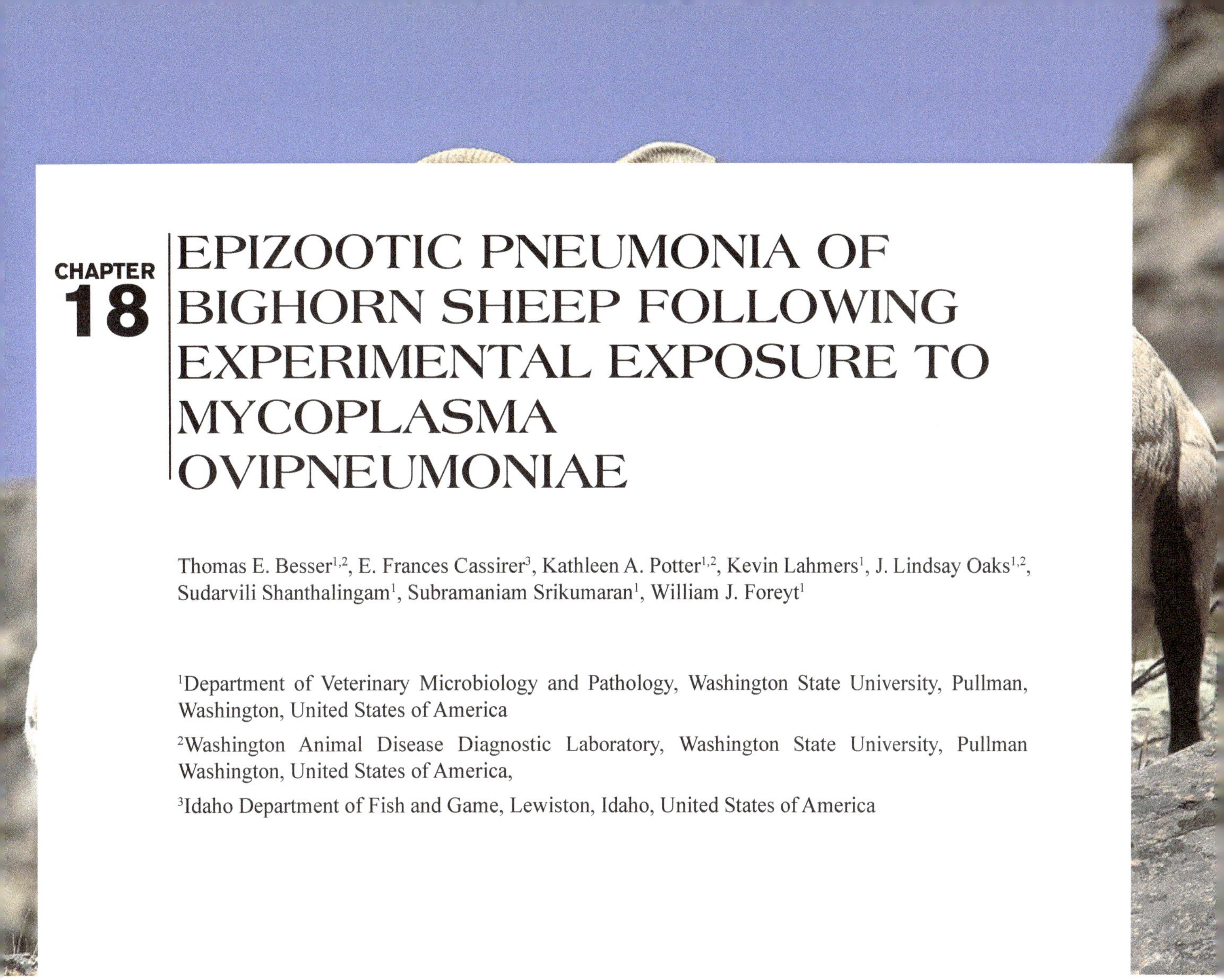

CHAPTER 18

EPIZOOTIC PNEUMONIA OF BIGHORN SHEEP FOLLOWING EXPERIMENTAL EXPOSURE TO MYCOPLASMA OVIPNEUMONIAE

Thomas E. Besser[1,2], E. Frances Cassirer[3], Kathleen A. Potter[1,2], Kevin Lahmers[1], J. Lindsay Oaks[1,2], Sudarvili Shanthalingam[1], Subramaniam Srikumaran[1], William J. Foreyt[1]

[1]Department of Veterinary Microbiology and Pathology, Washington State University, Pullman, Washington, United States of America

[2]Washington Animal Disease Diagnostic Laboratory, Washington State University, Pullman Washington, United States of America,

[3]Idaho Department of Fish and Game, Lewiston, Idaho, United States of America

ABSTRACT

Background

Bronchopneumonia is a population limiting disease of bighorn sheep (*Ovis canadensis*). The cause of this disease has been a subject of debate. Leukotoxin expressing *Mannheimia haemolytica* and *Bibersteinia trehalosi* produce acute pneumonia after experimental challenge but are infrequently isolated from animals in natural outbreaks. *Mycoplasma ovipneumoniae*, epidemiologically implicated in naturally occurring outbreaks, has received little experimental evaluation as a primary agent of bighorn sheep pneumonia.

Methodology/Principal Findings

In two experiments, bighorn sheep housed in multiple pens 7.6 to 12 m apart were exposed to*M. ovipneumoniae* by introduction of a single infected or challenged animal to a single pen. Respiratory disease was monitored by observation of clinical signs and confirmed by necropsy. Bacterial involvement in the pneumonic lungs was evaluated by conventional aerobic bacteriology and by culture-independent methods. In both experiments the challenge strain of *M. ovipneumoniae* was transmitted to all animals both within and between pens and all infected bighorn sheep developed bronchopneumonia. In six bighorn sheep in which the disease was allowed to run its course, three died with bronchopneumonia 34, 65, and 109 days after *M. ovipneumoniae* introduction. Diverse bacterial populations, predominantly including multiple obligate anaerobic species, were present in pneumonic lung tissues at necropsy.

Conclusions/Significance

Exposure to a single *M. ovipneumoniae* infected animal resulted in transmission of infection to all bighorn sheep both within the pen and in adjacent pens, and all infected sheep developed bronchopneumonia. The epidemiologic, pathologic and microbiologic findings in these experimental animals resembled those seen in naturally occurring pneumonia outbreaks in free ranging bighorn sheep.

Citation: Besser TE, Cassirer EF, Potter KA, Lahmers K, Oaks JL, Shanthalingam S, et al. (2014) Epizootic Pneumonia of Bighorn Sheep following Experimental Exposure toMycoplasma ovipneumoniae. PLoS ONE 9(10): e110039. doi:10.1371/journal.pone.0110039.

INTRODUCTION

Bighorn sheep are a North American species that has failed to recover from steep declines at the turn of the 20th century despite strict protections and intensive management, and two populations (Sierra Nevada and Peninsular) are currently classified as endangered [1]. Epizootic pneumonia is limiting bighorn sheep population restoration and as such, the etiology is of considerable interest. The first appearance of the disease in a population is typically in the form of epizootics that affect animals of all ages and is sometimes accompanied by high (>50%) mortality rates. Subsequently, epizootics affecting primarily lambs may occur for decades [2]. Various causes have been proposed for this disease, including lungworms (*Protostrongylus* sp.) [3]–[6], Pasteurellaceae, especially *Mannheimia (Pasteurella) haemolytica,* [7]–[12] and more recently, *Mycoplasma ovipneumoniae* [13]–[16]. In a recent comparative review of the evidence supporting each of these possible etiologies we concluded that *M. ovipneumoniae* was most strongly supported as the primary epizootic agent of bighorn sheep pneumonia [14]. However, the only two previous experimental challenge studies with *M. ovipneumoniae* either did not reproduce disease [13] or were confounded by challenges with other agents [16]. The objective of this study was to improve upon previous investigations to better assess the outcome of experimental introduction of *M. ovipneumoniae* to naïve bighorn sheep.

METHODS

Ethics Statement

This study was carried out in accordance with the recommendations in the Guide for the Care and Use of Laboratory Animals of the National Institutes of Health and in conformance with United States Department of Agriculture animal research guidelines, under protocols #03854 and #04482 approved by the Washington State University (WSU) Institutional Animal Care and Use Committee. As described in those protocols, euthanasia was performed by intravenous injection of sodium pentobarbital for animals observed to be in severe distress associated with pneumonia during the study and prior to necropsy examination for surviving animals at the end of each experiment.

Experimental Aims

Experiment 1 was conducted to investigate the transmission of *M. ovipneumoniae* to bighorn sheep and their subsequent development of disease, using an infected domestic sheep source. Experiment 2 was conducted to investigate experimental direct *M. ovipneumoniae*infection of a single bighorn sheep and the subsequent transmission of this agent to conspecifics. Both experiments were conducted in multiple pens separated by short distances, which allowed investigation of transmission to both commingled and non-commingled animals.

Experimental Animals

All experimental animals originated from herds and flocks unexposed to *M. ovipneumoniae* as determined by repeated testing with both serology on blood serum and PCR on enriched nasal swab cultures (using the methods described later in the 'Microbiological testing' section). In Experiment 1, three hand-reared bighorn sheep (yearling rams BHS #82 and #89 and yearling ewe BHS #07) that originated from a captive flock at WSU and three purchased domestic sheep (adult ewes DS #00 and #01 and yearling ewe DS #LA) were co-housed in three 46 m^{2}pens, with one domestic and one bighorn sheep per pen. Pens were separated by 7.6–12 m. Experiment 1 animals had all been commingled in a single pen for 104 days immediately prior to the beginning of this experiment, as previously described [15]. One of the four bighorn sheep used in that prior study had died of *M. haemolytica* pneumonia, while the other three, which had demonstrated no signs of respiratory disease in that study, were used in experiment 1. In Experiment 2, wild bighorn sheep captured from the Asotin Creek population in Hells Canyon were housed in two 700 m^2 pens, 7.6 m apart, with three animals per pen (Pen #1: adult ewe BHS #40, yearling ewe BHS #38, and yearling ram BHS #39; Pen #2: adult ewes BHS #41 and #42 and adult ram BHS #C). The study pens had either never previously housed domestic or bighorn sheep (pen 1 in experiment 1; both pens in experiment 2) or had been rested for greater than one year since their previous occupancy by any *M. ovipneumoniae*infected sheep (pens 2 and 3 in experiment 1) prior to these experiments.

Experimental Design

Experiment 1.

A domestic ewe (DS #00) was placed in isolation and experimentally infected with *M. ovipneumoniae.* The inoculum consisted of ceftiofur-treated (100 ug/ml, 2 hrs, 37°C; Pfizer, Florham Park, NJ) nasal wash fluids from a domestic sheep naturally colonized with *M. ovipneumoniae* [16]. Following ceftiofur treatment, no aerobic bacterial growth was observed from the nasal wash fluids cultured under conditions expected to permit growth of *M. haemolytica, B. trehalosi,* or *P. multocida* (Columbia blood agar with 5% sheep blood, 35°C, overnight, 5% CO_2). DS #00 was then challenged with the treated nasal wash fluid by infusion of 15 ml in each nares, 10 ml orally and 5 ml into each conjunctival sac. Subsequent nasal swab samples obtained on days 1, 2, 4 and 7 post-challenge were all PCR positive for *M. ovipneumoniae* using the method described later in the 'Microbiological testing' section confirming that the experimental infection had been successful. On post challenge day 7, DS #00 was introduced into pen #1 with BHS #82. Following commingling, DS #00 and BHS #82 were restrained for collection of nasal swab samples on days 1, 2, 4, 7, 14, 21, 28, and subsequently at 30 day intervals until the experiment was terminated. Rectal temperatures were recorded from both sheep approximately twice each week. Sheep in pens #2 (BHS #89 and DS #01) and #3 (BHS #07 and DS #LA) were restrained for rectal temperature determination and collection of nasal swabs for microbiology at approximately monthly intervals. All pens were observed daily for clinical signs of respiratory disease. The experiment was conducted October 2009–January 2010.

Experiment 2.

BHS #39 was inoculated with *M. ovipneumoniae* just prior to its release into pen #1 with non-inoculated BHS #38 and

#40. Non-inoculated BHS #C, #41, and #42 were housed in pen #2 on the same day. The inoculum for BHS #39 was prepared as described for that used in experiment 1 but originated from a different domestic sheep source. In lieu of computation of colony forming units, which is not possible for *M. ovipneumoniae* due to inconsistent growth on plated media, viable *M. ovipneumoniae* counts in the inoculum were determined using most probable number (MPN) using a custom 3×4 format: Triplicate enrichment broth tubes were inoculated at each of four decimal dilutions (10^{-2}–10^{-5}) of the treated nasal wash fluid [17], incubated (72 hrs, 35C) then PCR was used to detect growth of viable *M. ovipneumoniae*. The treated fluid was determined to contain 930 MPN/ml (95% confidence interval, 230 to 3800 MPN). Two of the bighorn sheep (BHS #38 and #39) in pen 1 were recaptured by drive net on day 21 of the experiment for nasal swab sampling to detect *M. ovipneumoniae* infection; otherwise, no live animal sampling was conducted in experiment #2 to reduce the risk of traumatic injury of the wild bighorn sheep involved. The experiment was conducted December 2011–June 2012.

Biosecurity.

In both experiments, routine biosecurity measures included: 1) the pens containing the single*M. ovipneumoniae*-challenged animals (exposed pens) were located downwind of the prevailing wind direction from the pens containing no experimentally *M. ovipneumoniae* exposed animals (clean pens), 2) order of entry rules were established so that on any single day exposed pens were routinely entered by animal care staff for feeding and cleaning only after all work in clean pens had been completed, and 3) personal protective equipment (coveralls and boots) used in exposed pens were either not reused, or were sanitized prior to use in clean pens.

Clinical Scores.

Clinical score data were determined using the following cumulative point system: observed anorexia (1), nasal discharge (1), cough (2), dyspnea (1), head shaking (1), ear paresis (1) and weakness/incoordination (1).

Microbiological Testing.

Routine diagnostic testing performed by the Washington Animal Diagnostic Laboratory (fully accredited by the American Association of Veterinary Laboratory Diagnosticians) included detection of *M. ovipneumoniae*-specific and small ruminant lentivirus-specific antibodies in serum samples using competitive enzyme-linked immunosorbent assays (cELISA) [14], [18],[19], detection of *M. ovipneumoniae* colonization by broth enrichment of nasal swabs followed by *M. ovipneumoniae*-specific PCR testing of the broths [20], [21], detection of Pasteurellaceae in pharyngeal swab samples by aerobic bacteriologic cultures, and detection of exposure to parainfluenza-3, border disease, and respiratory syncytial viruses by virus neutralization antibody assays applied to serum samples.

PCR tests specific for detection of *M. haemolytica*, *B. trehalosi*, and *P. multocida*, and *lktA*(the gene encoding the principal virulence factor of *M. haemolytica* and *B. trehalosi)* were applied to DNA extracted from pneumonic lung tissues using previously described primers (Table 1) and methods with minor modifications. All reactions were conducted individually in 20 µL volumes containing 80–300 ng of template DNA. For *M. haemolytica*, *B. trehalosi*, *lktA* and*P. multocida*, reactions contained 0.5 units of HotStar Taq DNA polymerase (Qiagen), 2 µL 10x PCR buffer (Qiagen), 4 µL Q-solution (Qiagen), 40 µM of each dNTP (Invitrogen). The *M. ovipneumoniae* reaction used QIAGEN Multiplex PCR mix. Primers were used at final concentrations of 0.2 µM (*M. haemolytica*, *B. trehalosi*, *P. multocida*, and *M. ovipneumoniae*) or 0.5 µM (leukotoxin A). Each reaction included an initial activation and denaturation step (95°C, 15 min) and a final 72°C extension step (10 min for Mhgcp-2, lktA, lktA set-1, and LM primers; 9 min for KMT primers; 5 min for Btsod and Mhgcp primers). Cycling conditions were as follows: *M. ovipneumoniae*, 30 cycles of 95°C for 30 s, 58°C for 30 s, 72°C for 30 s; *B. trehalosi* and *M. haemolytica* (Mhgcp and Btsod primers), 35 cycles of 95°C for 30 s, 55°C for 30 s, 72°C for 40 s; *P. multocida* and *lktA* (lktA primers), 30 cycles of 95°C for 60 s, 55°C for 60 s, 72°C for 60 s; *M. haemolytica* (Mhgcp-2 primers), 40 cycles of 95°C for 30 s, 54°C for 30 s, 72°C for 30 s; *lktA* (lktA set-1 primers), 40 cycles of 95°C for 30 s, 52°C for 30 s, 72°C for 40 s. Leukotoxin expression was detected in Pasteurellaceae isolates by MTT dye reduction cytotoxicity assay as described previously [22].

Table 1: Primers and PCR reaction targets used in these experiments

Pathogen/Virulence gene	Target	Primer Name	Sequence (5′ → 3′)	Size (bp)	Reference
M. haemolytica	*gcp*	MhgcpF	AGA GGC CAA TCT GCA AAC CTC G	267	[33]
		MhgcpR	GTT CGT ATT GCC CAA CGC CG		
M. haemolytica	*gcp*	MhgcpF2	TGG GCA ATA CGA ACT ACT CGG G	227	[34]
		MhgcpR2	CTT TAA TCG TAT TCG CAG		
B. trehalosi	*sodA*	BtsodAF	GCC TGC GGA CAA ACG TGT TG	144	[33]
		BtsodAR	TTT CAA CAG AAC CAA AAT CAC GAA TG		
P. multocida	*kmt1*	KMT1T7	ATC CGC TAT TTA CCC AGT GG	460	[35]
		KMT1SP6	GCT GTA AAC GAA CTC GCC AC		
Pasteurellaceae leukotoxin	*lktA*	lktAF	TGT GGA TGC GTT TGA AGA AGG	1,145	[36]
		lktAR	ACT TGC TTT GAG GTG ATC CG		
M. haemolytica leukotoxin	*lktA*	lktAF set-1	CTT ACA TTT TAG CCC AAC GTG	497	[34]
		lktAR set-1	TAA ATT CGC AAG ATA ACG GG		
Mycoplasma ovipneumoniae	16s rDNA	LMF	TGA ACG GAA TAT GTT AGC TT	361	[20,21]
		LMR	GAC TTC ATC CTG CAC TCT GT		
Mycoplasma ovipneumoniae	16S–23S IGS	MoIGSF	GGA ACA CCT CCT TTC TAC GG	Variable~490	[23]
		MoIGSR	CCA AGG CAT CCA CCA AAT AC		

The 16S–23S ribosomal operon intergenic spacer (IGS) regions of *M. ovipneumoniae*recovered from animals in these studies were PCR amplified (Table 1) and sequenced as previously described [23].

16S rDNA analyses to identify the predominant bacterial flora in pneumonic lung tissues.

In previous studies, culture-independent evaluation of the microbial flora of lung tissues in naturally occurring bighorn sheep pneumonia revealed a polymicrobial flora late in the disease course [13], [23]. For comparison, we applied the same methods to lung tissues of the experimentally challenged animals in this study. Note that more sensitive detection of specific respiratory pathogens was provided by the PCR assays described earlier, whereas these 16S studies were designed instead to identify the numerically predominant bacteria in affected lungs. The library size used was based on the binary distribution to provide a 95% chance of detection of each taxon comprising 10% or more of the ribosomal operon frequency in the source tissue. Two 1 g samples of pneumonic lung tissues were aseptically collected from sites at least 10 cm apart, homogenized by stomaching, and DNA was extracted (DNeasy tissue kit; Qiagen, Valencia, CA) from 100 uL aliquots of each homogenate. 16S rDNA segments were PCR amplified and cloned as described [13]. Insert DNA was sequenced from 16 clones derived from each of the two homogenates from each animal, and each sequence was attributed to species (≥99% identity) or genus (≥97% identity) based on BLAST GenBank similarity [24].

RESULTS

Experiment 1

M. ovipneumoniae infection of DS #00, introduced into pen 1 to start the experiment, was confirmed by positive nasal swab samples obtained on days 1, 4, and 7 after inoculation prior to its introduction into pen #1, and on days 1, 2, 4, 7, 14, 21, 28, 60 and 90 after its introduction into pen #1, confirming that the experimental colonization had been successful and maintained throughout experiment 1. *M. ovipneumoniae* was first detected in the bighorn sheep (BHS #82) commingled with DS #00 in pen #1 on day 28, and subsequent tests on days 60 and 90 were also positive. BHS #82 developed signs of respiratory disease including nasal discharge (onset day 37); coughing and fever (onset day 42); and lethargy and ear paresis (onset day 61) (Figure 1a). Signs of respiratory disease were observed in the bighorn sheep in pens #2 (BHS #89) and #3 (BHS #07) beginning on days 62 and 67, respectively; these signs also included fever, lethargy, paroxysmal coughing, nasal discharge, head shaking, and drooping ears. No signs of respiratory disease were observed in the commingled domestic sheep at any time during the experiment. *M. ovipneumoniae* was detected in nasal swab samples from all bighorn and domestic sheep in pens #2 and #3 when sampled on day 70. The bighorn sheep were euthanized for necropsy on days 93 (BHS #89) and 99 (BHS #82 and #07). At necropsy, significant abnormal findings were limited to the respiratory tract. Bronchopneumonia affecting 25–50% of the lung volume was observed in all three bighorn sheep (Figure 2). Histopathological examination revealed peribronchiolitis with large lymphoid cuffs, bronchiectasis with purulent exudates, pulmonary atelectasis, and hyperplastic bronchial epithelia lacking visible cilia (Figure 2).

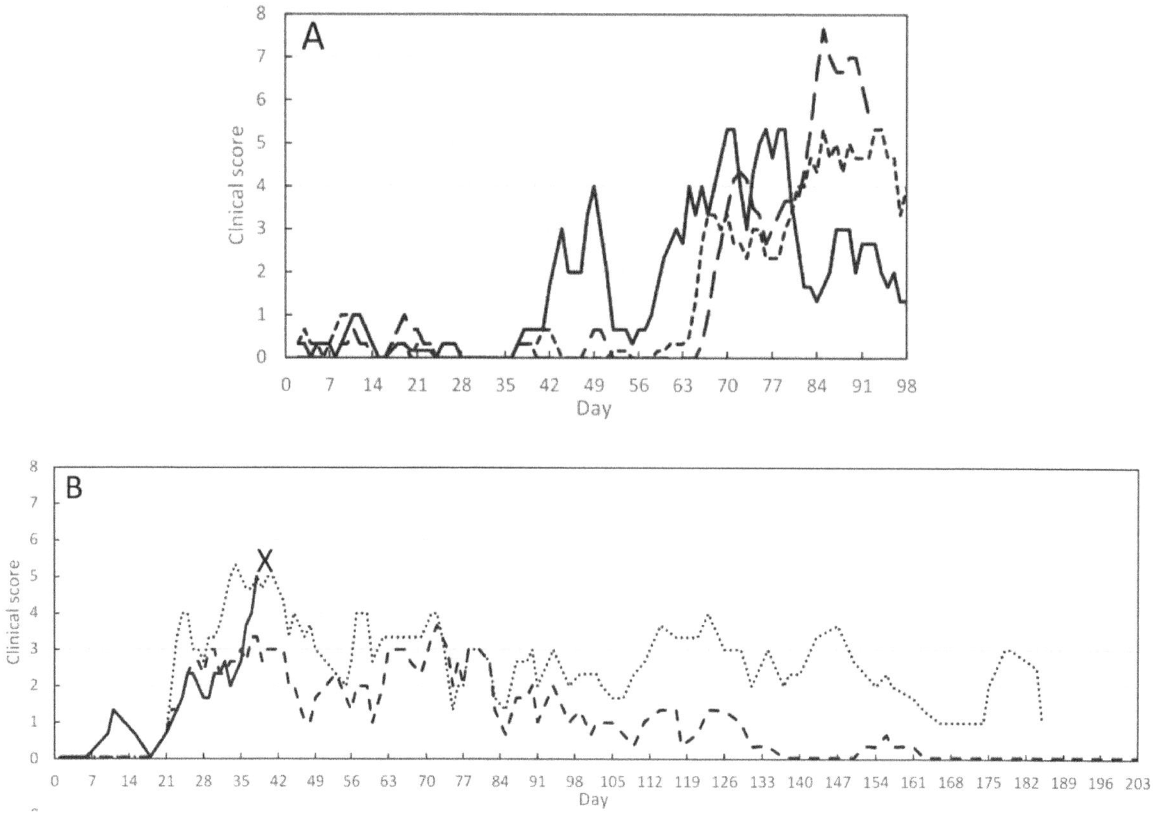

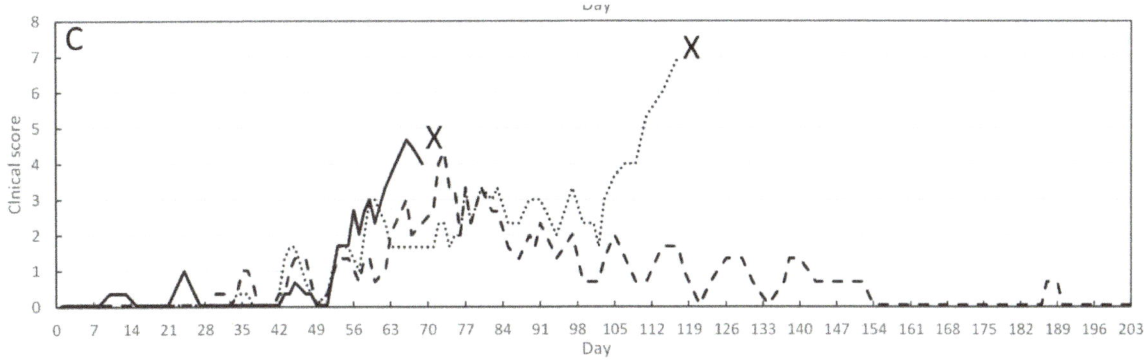

Figure 1: Clinical signs exhibited by *M. ovipneumoniae* **infected bighorn sheep.**

Clinical scores (3-day moving averages) of bighorn sheep following introduction of *M. ovipneumoniae*: A) Experiment 1, 3 separate pens; solid line, Pen 1, BHS #82; dashed line, Pen 2, BHS #89; dotted line, Pen 3, BHS #07; B) Experiment 2, Pen 1: solid line, BHS #39 (died day 34); dashed line, BHS #40; dotted line; BHS #38.; C) Experiment 2, Pen 2: solid line, BHS #42 (euthanized day 109); dotted line, BHS #41 (died day 65); dashed line, BHS #C.

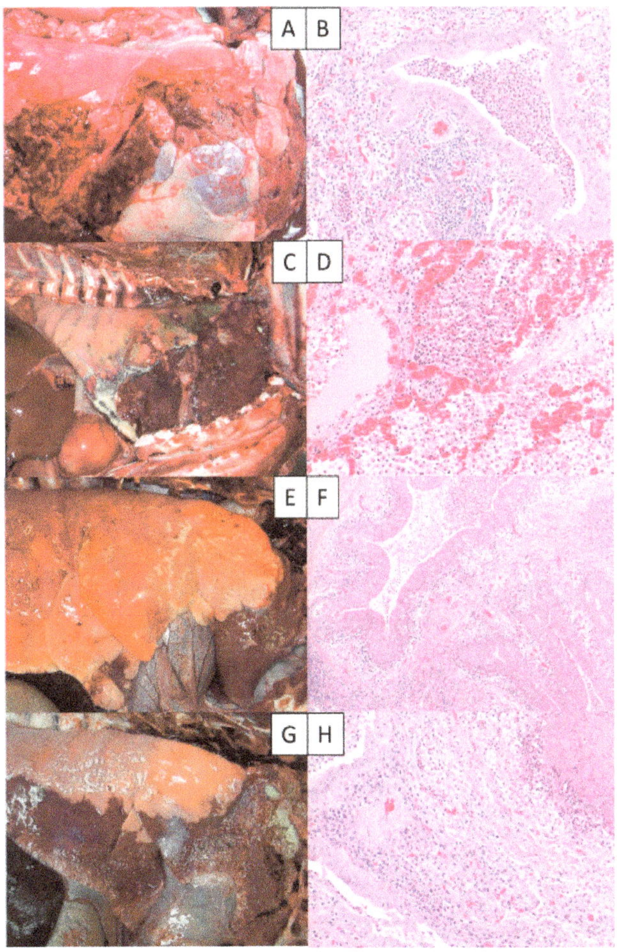

Figure 2: Gross and histologic lesions in lungs of bighorn sheep experimentally infected with *M. ovipneumoniae*.

Images of BHS #82 (A, B), BHS #39 (C, D), BHS #C (E, F) and BHS #42 (G, H). Original magnification of histologic images was 200X (B, D, H) or 100X (F).

Experiment 2

On day 21 following release of the inoculated bighorn into pen #1, *M. ovipneumoniae* was detected in the inoculated animal and one pen mate (BHS #38 and #39); the third animal (BHS #40) evaded capture and sampling on that day. The first signs of respiratory disease were observed in pen #1 animals on day 21 during drive net capture for sampling, apparently triggered by exertion (Figure 2a). On day 34, inoculated BHS #39 died in pen #1. On day 49, signs of respiratory disease were first observed in the bighorn sheep in pen #2 (Figure 2b). On days 65 and 109, #41, and #42 in pen #2 died or were euthanized *in extremis*. The surviving three bighorn sheep exhibited varying degrees of respiratory disease: BHS #38 showed persistent respiratory disease, while BHS #40 and #C showed decreasing respiratory disease over time, which became minimal after days 161 and 154, respectively. On day 204, the three surviving bighorn sheep were euthanized for necropsy. At necropsy, significant abnormal findings were limited to the respiratory tract. All six bighorn sheep had bronchopneumonia, with consolidation of lung tissue volumes ranging from an estimated 5% (BHS #40) to 80–100% (BHS #41) (Figure 2). Histopathological examination revealed severe peribronchiolitis with large lymphoid cuffs as seen in experiment 1. Animals that died or were euthanized in extremis had an overlying necrotizing bronchiolitis (#39) or abscessing bronchiolitis with bronchiectasis (BHS #41, #42) (Figure 2).

Microbiology

All bighorn sheep in both experiments seroconverted to *M. ovipneumoniae* (Table 2). Most experimental animals had neutralizing antibody to parainfluenza-3 virus, but no significant changes in antibody titers were observed during the experimental period. Detectable antibody to other ovine respiratory viruses, including border disease virus, ovine progressive pneumonia virus, and respiratory syncytial virus was occasionally observed in single samples.

Table 2: Antibody responses to *M. ovipneumoniae* and parainfluenza-3 (PI-3) virus

Experiment	ID	Pen	*M. ovipneumoniae*[1]		PI-3 virus[2]	
			Pre[3]	Post[3]	Pre[3]	Post[3]
1	82	1	−8%	93%	512	512
1	89	2	−7%	88%	128	128
1	07	3	−1%	92%	256	512
2	38	1	−6%	74%	Neg	64
2	39	1	−13%	67%	Neg	<32
2	40	1	−23%	75%	64	512
2	41	2	−19%	82%	512	NT
2	42	2	−11%	82%	256	NT
2	C	2	−4%	66%	256	512

[1]*M. ovipneumoniae* antibody detected by cELISA, expressed as percentage inhibition of the binding of an agent-specific monoclonal antibody [14,18].
[2]PI-3 virus neutralizing antibody detected by virus neutralization [37].
[3]Pre samples in experiment 1 were obtained on the day that the *M. ovipneumoniae* colonized domestic sheep was introduced to pen 1 and in experiment 2 were obtained on the day that BHS #39 was inoculated with *M. ovipneumoniae*. 'Post' samples in both experiments were obtained at necropsy. Neg = No titer detected. NT = Not tested, due to inadequate specimen volume.

Table 3: Microbiologic findings from pneumonic lung tissues, based on aerobic culture and species specific PCR

Expt.	ID	Bacterial pathogens identified in pneumonic lung tissues				
		B. trehalosi	*M. haemolytica*	*lktA*	*M. ovipneumoniae*	Other[5]
1	82	Cult, *sodA*[1]	Neg[2]	Pos[3]	16S[4]	None
1	89	Cult, *sodA*	Neg	Neg[3]	16S	*Pasteurella* sp.[5]
1	07	Cult, *sodA*	Neg	Pos	16S	*Pasteurella* sp.
2	38	Cult, *sodA*	Neg	Neg	16S	*Pasteurella* sp.
2	39	NT, *sodA*	NT, Neg[2]	Neg	16S	NT[5]
2	40	Cult	Neg	Neg	Neg[4]	*Trueperella pyogenes*[5]
2	41	Cult, *sodA*	Neg	Neg	16S	None
2	42	Cult	Neg	Neg	16S	None
2	C	Cult	Neg	Neg	16S	*Pasteurella* sp.

[1]Cult = *B. trehalosi* detected by bacterial culture; *sodA* = *B. trehalosi* detected by *sodA* species-specific PCR (Table 1); NT = Unable to test by bacterial culture (overgrowth by *Proteus* sp.).
[2]Neg = *M. haemolytica* not detected by either bacterial culture or by PCR with either *gcp* primer set (Table 1); NT = Unable to test by bacterial culture (overgrowth by *Proteus* sp.).
[3]Neg = Pasteurellaceae *lktA* not detected in DNA extracts from pneumonic lung tissues by two different *lktA* PCRs (Table 1) [34,36]. Pos = *lktA* detected in *B. trehalosi* isolates obtained from BHS #82 and #07 [36].
[4]16S = *M. ovipneumoniae* detected by PCR (Table 1) [20]; Neg = *M. ovipneumoniae* not detected by PCR.
[5]*Pasteurella* sp., *Trueperella pyogenes* = Bacteria isolated and identified by aerobic culture; *Pasteurella* sp. were determined not to be *B. trehalosi*, *M. haemolytica*, or *P. multocida*; NT = Unable to test by bacterial culture due to overgrowth by *Proteus* sp.

Culture Independent Survey of Bacteria in Pneumonic Bighorn Sheep Lung Tissues

DNA sequences of cloned 16S rDNA revealed that the predominant bacterial species in pneumonic sections of lung were diverse (Table 4). In experiment 1, *M. ovipneumoniae* was detected in the lung tissues of all animals. *B. trehalosi* also comprised substantial proportions of the pneumonic lung flora in two animals (BHS #82 and #07), while obligate anaerobic species, primarily Fusobacterium spp., predominated in the third animal (BHS #89). The flora identified in the pneumonic lungs of the animals in experiment 2 was also substantially comprised of mixed obligate anaerobes especially *Fusobacterium* spp. (Table 4).

Table 4: Microbiologic findings by 16S clone library (culture independent) method

Expt.	ID	Bacterial species identified in pneumonic lung tissues					
		Btre[1]	Movi[1]	Fuso[1]	Prev[1]	Porphyro[1]	Other[1]
1	82	20 (62.5)[2]	8 (25)	0	3 (9.4)	0	1 (3.1)
1	89	1 (3.1)	7 (21.9)	21 (65.6)	1 (3.1)	0	2 (6.3)
1	07	16 (50.0)	12 (37.5)	0	0	0	4 (12.5)
2	38	4 (7.1)	2 (3.6)	8 (14.3)	20 (35.7)	9 (16.1)	13 (23.2)
2	C	0	0	17 (30.4)	5 (8.9)	19 (33.9)	15 (26.8)
2	39	2 (6.3)	0	24 (75.0)	0	0	6 (18.8)
2	40	0	0	0	0	0	56 (100.0)
2	41	1 (3.1)	0	21 (65.6)	5 (15.6)	0	5 (15.6)
2	42	0	0	31 (96.9)	0	0	1 (3.1)

[1]Btre = *B. trehalosi*; Movi = *M. ovipneumoniae*; Fuso = *Fusobacterium* sp.; Prev = *Prevotella* sp.; Porphyro = *Porphyromonas* sp.; Other = taxa other than those previously listed, each comprising <5% of sequenced clones.
[2]N (%) of the sequenced 16S clones from each animal whose DNA sequences were identical to those of the tabulated bacterial species in each column.
doi:10.1371/journal.pone.0110039.t004

Molecular Epidemiology of Respiratory Pathogens.

Consistent with epidemic transmission, *M. ovipneumoniae* strains recovered from all experimental sheep within each experiment shared identical IGS DNA sequences with the respective challenge inoculum (GenBank HQ615162 in experiment 1; KJ551511 in experiment 2).

DISCUSSION

The most striking finding of these experiments was the high transmissibility of *M. ovipneumoniae* and the consistent development of pneumonia that followed infection of bighorn sheep. The bacterium was naturally transmitted from single experimentally inoculated animals (a domestic sheep in experiment 1 and a bighorn sheep in experiment 2) to all animals within and between pens up to 12 m distant. Eight of nine bighorn sheep exposed to *M. ovipneumoniae* developed severe bronchopneumonia and three died, while all the domestic sheep remained healthy.

Previous experimental challenge studies conducted with *M. haemolytica or B. trehalosi* in the absence of *M. ovipneumoniae* have not documented transmission. For example, Foreyt et al.[8] reported a series of three experiments in which commingled bighorn sheep were either challenged with intra-tracheal *M. haemolytica* or given sterile BHI as controls. Four of the five control bighorn sheep survived without evidence of disease while commingled with eight *M. haemolytica*-challenged bighorn sheep, of which seven died of pneumonia [8]. Commingled bighorn sheep also remained healthy in several other studies where individual bighorn sheep died with apparent *M. haemolytica* bronchopneumonia (confirmed by isolation of this bacterium from lung tissues) [15], [25], [26].

In addition to high transmissibility, the time course of disease development and the predominant microbiology of the pneumonic lung tissues following experimental introduction of*M. ovipneumoniae* differed from that seen in previous bighorn sheep challenge experiments with other respiratory pathogens. Bighorn sheep directly challenged with leukotoxin positive *M. haemolytica* or *B. trehalosi* develop peracute bronchopneumonia and >90% die within a week of challenges with 10^5 cfu or more [16], [27]–[30]. In contrast, disease following experimental*M. ovipneumoniae* exposures was considerably slower in onset (14–21 days post infection) and development (deaths occurring 34 to 109 days post infection; respiratory disease persisted up to 6 months post-infection); this slow time course closely resembles that documented previously in bighorn lamb pneumonia outbreaks [13]. After lethal *M. haemolytica* challenge, the agent is typically isolated from lung tissues in high numbers and pure cultures [15], [25]; in contrast in naturally occurring pneumonia outbreaks *M. ovipneumoniae* may be predominant early in the disease course but 16S library analyses have been used to document its overgrowth by diverse other bacteria later in the disease course [14], [23]. Although the numbers of animals in the experimental *M. ovipneumoniae* infection studies reported here are small, the results are consistent with the trend for early predominance of *M. ovipneumoniae*followed by overgrowth by diverse other bacterial later in the disease course (Tables 3 and 4)[13], [14], [23].

Our results also differ from our previous attempt to experimentally reproduce respiratory disease by challenge inoculation of 1-week-old bighorn lambs with *M. ovipneumoniae*, which produced minor lesions and seroconversion but no clinically significant respiratory disease[13]. However, laboratory passage of*M. ovipneumoniae* (as was performed in that experiment) has been reported to attenuate virulence in *M. ovipneumoniae* [31]. Challenge of bighorn sheep with un-passaged *M. ovipneumoniae* produced different results, as observed here in experiment #2. In another study [16], nasal washings from domestic sheep naturally colonized with *M. ovipneumoniae* or lung homogenates from a *M. ovipneumoniae*-infected bighorn sheep were used for challenge of bighorn sheep after ceftiofur treatment to eliminate detectable Pasteurellaceae. Consistent with increased virulence of un-passaged *M. ovipneumoniae*, infection and respiratory disease signs were observed in all four bighorn sheep, one of which died 19 days following challenge. The three surviving animals continued to exhibit respiratory disease signs for 42 days, at which time the experiment was terminated by challenge with *M. haemolytica* (using a dose documented to be rapidly fatal to bighorn sheep even in the absence of *M. ovipneumoniae*) [16]. As a result, the longer term effects of the mycoplasma infection were not determined in that study. Therefore, the experiments reported here are the first in which naïve bighorn sheep were exposed to un-passaged *M. ovipneumoniae* and then followed over a time period comparable with the naturally occurring disease course.

The possibility of viral agents contributing to the disease observed in this study cannot be completely ruled out, since the inoculum was derived from nasal washings from domestic sheep and no virucidal treatments were applied. However, a previous study using ultrafiltrates of bighorn sheep pneumonic lung tissues or nasal washings from domestic sheep failed to reproduce any respiratory disease in inoculated susceptible bighorn sheep [16]. In addition, serologic monitoring for the predominant domestic sheep respiratory viruses did not demonstrate seroconversion of the experimental animals in this study, as described in the Results and in Table 2. Therefore, the most parsimonious interpretation of the data presented here is that the disease observed resulted from *M. ovipneumoniae* infection and the sequelae of that infection.

The transmission of *M. ovipneumoniae* from pen-to-pen in these experiments strongly suggests that direct contact is not necessary for epizootic spread of pneumonia in bighorn sheep. Feeding, watering and other procedures involving animal care or research staff were designed to minimize the risk of human or fomite-mediated transmission of the pathogen from pen to pen, although we recognize it is impossible to completely rule out this possibility. On the other hand, since aerosolized droplet transmission is recognized as a transmission route for the closely related bacterium, *Mycoplasma hyopneumoniae* (the cause of atypical pneumonia of swine) [32], it is plausible that a similar transmission mode occurs with *M. ovipneumoniae*. Infectious aerosols generated by coughing animals would likely contribute to the explosive nature of the pneumonia outbreaks observed following initial introduction of *M. ovipneumoniae* into naïve bighorn sheep populations.

In conclusion, we demonstrated that experimental *M. ovipneumoniae* infection of naïve bighorn sheep induces chronic, severe bronchopneumonia associated with multiple secondary bacterial infections and that this infection spread rapidly to animals both within the same pen and to animals in nearby pens. The significance of these findings would be clarified by parallel experiments specifically designed to determine transmissibility and associated disease outcomes in other agents associated with bighorn sheep pneumonia, particularly *M. haemolytica,* in the absence of *M. ovipneumoniae.* Furthermore, the case-fatality rates of *M. ovipneumoniae* infected animals described here contrasts with the nearly 100% mortality that follows experimental commingling of bighorn sheep with presumptively or documented *M. ovipneumoniae*-positive domestic sheep and suggests an important role for polymicrobial secondary infections in determining mortality rates, which could be investigated in future studies. Finally, *M. ovipneumoniae* was still detected in nasal swab samples of several surviving bighorn sheep that were euthanized at the completion of these studies, suggesting that survivors of naturally occurring pneumonia outbreaks may continue to carry and shed this agent in nasal secretions. Such carriage may provide a mechanism for the post-invasion disease epizootics in lambs described in free-ranging populations. If so, this presumptive carrier state requires further study to characterize the factors that determine its occurrence and persistence, as these may be critical for the development of effective management control measures for this devastating disease.

ACKNOWLEDGMENTS

We thank Donald P. Knowles for his contribution to the design of experiment 1 and manuscript editing, Margaret Highland for skillful technical assistance and for manuscript editing, Glen Weiser for providing custom selective media for Pasteurellaceae, Duane Chandler and Amy Hetrick for assistance with animal care, handling and restraint and sample collection, George Barrington for providing access to *M. ovipneumoniae* free domestic sheep, the Washington Department of Fish and Wildlife for wild bighorn sheep, Katie Baker for skillful technical assistance, and Shannon Lee Swist for serving as Principal Investigator of the Wyoming Wildlife/Livestock Disease Partnership grant.

AUTHOR CONTRIBUTIONS

Conceived and designed the experiments: TEB EFC JLO S. Srikumaran WJF. Performed the experiments: TEB EFC JLO KAP KL S. Shanthalingam. Analyzed the data: TEB EFC KAP KL. Contributed reagents/materials/analysis tools: TEB EFC KAP KL S. Shanthalingam S. Srikumaran. Contributed to the writing of the manuscript: TEB EFC KAP S. Shanthalingam S. Srikumaran WJF.

REFERENCES

1. Festa-Bianchet M (2008) *Ovis canadensis*. The IUCN Red List of Threatened Species. Available: http://www.iucnredlist.org/details/summary/15735/0. Accessed 2014 Jul 24.
2. Cassirer EF, Plowright RK, Manlove KR, Cross PC, Dobson AP, et al. (2012) Spatio-temporal dynamics of pneumonia in bighorn sheep (*Ovis canadensis*). J Animal Ecol 82: 518–528. doi: 10.1111/1365-2656.12031
3. Marsh H (1938) Pneumonia in Rocky Mountain bighorn sheep. J Mammal 19: 214–219. doi: 10.2307/1374617
4. Buechner HK (1960) The bighorn sheep in the United States, its past, present, and future. Wildl Monog 4: 3–174.
5. Forrester DJ (1971) Bighorn sheep lungworm-pneumonia complex. In: Davis JW, Anderson RC, editors. Parasitic Diseases of Wild Mammals. Ames, IA: Iowa State University Press. 158–173.
6. Demartini JC, Davies RB (1977) An epizootic of pneumonia in captive bighorn sheep infected with *Muellerius* sp. J Wildl Dis 13: 117–124. doi: 10.7589/0090-3558-13.2.117
7. Miller MW (2001) Pasteurellosis. In: Williams ES, Barker, I K., editor. Infectious diseases of wild mammals. Ames IA USA: Iowa State University Press. 558.
8. Foreyt WJ, Snipes KP, Kasten RW (1994) Fatal pneumonia following inoculation of healthy bighorn sheep with *Pasteurella haemolytica* from healthy domestic sheep. J Wildl Dis 30: 137–145. doi: 10.7589/0090-3558-30.2.137
9. Kraabel BJ, Miller MW, Conlon JA, McNeil HJ (1998) Evaluation of a multivalent*Pasteurella haemolytica* vaccine in bighorn sheep: Protection from experimental challenge. J Wildl Dis 34: 325–333. doi: 10.7589/0090-3558-34.2.325
10. Rudolph KM, Hunter DL, Foreyt WJ, Cassirer EF, Rimler RB, et al. (2003) Sharing of*Pasteurella* spp. between free-ranging bighorn sheep and feral goats. J Wildl Dis 39: 897–903. doi: 10.7589/0090-3558-39.4.897
11. Rudolph KM, Hunter DL, Rimler RB, Cassirer EF, Foreyt WJ, et al. (2007) Microorganisms associated with a pneumonic epizootic in Rocky Mountain bighorn sheep (*Ovis canadensis canadensis*). J Zoo Wildl Med 38: 548–558. doi: 10.1638/2006-0027r.1
12. Weiser GC, DeLong WJ, Paz JL, Shafii B, Price WJ, et al. (2003) Characterization of*Pasteurella multocida* associated with pneumonia in bighorn sheep. J Wildl Dis 39: 536–544. doi: 10.7589/0090-3558-39.3.536
13. Besser TE, Cassirer EF, Potter KA, VanderSchalie J, Fischer A, et al. (2008) Association of *Mycoplasma ovipneumoniae* infection with population-limiting respiratory disease in free-ranging rocky mountain bighorn sheep (*Ovis canadensis canadensis*). J Clin Microbiol 46: 423–430. doi: 10.1128/jcm.01931-07
14. Besser TE, EF Cassirer, MA Highland, P Wolff, A Justice-Allen (2012) et.al (2012) Bighorn sheep pneumonia: Sorting out the cause of a polymicrobial disease. Prev Vet Med 108: 85–93. doi: 10.1016/j.prevetmed.2013.02.020
15. Besser TE, Cassirer EF, Yamada C, Potter KA, Herndon C, et al. (2012) Survival of Bighorn Sheep (*Ovis canadensis*) Commingled with Domestic Sheep (*Ovis aries*) in the Absence of *Mycoplasma ovipneumoniae*. J Wildl Dis 48: 168–172. doi: 10.7589/0090-3558-48.1.168
16. Dassanayake RP, Shanthalingam S, Herndon CN, Subramaniam R, Lawrence PK, et al. (2010) *Mycoplasma ovipneumoniae* can predispose bighorn sheep to

fatal*Mannheimia haemolytica* pneumonia. Vet Microbiol 145: 354–359. doi: 10.1016/j.vetmic.2010.04.011

17. Blodgett R (2010) Bacteriologic Analytical Manual Appendix 2: Most Probable Number from Serial Dilutions. Washington DC. Available: http://www.fda.gov/Food/FoodScienceResearch/LaboratoryMethods/ucm109656.htm. Accessed 2014 Jul 24.

18. Ziegler JC, Lahmers KK, Barrington GM, Parish SM, Kilzer K, et al. (2014) Safety and Immunogenicity of a Mycoplasma ovipneumoniae Bacterin for Domestic Sheep (*Ovis aries*). PLoS One 9(4): e95698. doi: 10.1371/journal.pone.0095698

19. Herrmann LM, Cheevers WP, Marshall KL, McGuire TC, Hutton MM, et al. (2003) Detection of serum antibodies to ovine progressive pneumonia virus in sheep by using a caprine arthritis-encephalitis virus competitive-inhibition enzyme-linked immunosorbent assay. Clin Diag Lab Immunol 10: 862–865. doi: 10.1128/cdli.10.5.862-865.2003

20. Lawrence PK, Shanthalingam S, Dassanayake RP, Subramaniam R, Herndon CN, et al. (2010) Transmission of *Mannheimia haemolytica* from domestic sheep (*Ovis aries*) to bighorn sheep (*Ovis canadensis*): unequivocal demonstration with green fluorescent protein-tagged organisms. J Wildl Dis 46: 706–717; erratum, J Wildl Dis 46: 1346. doi: 10.7589/0090-3558-46.3.706

21. McAuliffe L, Hatchell FM, Ayling RD, King AI, Nicholas RA (2003) Detection of*Mycoplasma ovipneumoniae* in *Pasteurella*-vaccinated sheep flocks with respiratory disease in England. Vet Rec 153: 687–688. doi: 10.1136/vr.153.22.687

22. Gentry MJ, Srikumaran S (1991) Neutralizing monoclonal antibodies to *Pasteurella haemolytica l*eukotoxin affinity purify the toxin from crude culture supernatants. Microb Pathog 10: 411–417. doi: 10.1016/0882-4010(91)90086-p

23. Besser TE, Highland M, Baker K, Anderson NJ, Ramsey JM (2012) Causes of pneumonia epizootics among bighorn sheep, western United States, 2008–2010. Emerg Infect Dis 18: 406–414. doi: 10.3201/eid1803.111554

24. Petti CA (2007) Detection and identification of microorganisms by gene amplification and sequencing. Clin Infect Dis 44: 1108–1114. doi: 10.1086/512818

25. Foreyt WJ, Jenkins EJ, Appleyard GD (2009) Transmission of lungworms (*Muellerius capillaris*) from domestic goats to bighorn sheep on common pasture. J Wildl Dis 45: 272–278. doi: 10.7589/0090-3558-45.2.272

26. Foreyt WJ, Lagerquist JE (1996) Experimental contact of bighorn sheep (*Ovis canadensis*) with horses and cattle, and comparison of neutrophil sensitivity to*Pasteurella haemolytica* cytotoxins. J Wildl Dis 32: 594–602.

27. Onderka DK, Rawluk SA, Wishart WD (1988) Susceptibility of Rocky Mountain bighorn sheep and domestic sheep to pneumonia induced by bighorn and domestic livestock strains of *Pasteurella haemolytica*. Can J Vet Res 52: 439–444. doi: 10.7589/0090-3558-24.4.663

28. Dassanayake RP, Shanthalingam S, Herndon CN, Lawrence PK, Cassirer EF, et al. (2009) *Mannheimia haemolytica* serotype A1 exhibits differential pathogenicity in two related species, *Ovis canadensis* and *Ovis aries*. Vet Microbiol 133: 366–371. doi: 10.1016/j.vetmic.2008.07.015

29. Subramaniam R, Shanthalingam S, Bavananthasivam J, Kugadas A, Potter KA, et al. (2011) A multivalent *Mannheimia-Bibersteinia* vaccine protects bighorn sheep against*Mannheimia haemolytica* challenge. Clin Vaccine Immunol 18: 1689–1694. doi: 10.1128/cvi.05276-11

30. Foreyt WJ, Snipes KP, Kasten RW (1994) Fatal pneumonia following inoculation of healthy bighorn sheep with *Pasteurella haemolytica* from healthy domestic sheep. J Wildl Dis 30: 137–145. doi: 10.7589/0090-3558-30.2.137

31. Alley MR, Ionas G, Clarke JK (1999) Chronic non-progressive pneumonia of sheep in New Zealand - a review of the role of *Mycoplasma ovipneumoniae*. N Z Vet J 47: 155–160. doi: 10.1080/00480169.1999.36135

32. Desrosiers R (2011) Transmission of swine pathogens: different means, different needs. Anim Health Res Rev 12: 1–13. doi: 10.1017/s1466252310000204

33. Dassanayake RP, Call DR, Sawant AA, Casavant NC, Weiser GC, et al. (2010)*Bibersteinia trehalosi* inhibits the growth of *Mannheimia haemolytica* by a proximity-dependent mechanism. Appl Environ Microbiol 76: 1008–1013. doi: 10.1128/aem.02086-09

34. Shanthalingam S, Goldy A, Bavananthasivam J, Subramaniam R, Batra SA, et al. (2014) PCR assay detects *Mannheimia haemolytica i*n culture-negative pneumonic lung tissues of bighorn sheep (*Ovis canadensis*) from outbreaks in the Western USA, 2009–2010. J Wildl Dis 50: 1–10.

35. Townsend KM, Frost AJ, Lee CW, Papadimitriou JM, Dawkins HJ (1998) Development of PCR assays for species- and type-specific identification of *Pasteurella multocida*isolates. J Clin Microbiol 36: 1096–1100.

36. Fisher MA, Weiser GC, Hunter DL, Ward ACS (1999) Use of a polymerase chain reaction method to detect the leukotoxin gene IktA in biogroup and biovariant isolates of *Pasteurella haemolytica* and *P. trehalosi*. Am J Vet Res 60: 1402–1406.

37. Rossi CR, Kiesel GK (1971) Microtiter tests for detecting antibody in bovine serum to parainfluenza 3 virus, infectious bovine rhinotracheitis virus, and bovine virus diarrhea virus. Appl Microbiol 22: 32–36.

CHAPTER 19

SEROEPIDEMIOLOGICAL STUDY OF Q FEVER IN DOMESTIC RUMINANTS IN SEMI-EXTENSIVE GRAZING SYSTEMS

Francisco Ruiz-Fons, Ianire Astobiza, Jesús F Barandika, Ana Hurtado, Raquel Atxaerandio, Ramón A Juste, Ana L García-Pérez

NEIKER- Instituto Vasco de Investigación y Desarrollo Agrario, Department of Animal Health, Berreaga 1, 48160 Derio, Bizkaia, Spain

ABSTRACT

Background

Q fever, a worldwide zoonotic disease caused by *Coxiella burnetii*, is endemic in northern Spain where it has been reported as responsible for large series of human pneumonia cases and domestic ruminants' reproductive disorders. To investigate pathogen exposure among domestic ruminants in semi-extensive grazing systems in northern Spain, a serosurvey was carried out in 1,379 sheep (42 flocks), 626 beef cattle (46 herds) and 115 goats (11 herds). Serum antibodies were analysed by ELISA and positive samples were retested by Complement Fixation test (CFT) to detect recent infections.

Results

ELISA anti-*C. burnetii* antibody prevalence was slightly higher in sheep (11.8 ± 2.0%) than in goats (8.7 ± 5.9%) and beef cattle (6.7 ± 2.0%). Herd prevalence was 74% for ovine, 45% for goat and 43% for bovine. Twenty-one percent of sheep flocks, 27% of goat and 14% of cattle herds had a *C. burnetii* seroprevalence ≥ 20%. Only 15 out of 214 ELISA-positive animals reacted positive by CFT. Age-associated seroprevalence differed between ruminant species with a general increasing pattern with age. No evidence of correlation between abortion history and seroprevalence rates was observed despite the known abortifacient nature of *C. burnetii* in domestic ruminants.

Conclusions

Results reported herein showed that sheep had the highest contact rate with *C. burnetii* in the region but also that cattle and goats should not be neglected as part of the domestic cycle of *C. burnetii*. This work reports basic epidemiologic patterns of *C. burnetii* in semi-extensive grazed domestic ruminants which, together with the relevant role of *C. burnetii* as a zoonotic and abortifacient agent, makes these results to concern both Public and Animal Health Authorities.

Citation: Francisco Ruiz-Fons, Ianire Astobiza, Jesús F Barandika, Ana Hurtado, Raquel Atxaerandio, Ramón A Juste, Ana L García-Pérez, Seroepidemiological study of Q fever in domestic ruminants in semi-extensive grazing systems, DOI: 10.1186/1746-6148-6-3.

BACKGROUND

Q fever is a worldwide distributed zoonosis caused by *Coxiella burnetii*, a ubiquitous Gram-negative bacterium that is able to infect humans and a wide range of animals, both aquatic and terrestrial [1, 2, 3]. Q fever is a polymorphic disease in humans with subclinic, acute and chronic forms [1, 3]. Several groups in Spain have studied the clinical aspects and the distribution of the disease in different regions [5, 6, 7]. The disease seems to be more prevalent in northern Spain than in the central and southern regions of the country, and it is especially high in the Basque Country (northern Spain) where large series of human pneumonia cases due to*C. burnetii* have been reported [1, 8]. It is proposed that *C. burnetii* is maintained in nature following two different cycles, the wild cycle in which ticks and wild animals are involved, and the domestic cycle, where ruminant and other animal species such as dogs and cats are the main reservoirs [1, 3]. Nonetheless, the link between both proposed cycles is currently weakly known, especially because the domestic cycle has been considered the main source for human infection [9] and has therefore been the focus of most studies.

Clinical outcome of *C. burnetii* infection in domestic ruminants consists of abortion and stillbirths in sheep and goats while it causes infertility and mastitis in cattle [10]. No clinical signs are evidenced in non-pregnant animals. When abortion occurs, or even when ewes lamb normally, animals shed a high number of *C. burnetii*through placenta, vaginal fluids, faeces and milk [1, 11, 12]. Infectious abortion in domestic ruminants is a multi-etiologic process that causes important losses in the livestock industry. Furthermore, the zoonotic nature of most of the abortifacient pathogens is a cause for concern from the perspective of Public Health. While attention has been paid to most of these pathogens, such as *Brucella*, *Chlamydophila* or *Toxoplasma* in sheep, others like *C. burnetii* have not been routinely investigated in cases of abortion. The recent application of molecular techniques to study fetal tissues and placenta indicates that *C. burnetii* could be more prevalent than previously thought [13, 14].

Serological surveys have been carried out in many countries to evaluate the distribution of *C. burnetii* in domestic ruminants. In some areas bovine seems to be the main reservoir [15, 16, 17] whereas in others, goats [18, 19] or sheep [20, 21, 22] are the main domestic reservoir. However in other studies, serological surveys indicate that the different domestic ruminant species can play together a relevant role in the domestic cycle of *C. burnetii* [3, 23, 24, 25]. In addition, different management systems showed different degree of exposure to infection [26]. Regarding Spain, few serological evidences have been reported both in domestic and wild ruminants [5, 27].

Under the current panorama of Q fever re-emergence and the lack of information on the current status of *C. burnetii* infection in domestic ruminants in one of the most traditional livestock producing regions in Spain, we aimed to determine the epidemiological situation of this pathogen in the framework of a larger project on coxiellosis in livestock and wildlife. This study updates the status of this zoonotic pathogen in the ruminants population of the Basque Country and highlights the main risks for human infection in a hyperendemic Q fever region. We also evaluated if the age of the animals might account for differences in exposure to *C. burnetii*. Moreover, relationships between *C. burnetii* contact rate and abortion history at the herd level were also investigated.

METHODS

Study Area

The Basque Country (7,234 km^2) is a region located in northern Spain (Figure 1). Livestock production is one of the pillars of the rural economy of the region, with a total amount of 344,288 sheep, 160,000 cattle (dairy and beef) and 28,500 goats [28]. Livestock production is widely scattered throughout the region and the number of herds is high, with approximately 5,300 sheep, 6,915 cattle (dairy and beef) and 2,000 goat herds. Semi-extensive production is predominant for sheep, beef cattle and goats, and it is characterized by housing in winter months until early spring, when parturition occurs, and extensive grazing the rest of the year.

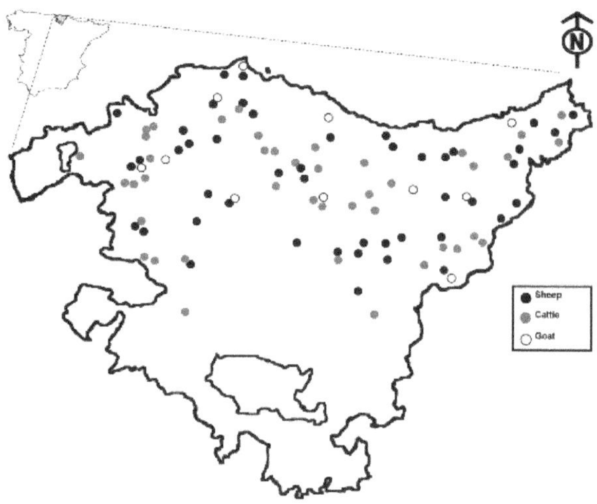

Figure 1: Geographic distribution of the sampled herds in the study area.

Sampling Approach

The survey was carried out from October 2007 to April 2008. Overall regional census was compiled for each ruminant species (data from the Basque Statistics Institute) and sample size was proportionally calculated according to the number of herds per county with a maximum number of 2,000 animals from 100 herds. Individuals (females) older than one year were randomly selected within herds to a maximum of 30 sheep, 15 beef cattle and 10 goats per herd. Finally, 1,379 sheep, 626 beef cattle and 115 goats from 46, 42 and 11 herds, respectively, were surveyed (Figure 1). Whole blood extractions were carried out by the veterinary practitioner groups in charge of the Official Sanitary Campaigns in the Basque Country, directed and supervised by the local Animal Health and Welfare Authorities (Diputaciones Forales).

After individual collection of blood into tubes without anticoagulant, sera were obtained by centrifugation and stored at -20°C until serological analyses were performed. History of recent abortion (*i.e.*, occurrence of abortions during the two previous breeding seasons) was obtained from a number of the surveyed herds by interviewing the farmers during sample collection.

Serological Analyses

Sera were tested for the presence of anti-*C. burnetii* antibodies by means of an ELISA test (ELISA Cox kit, LSI-Laboratoire Service International, Lyon, France) according to manufacturer's instructions. Sensitivity of this ELISA test reaches 100% whereas specificity was determined to be of 95% (manufacturer's data). ELISA positive sera were retested for anti-*C. burnetii* antibodies by means of the Complement Fixation test (CFT) following standard procedures [29]. *C. burnetii* antigen was provided by Dade Behring (Marburg, Germany) using Nine Mile and Henzerling strains produced on embryonated eggs. According to the standards of the OIE, samples with CFT titres ≤ 1/5 were considered negative. Titres between 1/10 and 1/40 were representative for latent infection while titres ≥ 1/80 revealed an evolutive phase of the infection [29].

Statistical Analyses

For statistical analysis purposes, two age categories were established for each animal species (Table 1) in relation to the age at first parturition. Sheep and goats were classified in two groups, yearlings (1-2 years old) and adults (>2 years old), while beef cattle was classified as heifer (1-3 years old) or adult (>3 years old). Several animals younger than 1 year-old (73 sheep, 8 cattle and 6 goats) were sampled but were not considered for age-associated seroprevalence pattern analyses because of the smaller sample size.

Table 1: Mean anti-*C. burnetii* antibody prevalence (Serop.) and its associated standard error (SE) throughout ruminant species-by-age class

	Age class	N	Pos	Serop. (%)	SE
Sheep	1-2 yr.	225	21	9.3	0.02
	Adult	1073	139	13.0	0.01
Subtotal sheep		*1298*	*160*	*12.3*	*0.01*
Beef cattle	Heifer	97	6	6.2	0.02
	Adult	521	35	6.7	0.01
Subtotal cattle		*618*	*41*	*6.6*	*0.01*
Goats	1-2 yr.	40	1	2.5	0.03
	Adult	69	8	11.6	0.04
Subtotal goats		*109*	*9*	*8.3*	*0.03*

N: Number of animals analyzed; Pos: Number of seropositive animals.

ELISA anti-*C. burnetii* antibody prevalence was calculated at individual and at herd level for each ruminant species. Rogan-Gladen correction (RGC) according to the sensitivity and specificity of the ELISA test was used for population seroprevalence calculation [30]. A herd was considered positive when at least one animal showed antibodies by ELISA. Thus, differences on antibody prevalence (continuous) between ruminant species, age classes (categorical) and abortion history (categorical, reported/non-reported) were statistically assessed by means of Chi-square tests. Statistical uncertainty was assessed by calculating the 95% confidence interval for each of the proportions according to the expression $S.E._{\cdot 95\% C.I.} = 1.96\ [p(1 - p)/n]^{1/2}$ [31].

RESULTS

ELISA test showed an average *C. burnetii* seroprevalence of 11.8 ± 2.0% (RGC: 7.1 ± 1.4%) in sheep, 8.7 ± 5.9% (RGC: 3.9 ± 3.5%) in goats and 6.7 ± 2.0% (RGC: 1.8 ± 1.0%) in beef cattle. Statistically significant differences were found between cattle and sheep seroprevalences ($\chi^2 = 11.7$, $p < 0.001$). The percentage of seropositive herds was 74% (34/46) for sheep, 43% (18/42) for cattle and 45% (5/11) for goats. Within-herd seroprevalence values ranged 0-80% for sheep, 0-53% for cattle and 0-30% for goats, with 21%, 14% and 27% of the herds, respectively, showing a *C. burnetii* seroprevalence ≥ 20%.

Eight out of 162 (4.9 ± 3.3%), 6 out of 42 (14.3 ± 10.6%) and 1 out of 10 (10.0 ± 18.6%) ELISA-positive sheep, cattle and goats, respectively, also reacted positive in the CFT giving titres ≥ 1/10. CFT positive ewes belonged to 5 herds (5/46, 8.7%) and antibody titres did not exceed 1/20. In cattle, CFT positive animals belonged to 3 herds (3/42, 7.1%) and antibody titres did not exceed 1/40. Finally, only one goat reacting positive in ELISA also reacted in the CFT showing a titre of 1/10.

ELISA seroprevalence-age associated patterns differed between ruminant species (Table 1). While *C. burnetii*seroprevalence tended to increase from yearlings to adults in sheep and goats, seroprevalence values remained similar for heifer and adult cattle. Nonetheless, no statistically significant differences between age class seroprevalence values were found. In addition, anti-*C. burnetii* antibody prevalence did not differ statistically in relation to herd abortion history, neither in sheep (9.1 ± 3.9% for flocks reporting abortion and 9.0 ± 2.0% for non-reporting flocks) nor in cattle (10.7 ± 7.8% and 9.4 ± 3.9%, respectively). Seven of the 23 interviewed sheep flock owners reported recent problems of abortion. Five of these flocks were positive for ELISA anti-*C. burnetii* antibodies, with seroprevalences ranging between 3.3% and 36.7%. Interestingly, CFT titres ≥ 1/10 were detected in only one of those flocks. Meanwhile, 5 of 18 cattle herds reported abortion problems and showed seroprevalences between 0% and 20%, but none of the ELISA positive animals from those herds reporting abortion had significant CFT titres.

Conversely, 6 of 13 cattle herds reporting no reproductive problems showed seroprevalences between 6.6% and 53.3% by ELISA, and in 2 of these herds several animals showed titres ≥ 1/10 against *Coxiella* by CFT. Recent abortion history could only be obtained from a small number of goat herds (n = 4) and consequently we did not considered them in the analysis.

DISCUSSION

Q fever is considered a strongly endemic disease in humans in the Basque Country [32, 33]. Contact with domestic ruminants was considered one of the most relevant risk factors for *C. burnetii* infection. Moreover,*C. burnetti* was found to be widespread in sheep flocks [34] and is known to be a relevant agent for ovine abortion [13] that causes important economic losses to livestock producers. Nevertheless, very scarce information on the current status of this pathogen in other ruminant species, such as cattle or goats, was available for this region. As a first approach to improve knowledge on the current status of *C. burnetii* among livestock in the Basque Country, we studied the seroprevalence in beef cattle, sheep and goats, which are reared in semi-extensive conditions, while intensively managed species (dairy cattle) will be the subject of a future study.

Comparison of herein reported ELISA results with other epidemiological surveys has to be carefully considered due to the different serological techniques employed. While recent studies tend to use the indirect fluorescence assay (IFA) or ELISA, those carried out some decades ago used mainly CFT. Whereas IFA and ELISA tests on ruminant sera showed similar results, low agreement was observed between ELISA and CFT [35,36], which agrees with our observations in sheep (unpublished data). CFT has a good specificity but a low sensitivity [29]; in fact, only 15 out of 214 ELISA positive animals gave CFT titres ≥ 1/10. The highest sensitivity associated to the ELISA test together with the high duration of detectable levels of circulating anti-*C. burnetii*antibodies were the reasons for using this technique for epidemiological purposes in the current study. Although ELISA test can fail to detect *C. burnetii* contact at an individual level [36], it becomes very useful for studies at the population level like the one presented herein. On the other hand, molecular methods are highly sensitive tools for detecting *C. burnetii* infected animals. Nonetheless, the high variability of *C. burnetii*excretion by animals throughout the year limits the reliability of molecular methods for epidemiological purposes, especially if sampling takes place outside of the reproductive season.

The seroprevalence found in sheep was comparable to that reported in other Spanish regions where seroprevalence ranged between 1.7% and 18.8% [5] or in some Mediterranean regions, with values between 9% and 25% [19, 22, 24, 37, 38]. These data highlight the risk of *C. burnetii* zoonosis associated to sheep in all the Mediterranean countries. Nevertheless, seroprevalence of cattle and goats in some of these countries suggest that these species would also represent a potential risk. In fact, cattle seropositivity ranged between 5.8% and 25% [24, 37], and in goats between 13% and 51% [19, 24, 38]. In Spain, the highest prevalences found in these species were 66.9% for cattle and 32.7% for goats in different production systems from central and southern Spain, respectively [5], and more recently, 35% of southern Spanish cattle in extensive production have been found to have contact with *C. burnetii* [27].

The lower seroprevalence observed in the present study in cattle and goats could be explained by the semi-extensive management conditions in which animals are moving during part of the year in large land surfaces thus reducing the contact between animals. Therefore, the different prevalences of *C. burnetii* in livestock suggest that local productive system and management factors might influence the life cycle of *C. burnetii*. Moreover, wildlife could play a relevant role as reservoir for livestock [27], especially where extensive productive systems are predominant, which increases the risk of wildlife/livestock contact. The significantly higher seroprevalence observed in sheep with regard to beef cattle could not be explained by differences in the sampling dates in relation to the lambing/calving season. Both beef cattle and sheep were surveyed coinciding with the end of the gestation period, when the excretion of *C. burnetii* by infected animals is higher because of parturition [10]. Interestingly, when CFT was analysed in ELISA positive animals, beef cattle had a higher percentage of reactors (14.3%) compared to sheep (4.9%) indicating a higher number of latent infections in cattle than in sheep. Nevertheless, the small size of the sample and the concentration of CFT-positive animals in a reduced number of herds make it difficult to reach a definitive explanation. Other management factors, like closer contact among ewes during milking, which implies overnight housing, could be the reason for a higher overall ELISA seroprevalence in sheep than in cattle.

Age-related *C. burnetii* serological patterns have been seldom reported in the scientific literature in regard to domestic ruminants [24, 34]. Pathogen contact rate tends to increase with age simply as a consequence of a higher probability of contact with life span, a feature that herein was observed for sheep and goats.

Long-time contact with *C. burnetii* in the surveyed herds together with the random selection of sampled animals could explain the lack of association found between herd seroprevalence and abortion reports. Different results have been reported in this regard, with significant associations between seroprevalence and abortion reported for cattle and sheep in several studies [16, 37], whereas in other reports infection with *C. burnetii* in cattle did not result in abortion, suggesting that infection sometimes can pass unnoticed [39]. In the current study, in 6 cattle herds without reproductive problems within-herd seroprevalence by ELISA ranged between 6.6 and 53% and in 2 of these herds several animals had CFT titers ≥ 1/10 indicating a recent contact with *C. burnetii*. Although several farmers did not report abortion or reproductive problems, high seroprevalences can be associated with the presence of *C. burnetii* in the herd. Similarly, Astobiza et al. [12] found a high within-flock seroprevalence (54%) and a high percentage of *C. burnetii* shedders at lambing (55-79%) in a sheep flock with a low rate of abortion (3.4%). These observations indicate that there are several epidemiological and clinical aspects of *C. burnetii* infection that need to be elucidated and require further investigation.

CONCLUSIONS

The results reported herein showed that sheep had the highest contact rate with *C. burnetii* in the region, but also that cattle and goats should not be neglected as part of the domestic cycle of *C. burnetii*. Based on our observations, we can conclude that measures are to be implemented for the control of *C. burnetii* and Q fever in the study region along the line of those currently in operation in other European countries. Moreover, further epidemiological research on herd, local and regional factors influencing *C. burnetii* life cycle is needed in order to establish more efficient control measures that prevent spread of the infection and its associated effects on livestock and humans. At present, a control programme based on vaccination using a Phase I vaccine is in progress and its efficacy will be assessed in the near future.

ACKNOWLEDGEMENTS

We acknowledge the collaboration of farmers from the different Breed Farmers Associations. This work was supported by funding from INIA (FAU2006-00002-C04-01), FEDER, and the Department of Agriculture, Fisheries and Food of the Basque Government. F. Ruiz-Fons is supported by a research contract from the 'Instituto de Salud Carlos III' of the Spanish Ministry for Health.

AUTHORS' CONTRIBUTIONS

FR was responsible for data collection and statistical analysis, and wrote the manuscript; JFB, JA and RA helped in the samplings and performed the serological tests; AH assisted with the interpretation and discussion of results and correcting the manuscript; RAJ advised on statistical analysis and critically revised the manuscript. ALG is head of the project and had primary responsibility for the investigations reported here. All authors revised the manuscript and approved it in its final version.

REFERENCES

1. Maurin M, Raoult D: Q fever. Clin Microbiol Rev. 1999, 12: 518-553.
2. Lapointe JM, Gulland FM, Haines DM, Barr BC, Duignan PJ: Placentitis due to *Coxiella burnetii* in a Pacific harbour seal (*Phoca vitulina richardsi*). J Vet Diagn Invest. 1999, 11: 541-543.
3. Arricau-Bouvery N, Rodolakis A: Is Q Fever an emerging or re-emerging zoonosis?. Vet Res. 2005, 36: 327-349. 10.1051/vetres:2005010.
4. Kovácová E, Kazar J: Q fever--still a query and underestimated infectious disease. Acta Virol. 2002, 46: 193-210.
5. Pascual-Velasco F: [Fiebre Q]. Zamora: Junta de Castilla y León Press 1996.
6. Bolaños M, Santana OE, Pérez-Arellano JL, Ángel-Moreno A, Moreno G, Burgazzoli JL, Martín-Sánchez AM: Q fever in Gran Canaria: 40 new cases. Enferm Infecc Microbiol Clin. 2003, 21: 20-23. 10.1157/13042133.
7. Cardenosa N, Sanfeliu I, Font B, Muñoz T, Nogueras MM, Segura F: Short report: seroprevalence of human infection by*Coxiella burnetii* in Barcelona (northeast of Spain). Am J Trop Med Hyg. 2006, 75: 33-35.
8. Sobradillo V, Ansola P, Baranda F, Corral C: Q fever pneumonia: a review of 164 community-acquired cases in the Basque country. Eur Respir J. 1989, 2: 263-266.
9. Lang GH: Coxiellosis (Q fever) in animals. Q fever: The disease. Edited by: Marrie TJ. Boca Raton: CRC Press, 1990, 1: 24-42.
10. Woldehiwet Z: Q fever (coxiellosis): epidemiology and pathogenesis. Res Vet Sci. 2004, 77: 93-100. 10.1016/j.rvsc.2003.09.001.
11. Rodolakis A, Berri M, Hechard C, Caudron C, Souriau A, Bodier CC, Blanchard B, Camuset P, Devillechaise P, Natorp JC, Vadet JP, Arricau-Bouvery N: Comparison of *Coxiella burnetii* shedding in milk of dairy bovine, caprine, and ovine herds. J Dairy Sci. 2007, 90: 5352-5360. 10.3168/jds.2006-815.
12. Astobiza I, Barandika JF, Hurtado A, Juste RA, García-Pérez AL: Kinetics of *Coxiella burnetii*excretion in a commercial dairy sheep flock after treatment with oxytetracycline. Vet J.
13. Oporto B, Barandika JF, Hurtado A, Adúriz G, Moreno B, García-Pérez AL: Incidence of ovine abortion by *Coxiella burnetii*in northern Spain. Ann N Y Acad Sci. 2006, 1078: 498-501. 10.1196/annals.1374.095.
14. Perugini AG, Capuano F, Esposito A, Marianelli C, Martucciello A, Iovane G, Galiero G: Detection of *Coxiella burnetii* in buffaloes aborted fetuses by IS111 DNA amplification: A preliminary report. Res Vet Sci. 2009, 87: 189-191. 10.1016/j.rvsc.2009.01.005.
15. To H, Htwe KK, Kako N, Kim HJ, Yamaguchi T, Fukushi H, Hirai K: Prevalence of *Coxiella burnetii* infection in dairy cattle with reproductive disorders. J Vet Med Sci. 1998, 60: 859-861. 10.1292/jvms.60.859.
16. Cabassi CS, Taddei S, Donofrio G, Ghidini F, Piancastelli C, Flammini CF, Cavirani S: Association between *Coxiella burnetii*seropositivity and abortion in dairy cattle of Northern Italy. New Microbiol. 2006, 29: 211-214.
17. Kim WJ, Hahn TW, Kim DY, Lee MG, Jung KS, Ogawa M, Kishimoto T, Lee ME, Lee SJ: Seroprevalence of *Coxiella burnetii*infection in dairy cattle and non-symptomatic people for routine health screening in Korea. J Korean Med Sci. 2006, 21: 823-826. 10.3346/jkms.2006.21.5.823.
18. Hatchette TF, Hudson RC, Schlech WF, Campbell NA, Hatchette JE, Ratnam S, Raoult D, Donovan C, Marrie TJ: Goat-associated Q fever: a new disease in Newfoundland. Emerg Infect Dis. 2001, 7: 413-419.
19. Loukaides F, Hadjichristodoulou C, Soteriades ES, Kolonia V, Ioannidou MC, Psaroulaki A, Tselentis Y: Active surveillance of Q fever in human and animal population of Cyprus. BMC Infect Dis. 2006, 6: 48-10.1186/1471-2334-6-48.
20. Hellenbrand W, Breuer T, Petersen L: Changing epidemiology of Q fever in Germany, 1947-1999. Emerg Infect Dis. 2001, 7: 789-796. 10.3201/eid0705.010504.
21. Tissot-Dupont H, Amadei MA, Nezri M, Raoult D: Wind in November, Q fever in December. Emerg Infect Dis. 2004, 10: 1264-1269.
22. Kennerman E, Rousset E, Gölcü E, Dufour P: Seroprevalence of Q fever (coxiellosis) in sheep from

the southern Marmara Region, Turkey. Comp Immunol Microbiol Infect Dis. 2010, 33: 37-45. 10.1016/j.cimid.2008.07.007.

23. Hatchette T, Campbell N, Whitney H, Hudson R, Marrie TJ: Seroprevalence of *Coxiella burnetii* in selected populations of domestic ruminants in Newfoundland. Can Vet J. 2002, 43: 363-364.

24. Psaroulaki A, Hadjichristodoulou C, Loukaides F, Soteriades E, Konstantinidis A, Papastergiou P, Ioannidou MC, Tselentis Y: Epidemiological study of Q fever in humans, ruminant animals, and ticks in Cyprus using a geographical information system. Eur J Clin Microbiol Infect Dis. 2006, 25: 576-586. 10.1007/s10096-006-0170-7.

25. Çekani M, Papa A, Kota M, Velo E, Berxholi K: Report of a serological study of *Coxiella burnetii* in domestic animals in Albania. Vet J. 2008, 175: 276-278. 10.1016/j.tvjl.2007.01.005.

26. Capuano F, Landolfi MC, Monetti DM: Influence of three types of farm management on the seroprevalence of Q fever as assessed by an indirect immunofluorescence assay. Vet Rec. 2001, 149: 669-671.

27. Ruiz-Fons F, Rodriguez O, Torina A, Naranjo V, Gortázar C, de la Fuente J: Prevalence of *Coxiella burnetti* infection in wild and farmed ungulates. Vet Microbiol. 2008, 126: 282-286. 10.1016/j.vetmic.2007.06.020.

28. Eustat: Basque Statistics Institute. [http://www.eustat.es/bancopx/spanish/Economía/Sector%20primario/Censo%20agrario/Ganadería/Ganadería.html]

29. World Organization for Animal Health. [http://www.oie.int/eng/normes/mmanual/2008/pdf/2.01.12_Q-FEVER.pdf]

30. Rogan WJ, Gladen B: Estimating prevalence from the results of a screening test. Am J Epidemiol. 1978, 107: 71-76.

31. Martin SW, Meek AH, Willeberg P: Veterinary Epidemiology. Measures of disease frequency. Ames: Iowa State University Press 1987.

32. Sanzo JM, García MA, Sáez MP, Sarobe V, Audikana A, Dehesa V: [Fiebre Q]. Vitoria-Gasteiz: Servicio Central de Publicaciones del Gobierno Vasco Press 1991.

33. Montes M, Cilla G, Vicente D, Nieto D, Ercibengoa M, Pérez-Trallero E: Gipuzkoa, Basque Country, Spain (1984-2004): A hyperendemic area of Q fever. Hospital Donostia. Ann N Y Acad Sci. 2006, 1078: 129-132. 10.1196/annals.1374.020.

34. García-Pérez AL, Astobiza I, Barandika JF, Atxaerandio R, Hurtado A, Juste RA: Investigation of *Coxiella burnetii*occurrence in dairy sheep flocks by bulk-tank milk analysis and antibody levels determination. J Dairy Sci. 2009, 92: 1581-1584. 10.3168/jds.2008-1672.

35. Kovácová E, Kazar J, Spanelova D: Suitability of various *Coxiella burnetii* antigen preparations for detection of serum antibodies by various tests. Acta Virol. 1998, 42: 365-368.

36. Rousset E, Durand B, Berri M, Dufour P, Prigent M, Russo P, Delcroix T, Touratier A, Rodolakis A, Aubert M: Comparative diagnostic potential of three serological tests for abortive Q fever in goat herds. Vet Microbiol. 2007, 124: 286-297. 10.1016/j.vetmic.2007.04.033.

37. Cetinkaya B, Kalender H, Ertas HB, Muz A, Arslan N, Ongor H, Gurcay M: Seroprevalence of coxiellosis in cattle, sheep and people in the east of Turkey. Vet Rec. 2000, 146: 131-136.

38. Masala G, Porcu R, Sanna G, Chessa G, Cillara G, Chisu V, Tola S: Occurrence, distribution, and role in abortion of *Coxiella burnetii* in sheep and goats in Sardinia, Italy. Vet Microbiol. 2004, 99: 301-305. 10.1016/j.vetmic.2004.01.006.

39. Paiba GA, Lloyd G, Bewley K, Webster GJ, Green LE, Morgan KL: An investigaton of *Coxiella burnetii* infection at calving within a herd of dairy cows in England using PCR. Rickettsiae and rickettsial diseases at the turn of the third millennium. Edited by: Brouqui P, Raoult D. Amsterdam: Elsevier, 1999:387-392.

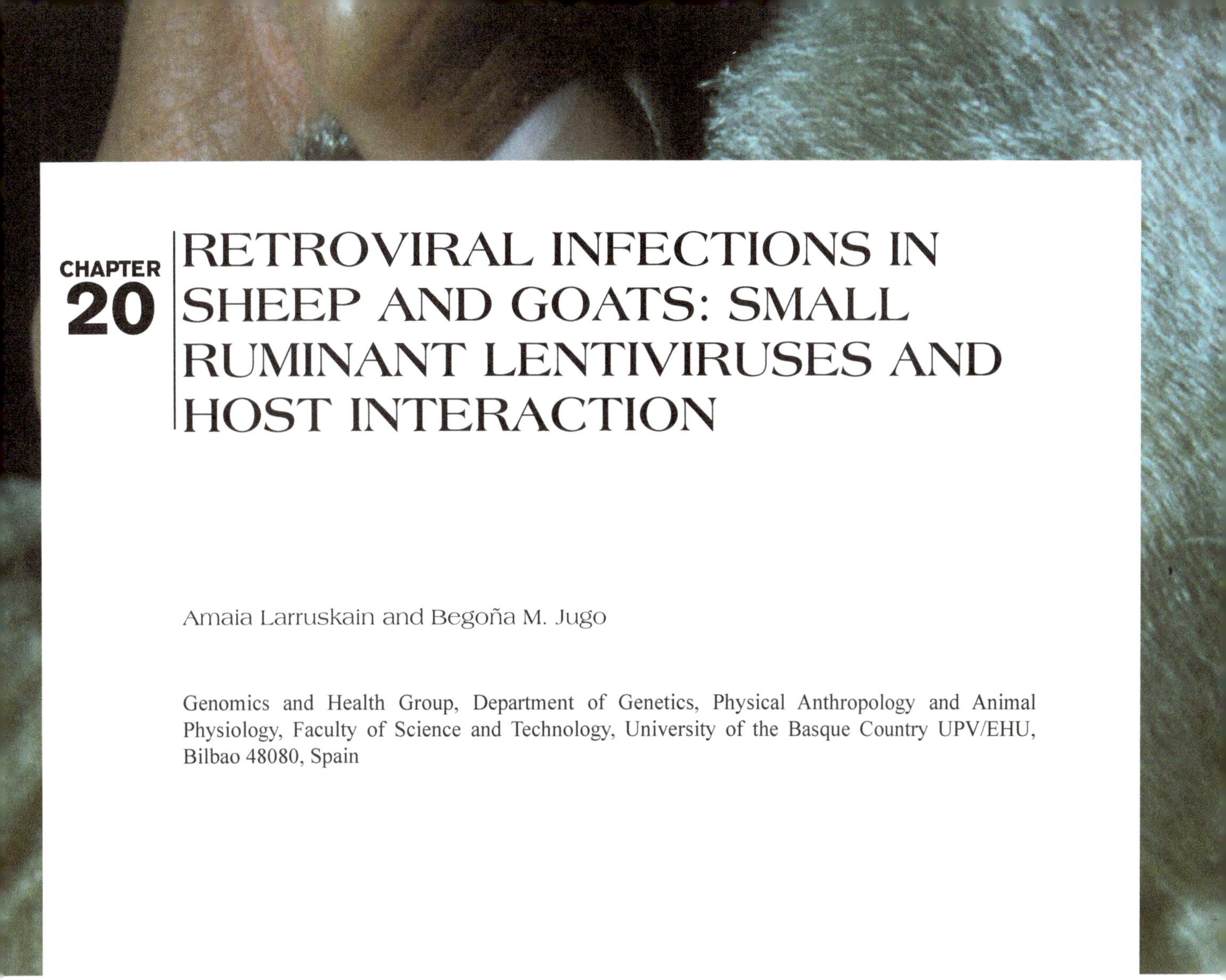

CHAPTER 20 RETROVIRAL INFECTIONS IN SHEEP AND GOATS: SMALL RUMINANT LENTIVIRUSES AND HOST INTERACTION

Amaia Larruskain and Begoña M. Jugo

Genomics and Health Group, Department of Genetics, Physical Anthropology and Animal Physiology, Faculty of Science and Technology, University of the Basque Country UPV/EHU, Bilbao 48080, Spain

ABSTRACT

Small ruminant lentiviruses (SRLV) are members of the Retrovirus family comprising the closely related Visna/Maedi Virus (VMV) and the Caprine Arthritis-Encephalitis Virus (CAEV), which infect sheep and goats. Both infect cells of the monocyte/macrophage lineage and cause lifelong infections. Infection by VMV and CAEV can lead to Visna/Maedi (VM) and Caprine Arthritis-Encephalitis (CAE) respectively, slow progressive inflammatory diseases primarily affecting the lungs, nervous system, joints and mammary glands. VM and CAE are distributed worldwide and develop over a period of months or years, always leading to the death of the host, with the consequent economic and welfare implications. Currently, the control of VM and CAE relies on the control of transmission and culling of infected animals. However, there is evidence that host genetics play an important role in determining Susceptibility/Resistance to SRLV infection and disease progression, but little work has been performed in small ruminants. More research is necessary to understand the host-SRLV interaction.

SMALL RUMINANT LENTIVIRUSES (SRLVS)

Lentiviruses are a subgroup of the Retrovirus family, which infect a wide range of species including humans and livestock species, causing slow infections that may lead to progressive degenerative diseases. Visna/Maedi Virus (VMV) and Caprine Arthritis-Encephalitis Virus (CAEV) infect sheep and goats. Phylogenetic analyses have established that they are part of a viral continuum and therefore are grouped together as Small Ruminant Lentiviruses (SRLVs) [1,2,3].

Citation: Amaia Larruskain and Begoña M. Jugo, Retroviral Infections in Sheep and Goats: Small Ruminant Lentiviruses and Host Interaction, doi:10.3390/v5082043.

SRLV Infection and Disease

Although SRLVs can infect a variety of cells, their target cells are of the monocyte/macrophage lineage where viral expression is closely dependent on the monocyte to macrophage maturation [4,5,6,7].

SRLVs are mainly transmitted horizontally or from dam to offspring via the respiratory and lactogenic routes. Both asymptomatic and diseased animals are a source of viruses for naive animals [8,9,10,11,12,13,14,15,16].

Lesions induced by SRLVs are characterized by mononuclear infiltration in target organs and persistent inflammation [17,18]. SRLVs cause Visna/Maedi (VM) in sheep and Caprine Arthritis-Encephalitis (CAE) in goats, multisystemic inflammatory diseases affecting lungs, the central nervous system (CNS), joints and mammary glands. In both cases, symptoms take several months to years to develop (see Figure 1 for disease timeline). The syndromes may be present to varying degrees in the same animal or occur independently [6,10,19,20,21,22].

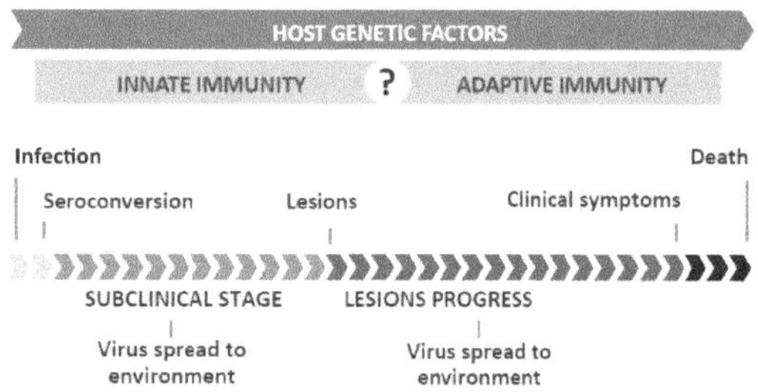

Figure 1: Small Ruminant Lentivirus (SRLV) timeline. SRLVs are transmitted via the respiratory or lactogenic route. Proviral DNA transcription and gene expression is suppressed until infected monocytes mature into macrophages. Once in the target organs, infected macrophages initiate viral replication, which induces an inflammatory cascade. Despite a vigorous immune response, the virus is not cleared and the animal will remain a carrier for life. Most animals remain asymptomatic, but a certain percentage of the animals develop the clinical disease in one or several target organs. Subclinical infection and disease progression may range from months to years. Both Visna/Maedi (VM) and Caprine Arthritis-Encephalitis (CAE) are ultimately fatal. Host genetic factors, infecting viral strain and management influence the occurrence, length and spectrum of affected target organs.

Relevance and Control of SRLVs

SRLV infection and associated diseases are present in most sheep-rearing countries worldwide, negatively affecting production and animal welfare [1,17]. The economic impact depends on the breed, management system and type of production [6,10,11,23].

SRLV infections are difficult to control due to the ability of the virus to integrate into the host's genome, induce persistent infections and elude neutralization. Vaccination attempts have occasionally caused increased viremia and more severe disease [1,6,18,24,25,26,27,28,29]. Currently, the control of VM and CAE relies on the control of transmission and test and cull schemes of infected animals and their progeny [30,31,32].

The development of disease-resistant breeding stock has been undertaken in other diseases due to lack of effectiveness of vaccines and development of resistance of pathogens to drugs and chemicals, which are becoming increasingly common [33]. However, the detection of SRLV-resistant animals remains problematic since DNA markers have to be identified and the interaction of SRLVs with the host and the pathogenesis of VM and CAE are not fully understood. It is therefore necessary to dissect the antigen and immune response if appropriate control methods are to be developed [34].

HOST GENETIC RESOURCES

Since the domestication of sheep and goats human-mediated breeding has generated specialized animals suitable for a wide range of purposes, and hundreds of breeds exist worldwide which often have their own genetic signature [35,36].

There has been a huge increase in the research and application of disease genetics in small ruminants due to the growing knowledge of the influence of host genetics on disease control and the increase in available genetic and genomic tools. Apart from the scientific interest, there is a growing pressure on breeders to select animals that are healthier and more resistant both to infectious and metabolic diseases, which could be feasible with the available biotechnology tools and quickly augmenting knowledge on lentivirus molecular biology/pathogenesis [32,33].

However, in general the development of small ruminant genetic and genomic resources lags behind that of other domestic species such as cattle [37,38,39].

Different markers and strategies can be used to discover disease-associated loci, including microsatellites, single nucleotide polymorphisms (SNP), copy number polymorphisms or variants, *etc.*, which in addition can be complemented with expression assays [38,40]. Current high-throughput techniques allow the rapid genotyping of markers such as SNPs. (see Table 1 for limitations of association studies).

HOST-VIRAL PATHOGEN INTERACTION

The interaction between retroviruses (RV) and their hosts is complex. RVs are obligate pathogens that require the host's cellular machinery to complete their cycle. In response, the hosts have developed sophisticated mechanisms to fight viral infections, including innate and adaptive immune systems [50,51]. Observation of retroviral diseases in various species has shown that even in a population infected by a particular virus strain there are usually differences in the outcome of infection and disease of individual animals [52], and studies on host immune response, gene variability and expression could reveal why.

In humans, host genetic factors are important determinants that influence susceptibility to HIV infection and subsequent progression to AIDS, which has been thoroughly studied. Inter-individual variability in susceptibility to HIV-1 infection, transmission, disease progression, and response to antiviral therapy have been attributed to host determinants and variability in multiple genes [53,54].

SRLVs share many characteristics with HIV and indeed, in small ruminants, differences in susceptibility have been observed as well. However, a characteristic that differentiates SRLVs from other lentiviruses is that they do not cause immunodeficiency. In fact, one of the unresolved issues in SRLV infections is the fact that the virus is not cleared despite the host mounting an immune response. It is believed that SRLV proviral DNA escapes detection by the immune system by persisting in monocytes, thus allowing viral dissemination to target tissues. Furthermore, SRLVs may interfere with the function of effector cells implicated in the defense against the virus, such as macrophages and dendritic cells, altering the type of immune responses that are induced [5,11,17,55,56].

Table 1: Limitations of genetic association studies in complex multifactorial diseases such as SRLV-induced pathologies. Factors leading to confounding that may be encountered as well as their consequences are shown (information compiled from [41,42,43,44,45,46,47,48,49]

HOST		**GENOTYPING**	
Population stratification	Often present in livestock due to breeding practices	**Bias/Partiality**	Case samples are treated with preference
Sample size	Affects power to detect association	**Marker density**	Often few markers are analyzed per gene
Phenotype	Description must be accurate	**Marker frequency**	Frequency of marker variants affect odds of detecting association
Age	Older animals have been exposed for a longer time	**STATISTICAL ANALYSIS**	
Gene effect	Genes involved have small/moderate effects	**Power**	Depends on sample size, marker frequency and gene effect
Presence of other diseases	May facilitate SRLV pathogenesis	**Gene interaction**	Often unaccounted for
SRLVs		**Confounding factors**	Failure to account for them may lead to erroneous interpretations
Different virus strains	Different virulence and host/organ spectrum complicates research; Strain variability may affect detection of infected individuals	**Multiple corrections**	Necessary yet may lead to reject real associations
ENVIRONMENTAL FACTORS		**Consistency/ replicability**	Results must be replicated in different populations/ Can results be replicated in a different population?
Husbandry	Prolonged and crowded housing enhances infection		

Other lentivirus species, although not as extensively studied as HIV, have added information on host genetic factors that may influence lentiviral pathogenesis including Equine Infectious Anemia Virus (EIAV), bovine immunodeficiency virus (BIV), Jembrana disease virus (JDV) and feline immunodeficiency virus (FIV). Among these species, SRLVs, EIAV and BIV/JDB have a tropism for cells of the monocyte/macrophage lineage, while the others also infect lymphocytes. In these non-primate lentivirus species differential susceptibility and associated genes may be found as well [1,7,57].

EVIDENCE POINTING TO THE EXISTENCE OF HOST GENETICS CONTROLLING SRLV PATHOGENESIS

SRLV-induced pathogenesis is a complex process determined by multiple factors (See Table 1 for more details) such as host genetics, virus strain, management practices and presence of other diseases [10,17,32,58,59,60,61,62,63].

The above factors must be accounted for, but do not rule out genetic susceptibility. There is evidence that host genetics play an important role in determining susceptibility/resistance to SRLV infection and pathogenesis, but little work has been performed in small ruminants [64].

Research indicates that a breed (or genetic) predisposition may exist regarding infection susceptibility, provirus levels and lesion occurrence and progression, and thus the influence of the host's genetics can be studied at different levels. The VMV-infected asymptomatic Karakul sheep imported to Iceland in the 1930s never developed signs of the disease but their importation resulted in a widespread dissemination of VM to the extremely susceptible native Icelandic sheep [34]. The research carried out by Icelandic scientists showed that some flocks/family lines had a slower disease progression. In addition, progression of Maedi was delayed in Icelandic x Border Leicester cross individuals [17,32,65]. Research carried out in other countries/breeds has provided further evidence of differential individual and breed susceptibility as well [55,66,67,68,69].

Infection

Resistance to SRLV infection despite repeated exposure could be interpreted as an innate resistance to infection [64,70]. Significant breed effects on seroprevalence have been observed in comingled flocks, with some sheep and goat breeds being more likely to seroconvert, indicating a possible host genetic restriction. For instance, a higher seroprevalence has been demonstrated in Texel, Border Leicester and Finnish sheep breeds as opposed to Ile de France, Rambouillet and Suffolk [10,23,32,68,71,72]. Saanen and Toggenburg goats are more likely to seroconvert whereas Bedouin Black could be resistant to infection under natural conditions [73,74].

In Latxa dairy-sheep, seroconversion was strongly associated with lifetime maternal VMV-serological status. Offspring of consistently seronegative ewes (>4 years old) were less likely to become infected, suggesting the existence of an inheritable factor of VMV-infection resistance [31].

Herrmann-Hoesing *et al.* [64] detected breed differences in seroprevalence and provirus levels (Rambouillet had lower values in both characters in comparison with Columbia and Polipay), which could imply mechanisms preventing infection and/or aiding in virus control after infection occurs. Interestingly, a correlation has been observed between virus load and the severity of lesions in both sheep and goats

[17,21,26,34,75,76] suggesting that breeds/individuals able to control virus levels may be less likely to develop VM and CAE. After infection, there is an acute viremia followed by an immune response that restricts virus replication to low levels; although the infection is not cleared, virus replication is kept at a low level [77]. Some hosts may be better at regulating the extent of viral gene expression in macrophages and perhaps disease progression [1,64]. Latency appears to be controlled by an interaction of cellular and viral transcription factors that regulate viral RNA expression [32,78,79].

Clinical Disease

Concerning disease progression, it does not progress uniformly in all individuals and rapid progressors have been observed [19,56]. Furthermore, the extent of SRLV-induced lesions and the spectrum of affected organs may depend on the host's genetics as well as the infecting virus strain [10,80]. Certain breeds seem to be more likely to develop the clinical signs, while others remain in a subclinical infection stage. Coarse wool type sheep may be more susceptible than fine wool type sheep [66]. Border Leicester sheep could be more likely than Columbia to develop SRLV-specific lesions [66,67]. Chios and Awassi sheep seem to be highly susceptible to infection but resistant to the development of the clinical disease [32,74,81]. Interestingly, Assaf sheep, a stabilized Awassi x East Friesian cross, show high SRLV seroprevalence and VM clinical disease occurrence including the neurological manifestation [82].

Further evidence is provided by experiments carried out with isogenic twin lambs, which showed that the host's genetics influence the extent and severity of SRLV-induced pulmonary lesions [70].

HOST GENETIC FACTORS INVOLVED IN SRLV-INDUCED PATHOGENESIS

SRLV pathogenesis is difficult to analyze due to the strains, different host species and breeds, differential disease progression and affected organ spectrums. It seems that the relationship between small ruminants and SRLVs is complex and that the pathogenesis is likely induced by a number of genes with small or moderate effects [7,56].

The cellular receptor(s) for SRLVs has not been conclusively identified and therefore that information cannot be exploited yet. Most likely it is a common cell membrane molecule as SRLVs can enter other cells apart from target cells, and thus the receptor does not dictate cell tropism [17,34,83,84]. However, classical VMV and CAEV strains appear to use different receptors [7,85,86]. The mannose receptor (MR) is a putative receptor for SRLVs. Crespo *et al.* [87] characterized the ovine MR nucleotide and protein sequence, and its role in VMV infection is currently being studied.

Both innate and adaptive (humoral and cellular) immune responses are induced by SRLVs and various works have identified immune response loci that could influence resistance/susceptibility to SRLV infection and disease, providing evidence that genetic factors might modulate the outcome. Below are some host genetic factors that have been involved in SRLV infection and disease.

Major Histocompatibility Complex (MHC)

The major histocompatibility complex (MHC) region, a polymorphic multi-gene complex located on chromosome 20 in sheep and chromosome 23 in goats [88,89], has been implicated in SRLV infection and SRLV-induced disease. The MHC Class I and II genes encode receptor glycoproteins that bind and present antigenic peptides to T cells initiating the immune response. The MHC is one of the few polymorphic systems for which it has been possible to establish a functional significance for the observed genetic variation [90]. Its polymorphism and association with infectious disease has been intensely studied in a myriad of diseases with viral etiology, although such studies are scarce in small ruminants.

In the ovine species, VMV infection increases the expression level of the MHC Class II in the lung, the CNS and the synovium [76,91,92,93,94]. In addition, Class I and II polymorphic gene variants have been linked to SRLV provirus levels and disease progression (See Table 2 for more details; [64,95,96]).

Table 2: Major histocompatability complex (MHC) genes/variants associated with VM or CAE pathogenesis

Region	Variant	Typing method/marker	Species/Breed(s) studied	Reference
Class I	allele CLA Be7	Alloantisera	Goat/Saanen	[97]
	Allele OMHC1* 205	Microsatellite	Sheep/Latxa	[96]
Class II	Alleles DRB1*0403- and DRB1*07012 and various amino acid positions	Cloning and direct sequencing	Sheep/Rambouillet, Polipay & Columbia	[64]
	DRB1*0325	PCR-Sequence-Based Typing	Sheep/Latxa	[95]
	Allele DRB2* 275	Microsatellite	Sheep/Latxa	[96]

The highly polymorphic nature of many loci in the MHC, among which the DR beta 1 (DRB1) gene is a clear example (over 100 alleles identified to date in sheep [64]), makes it difficult to investigate its involvement in SRLV pathogenesis [90]. Genotyping methods with enough resolution are necessary to type MHC loci, and sample sizes are often inadequate to test rare variants. The effect of different MHC alleles remains to be elucidated but it is possible that polymorphisms, depending on the location, may alter the ability of MHC molecules to bind and present antigens, affect the interaction with T cells or elicit differential immune responses [98,99].

Antibody and T Cell Response

SRLV infection induces antibody response, which has been well studied due to its use in SRLV serologic diagnostics [100]. However, neutralizing antibodies are slow to be induced or have low affinity and relatively low titers. A small amount of free viruses combined with the ability to spread from cell to cell means that propagation and spread cannot be fully stopped by antibodies [7,101].

Nevertheless, some antibody responses may be better at controlling SRLV. Data indicates that the antibody response is skewed in SRLV-infected sheep and goats. Only immunoglobulin G1 (IgG1) subtype responses are detected in sheep whilst in goats IgG1 dominates the humoral response [19,102,103,104,105].

Concerning T cells, both T cell proliferative and cytotoxic responses are induced after SRLV infection [7]. However, the $CD4^+/CD8^+$ cell ratio is decreased in the bronchoalveolar fluid (BALF), synovial fluid and cerebrospinal fluid of diseased animals because of higher levels of $CD8^+$ cells, which could be correlated with the severity of lung lesions [93,94,106,107,108]. Cytotoxic T lymphocytes (CTLs) appear to be important effector cells, for they may inhibit viral replication but also contribute to lesions through cytokine production or cytotoxicity [34,76,109,110].

In ruminants, IgG1 induces a type-2 T helper cell (Th2) response, while production of IgG2 is indicative of a Th1 response [111]. Interestingly, goats with a Th2-biased $CD4^+$ T cell response are known to develop arthritis, but those with a mixed IgG1 and IgG2 response remain without clinical signs, suggesting that anti-SRLV IgG2 antibodies protect against disease induction [7,19,104,112]. In addition, CD80 levels, which favor Th1 cell differentiation, were low in clinically affected sheep compared with asymptomatic and seronegative controls [80].

Cytokines and Receptors

Cytokines are important signaling proteins that act as important mediators of the immune system, which initiate and modulate many processes. Studies in diverse species have revealed that cytokine and cytokine receptor expression levels, polymorphisms and profiles in the host can affect the pathogenesis of virus-induced diseases.

Cytokines seem to have an important role in SRLV induced pathogenesis, including the modulation of the ongoing immune activation in target organ lesions with some cytokines favoring the appearance of lesions. Cytokines induce the recruitment and differentiation of monocytes to macrophages as well, favoring additional infection by attracting target cells and thus creating a vicious circle. Indeed, several cytokines have been found up or down regulated (See Table 3) in VM and CAE, although more data on cytokines are necessary [7,10,19, 20,112,113,114,115,116,117,118,119,120].

Although most research has focused on expression, a few works have explored the influence of polymorphisms. Cytokine polymorphisms are known to affect cytokine gene transcription [121,122], or they may affect cytokine function thus influencing the outcome of infection and disease. Chemokine receptor 5 (CCR5) is an example of how polymorphisms could affect SRLV pathogenesis. CCR5 participates in leukocyte recruitment against different pathogens, including ovine lentiviruses. A deletion in this locus causes an almost four-fold reduction in transcription in animals carrying the deletion allele, as well as showing association with a decreased provirus-burden. Considering that monocytes/macrophages are the main target cells of VMV, it has been suggested that a reduced chemotactic ability of CCR5 could result in reduced influx of such cells to the site of infection, which could also slow the rate of cellular infection [120,121,123].

Alteration of cytokine profile has been suggested in both sheep, and goats and it is suspected that SRLVs induce a switch to a Type 2 (Th2 type) cytokine response. Evidence backing this is the up regulation of Type 2 cytokines such as anti-inflammatory cytokines IL4 and IL10 [20,80,102,105].

Innate Immunity and Restriction Factors

The role of innate immunity is gaining interest in the field of lentiviral infections [7]. Genes of the innate immune response are being characterized in small ruminants and their association with SRLV pathogenesis is being tested.

Since the innate immunity senses highly conserved pathogen-associated molecular patterns (PAMPs) via a number of receptors and signaling molecules, polymorphisms in innate immune genes are very likely to affect the host susceptibility to infections. Indeed, such an effect has been observed in a number of species and diseases, and thus genes such as Toll-like receptors (TLRs) and their variation have been suggested to be good candidate prospects in various diseases affecting domestic livestock [124,125].

TLRs are a family of transmembrane signaling molecules that trigger both the innate and the adaptive immune response mechanisms in response to PAMPs, including viral components [50,126].

Mikula *et al.* [127] suggested that individual susceptibility existed in the Tsigai breed that may be defined by the presence of SNPs in TLR7 and TLR8, which sense double stranded viral RNA. Mutations at the TLR7 locus may affect PAMP binding onto the TLR molecule [127,128]. In addition, these two genes have recently been found to be up regulated in diseased sheep [120]. Furthermore, different Toll-like receptors may activate different signaling pathways, with different biological consequences, and thus merit additional research [50].

In response to retroviruses and other transposable elements, which invade the host's genome, hosts have developed intracellular defenses known as restriction factors. These proteins block the viral cycle using different strategies, such as directly attacking viral structures or editing viral genetic material during reverse transcription [129,130]. In recent years there has been a notable increase in this research area.

Table 3: Cytokine and cytokine receptor genes implicated in SRLV pathogenesis in sheep and goats

Gene symbol	Gene	Species	Methods	Analyzed material	Parameter analysed	References
IL1β	*Interleukin-1beta*	Sheep	Semiquantitative RT-PCR [1]	Lung	Clinical disease	[114]
IL2/IL2R	*Interleukin-2/ Interleukin-2 receptor*	Sheep	Semiquantitative RT-PCR, qPCR [2]	Lung, PBMCs [3], lymph node leukocytes	Infection, Clinical disease	[114,118,120]
		Goat	*In situ* hybridization	Joints	Infection, Clinical disease	[113]
IL4	*Interleukin-4*	Sheep	Semiquantitative RT-PCR	Lung	Clinical disease	[114]
		Goat	Semiquantitative RT-PCR	PBMCs	Clinical disease	[20]
IL6	*Interleukin-6*	Sheep	RT-PCR	Alveolar macrophages	Infection, Clinical disease	[116]
IL8	*Interleukin-8*	Sheep	RT-qPCR, *in situ* hybridization, Northern blot, Semiquantitative RT-PCR	BALF, alveolar macrophages,	Infection, Clinical disease	[115,117,119]
		Goat	*In situ* hybridization	Macrophages	Infection	[20]
IL10	*Interleukin-10*	Sheep	Semiquantitative RT-PCR	Lung, alveolar macrophages	Infection, Clinical disease	[114,116]
IFNγ	*Interferon-gamma*	Sheep	Semiquantitative RT-PCR	Lung	Clinical disease	[114]
		Goat	Semiquantitative RT-PCR, *in situ* hybridization	PBMCs, joints	Clinical disease	[19,113]
TNFα	*Tumor Necrosis factor-alpha*	Sheep	qPCR	Lung, udder	Clinical disease	[120]
TGF-β1	*Tumor growth factor beta-1*	Sheep	Semiquantitative RT-PCR	Alveolar macrophages	Infection, Clinical disease	[116]
		Goat	*In situ* hybridization	Macrophages	Infection	[20]
MCP-1	*Monocyte chemoattractant protein 1*	Goat	*In situ* hybridization	Macrophages, joints	Infection ,Clinical disease	[20,113]
GM-CSF	*Granulocyte macrophage stimulating factor*	Sheep	Semiquantitative RT-PCR	Lung, alveolar macrophages	Infection, Clinical disease	[114,116]
		Goat	*In situ* hybridization	Macrophages	Infection	[20]
CCR5	*Chemokine (C-C motif) Receptor 5*	Sheep	Cloning & sequencing, qPCR	PBMCs, lung	Infection, Clinical disease	[120,121]

[1] RT-PCR: Reverse Transcriptase PCR; [2] qPCR: Quantitative PCR; [3] PBMCs: Peripheral Blood Mononuclear Cells.

Ovine TRIM5α seems to be able to restrict VMV DNA synthesis [131]. This intracellular factor restricts retroviral replication by interacting with the capsid and preventing uncoating. A recent study has suggested an association between a tripartite motif protein 5 alpha (TRIM5α) polymorphism that inactivates antiviral activity and accelerates AIDS disease progression [56,132]. Whether such an effect is also present in sheep and goats will still have to be investigated.

Research is needed concerning additional innate immunity genes. Apolipoprotein B mRNA-editing enzyme (APOBEC3) proteins, which act against a wide variety of retroviruses including HIV, have been studied in sheep and they could be good candidates for SRLVs [7,130,133,134,135]. A human APOBEC3G variant has been associated with rapid HIV-1 disease progression [50].

Recently, allele and haplotype variants of the transmembrane protein gene 154 (TMEM154) locus have been associated with SRLV infection, which has been proposed as a locus that could be used for genetic marker-based selection [23]. Sheep with the ancestral variant haplotypes of this gene had an increased risk of becoming infected compared with individuals with mutant forms. However, the function of TMEM14 has not been established yet.

CONCLUSIONS

So far, a number of genes implicated in SRLV infection and disease have been identified, but more research is necessary to understand the host-SRLV interaction. A better understanding of loci involved in SRLV infection and pathology and their polymorphism could lead to the identification and selective breeding of naturally resistant animals, thus avoiding culling and reducing viral load and disease development [23,131]. There are encouraging examples where breeding programs have successfully selected animals with enhanced resistance, for example nematodes, mastitis, foot rot and scrapie in sheep; nowadays genetic tools are being employed to aid this selection, as seen in scrapie. However, a critical question will be if there is also a correlation between disease resistance and production traits. Breeding for resistance as a sole objective may not be desirable due to the potential negative impact it may have on other desirable production traits [33,90]. In addition, the molecular characterization of host genetic factors involved in SRLV infection and disease could detect new targets, which could uncover new host pathways leading to opportunities to develop antiviral therapies.

ACKNOWLEDGMENTS

We are grateful to the editorial board of this journal for the opportunity to write this review. The research of Genomics and Health group is funded by the Basque Government Industry Dpt. (grant SA-10/00120 to B.M.J.) and UPV/EHU (grants GIU07/62 and GIU10/22 to B.M.J. and UFI 11/20). We are also grateful to the four anonymous reviewers for their suggestions and constructive criticism.

REFERENCES AND NOTES

1. Patel, J.R.; Heldens, J.G.M.; Bakonyi, T.; Rusvai, M. Important mammalian veterinary viral immunodiseases and their control. *Vaccine* 2012, *30*, 1767–1781.
2. Leroux, C.; Cruz, J.C.M.; Mornex, J.F. SRLVs: A genetic continuum of lentiviral species in sheep and goats with cumulative evidence of cross species transmission. *Curr. HIV Res.* 2010, *8*, 94–100.

3. Leroux, C.; Vuillermoz, S.; Mornex, J.F.; Greenland, T. Genomic heterogeneity in the pol region of ovine lentiviruses obtained from bronchoalveolar cells of infected sheep from France. *J. Gen. Virol.* 1995, *76*, 1533–1537.
4. Gorrell, M.D.; Brandon, M.R.; Sheffer, D.; Adams, R.J.; Narayan, O. Ovine lentivirus is macrophagetropic and does not replicate productively in T lymphocytes. *J. Virol.* 1992, *66*, 2679–2688.
5. Ryan, S.; Tiley, L.; McConnell, I.; Blacklaws, B. Infection of dendritic cells by the Maedi-Visna lentivirus. *J. Virol.* 2000,*74*, 10096–10103.
6. Christodoulopoulos, G. Maedi-Visna: Clinical review and short reference on the disease status in Mediterranean countries. *Small Rumin. Res.* 2006, *62*, 47–53.
7. Blacklaws, B.A. Small ruminant lentiviruses: Immunopathogenesis of Visna-Maedi and caprine arthritis and encephalitis virus. *Comp. Immunol. Microbiol. Infect.Dis.* 2012, *35*, 259–269.
8. Rowe, J.D.; East, N.E. Risk factors for transmission and methods for control of caprine arthritis-encephalitis virus infection. *Vet. Clin. North Am. Food Anim. Pract.* 1997, *13*, 35–53.
9. Blacklaws, B.A.; Berriatúa, E.; Torsteinsdottir, S.; Watt, N.J.; De Andrés, D.; Klein, D.; Harkiss, G.D. Transmission of small ruminant lentiviruses. *Vet. Microbiol.* 2004, *101*, 199–208.
10. Pépin, M.; Vitu, C.; Russo, P.; Mornex, J.F.; Peterhans, E. Maedi-Visna Virus infection in sheep: A review. *Vet. Res.*1998, *29*, 1–53.
11. Peterhans, E.; Greenland, T.; Badiola, J.; Harkiss, G.; Bertoni, G.; Amorena, B.; Eliaszewicz, M.; Juste, R.A.; Krassnig, R.; Lafont, J.P.; *et al.* Routes of transmission and consequences of small ruminant lentiviruses (SRLVs) infection and eradication schemes. *Vet. Res.* 2004, *35*, 257–274.
12. Leginagoikoa, I.; Daltabuit-Test, M.; Alvarez, V.; Arranz, J.; Juste, R.A.; Amorena, B.; de Andrés, D.; Luján, L.L.; Badiola, J.J.; Berriatúa, E. Horizontal Maedi-Visna Virus (MVV) infection in adult dairy-sheep raised under varying MVV-infection pressures investigated by ELISA and PCR. *Res. Vet. Sci.* 2006, *80*, 235–241.
13. Gufler, H.; Gasteiner, J.; Lombardo, D.; Stifter, E.; Krassnig, R. Serological study of small ruminant lentivirus in goats in Italy. *Small Rumin. Res.* 2007, *73*, 169–173.
14. Herrmann-Hoesing, L.M.; Palmer, G.G.H.; Knowles, D.P.D. Evidence of proviral clearance following postpartum transmission of an ovine lentivirus. *Virology* 2007, *362*, 226–234.
15. Broughton-neiswanger, L.E.; White, S.N.; Knowles, D.P.; Mousel, M.R.; Lewis, G.S.; Herndon, D.R.; Herrmann-Hoesing, L.M. Non-maternal transmission is the major mode of ovine lentivirus transmission in a ewe flock: A molecular epidemiology study. *Infect. Genet. Evol.* 2010, *10*, 998–1007.
16. Álvarez, V.; Arranz, J.; Daltabuit-Test, M.; Leginagoikoa, I.; Juste, R.A.; Amorena, B.; de Andrés, D.; Luján, L.L.; Badiola, J.J.; Berriatúa, E. Relative contribution of colostrum from Maedi-Visna Virus (MVV) infected ewes to MVV-seroprevalence in lambs. *Res. Vet. Sci.* 2005, *78*, 237–243.
17. Thormar, H. Maedi-Visna Virus and its relationship to human immunodeficiency virus. *AIDS Rev.* 2005, *7*, 233–245.
18. Leroux, C.; Mornex, J.F. Retroviral infections in sheep and the associated diseases. *Small Rumin. Res.* 2008, *76*, 68–76.
19. Cheevers, W.P.; Beyer, J.C.; Knowles, D.P. Type 1 and type 2 cytokine gene expression by viral gp135 surface protein-activated T lymphocytes in caprine arthritis-encephalitis lentivirus infection. *J. Virol.* 1997, *71*, 6259–6263.
20. Lechner, F.; Machado, J.; Bertoni, G.; Seow, H.F.; Dobbelaere, D.A.E.; Peterhans, E. Caprine arthritis encephalitis virus dysregulates the expression of cytokines in macrophages. *J. Virol.* 1997, *71*, 7488–7497.
21. Ravazzolo, A.P.; Nenci, C.; Vogt, H.R.; Waldvogel, A.; Obexer-Ruff, G.; Peterhans, E.; Bertoni, G. Viral load, organ distribution, histopathological lesions, and cytokine mRNA expression in goats infected with a molecular clone of the caprine arthritis encephalitis virus. *Virology* 2006, *350*, 116–127.
22. Benavides, J.; García-Pariente, C.; Fuertes, M.; Ferreras, M.C.; García-Marín, J.F.; Juste, R.A. Maedi-Visna: The meningoencephalitis in naturally occurring cases. *J. Comp. Pathol.* 2009, *141*, 1–11.
23. Heaton, M.P.M.; Clawson, M.L.M.; Chitko-Mckown, C.G.; Leymaster, K.A.; Smith, T.P.L.; Harhay, G.P.; White, S.N.; Herrmann-Hoesing, L.M.; Mousel, M.R.; Lewis, G.S.; *et al.* Reduced lentivirus susceptibility in sheep with TMEM154 mutations. *PLoS Genet.* 2012, *8*, e1002467.
24. Cheevers, W.P.; Ho, I.; Beyer, J.C. Immune response to caprine arthritis/encephalitis virus surface protein induced by coimmunization with recombinant vaccinia viruses expressing the caprine arthritis/encephalitis virus envelope gene and caprine interleukin-12. *Vaccine* 2000, *18*, 2494–2503.
25. Torsteinsdóttir, S.; Carlsdóttir, H.M.; Svansson, V.; Matthíasdóttir, S.; Pétursson, G. Vaccination of sheep with Maedi-Visna Virus gag gene and protein, beneficial or harmful? *Vaccine* 2007, *25*, 6713–6720.
26. Brodie, S.J.; Marcom, K.A.; Pearson, L.D.; Anderson, B.C.; de la Concha-Bermejillo, A.; Ellis, J.A.; DeMartini, J.C. Effects of virus load in the pathogenesis of lentivirus-induced lymphoid interstitial pneumonia. *J. Infect. Dis.* 1992,*166*, 531–541.
27. Pétursson, G.; Matthíasdóttir, S.; Svansson, V.; Andrésdóttir, V.; Georgsson, G.; Martin, A.H.; Agnarsdóttir, G.; Gísladóttir, E.; Arnadóttir, S.; Högnadóttir, S.; *et al.* Mucosal vaccination with an attenuated Maedi-Visna Virus clone.*Vaccine* 2005, *23*, 3223–3228.
28. Cheevers, W.P.; Snekvik, K.R.; Trujillo, J.D.; Kumpula-McWhirter, N.M.; Pretty On Top, K.J.; Knowles, D.P. Prime-boost vaccination with plasmid DNA encoding

caprine-arthritis encephalitis lentivirus *env* and viral SU suppresses challenge virus and development of arthritis. *Virology* 2003, *306*, 116–125.

29. Nenci, C.; Zahno, M.L.; Vogt, H.R.; Obexer-Ruff, G.; Doherr, M.G.; Zanoni, R.; Bertoni, G. Vaccination with a T-cell-priming Gag peptide of caprine arthritis encephalitis virus enhances virus replication transiently *in vivo*. *J. Gen. Virol.*2007, *88*, 1589–1593.
30. Blacklaws, B.; Bird, P.; McConnell, I. Early events in infection of lymphoid tissue by a lentivirus, Maedi-Visna. *Trends Microbiol.* 1995, *3*, 434–440.
31. Berriatúa, E.; Álvarez, V.; Extramiana, B.; González, L.; Daltabuit, M.; Juste, R. Transmission and control implications of seroconversion to Maedi-Visna Virus in Basque dairy-sheep flocks. *Prev. Vet. Med.* 2003, *60*, 265–279.
32. DeMartini, J.; de la Concha-Bermejillo, A.; Carlson, J.; Bowen, R. Diseases caused by Maedi-Visna and other ovine lentiviruses. In *Breeding for Disease Resistance in Farm Animals*; Axford, R.F.E., Bishop, S.C., Nicholas, F.W., Owen, J.B., Eds.; CAB International: Oxon, UK, 2000; pp. 301–324.
33. Bishop, S.; Morris, C. Genetics of disease resistance in sheep and goats. *Small Rumin. Res.* 2007, *70*, 48–59.
34. Torsteinsdottir, S.; Andresdottir, V.; Arnarson, H.; Petursson, G. Immune response to Maedi-Visna Virus. *Front Biosci.*2007, *12*, 1532–1543.
35. Lawson-Handley, L.; Byrne, K.; Santucci, F.; Townsend, S.; Taylor, M.; Bruford, M.W.; Hewitt, G.M. Genetic structure of European sheep breeds. *Heredity* 2007, *99*, 620–631.
36. Kijas, J.W.; Townley, D.; Dalrymple, B.P.; Heaton, M.P.; Maddox, J.F.; Wilson, P.; Ingersoll, R.G.; Mcculloch, R.; Mcwilliam, S.; Tang, D.; *et al.* A Genome wide survey of SNP variation reveals the genetic structure of sheep breeds.*PLoS One* 2009, *4*, e4668.
37. The International Sheep Genomics Consortium; Archibald, A.; Cockett, N.; Dalrymple, B.P.; Faraut, T.; Kijas, J.W.; Maddox, J.F.; Mcewan, J.C.; Oddy, V.H.; Raadsma, H.W.; *et al.* The sheep genome reference sequence: A work in progress. *Anim. Genet.* 2010, *2009*, 449–453.
38. Ibeagha-Awemu, E.M.; Kgwatalala, E.M.I.P.; Ibeagha, A.E.; Zhao, X. A critical analysis of disease-associated DNA polymorphisms in the genes of cattle, goat, sheep, and pig. *Mamm. Genome* 2008, *19*, 226–245.
39. Becker, D.; Tetens, J.; Brunner, A.; Bürstel, D.; Ganter, M.; Kijas, J.; International Sheep Genomics Consortium; Drögemüller, C. Microphthalmia in Texel sheep is associated with a missense mutation in the paired-like homeodomain 3 (PITX3) gene. *PLoS One* 2010, *5*, e8689.
40. Purdie, A.C.; Plain, K.M.; Begg, D.J.; de Silva, K.; Whittington, R.J.; de Silva, K. Candidate gene and genome-wide association studies of *Mycobacterium avium* subsp. paratuberculosis infection in cattle and sheep: A review. *Comp. Immunol. Microbiol. Infect. Dis.* 2011, *34*, 197–208.
41. Silverman, E.K.; Palmer, L.J. Case-control association studies for the genetics of complex respiratory diseases. *Am. J. Respir. Cell Mol. Biol.* 2000, *22*, 645–648.
42. Daly, A.K.; Day, C.P. Candidate gene case-control association studies: Advantages and potential pitfalls. *Br. J. Clin. Pharmacol.* 2001, *52*, 489–499.
43. Campbell,H.;Rudan,I.Interpretationofgeneticassociation studies in complex disease. *Pharmacogenomics J.* 2002, *2*, 349–360.
44. Hirschhorn, J.N.; Lohmueller, K.; Byrne, E.; Hirschhorn, K. A comprehensive review of genetic association studies.*Genet. Med.* 2002, *4*, 45–61.
45. Cardon, L.R.; Palmer, L.J. Population stratification and spurious allelic association. *Lancet* 2003, *361*, 598–604.
46. Colhoun, H.M.; McKeigue, P.M.; Smith, G.D. Problems of reporting genetic associations with complex outcomes. *Lancet* 2003, *361*, 865–872.
47. Cordell, H.J.; Clayton, D.G. Genetic association studies. *Lancet* 2005, *366*, 1121–1131.
48. Balding, D.J. A tutorial on statistical methods for population association studies. *Nat. Rev. Genet.* 2006, *7*, 781–791.
49. Narum, S.R. Beyond bonferroni: Less conservative analyses for conservation genetics. *Conserv. Genet.* 2006, *7*, 783–787.
50. Bochud, P.Y.; Bochud, M.; Telenti, A.; Calandra, T. Innate immunogenetics: A tool for exploring new frontiers of host defence. *Lancet Infect. Dis.* 2007, *7*, 531–542.
51. Abbas, A.K.; Lichtman, A.H. *Basic Immunology, Updated Edition*; Saunders Elsevier: Philadelphia, PA, USA, 2006.
52. Maclachlan, N.; Dubovi, E.J. *Fenner's Veterinary Virology*, 4th ed.; Elsevier: London, UK, 2011.
53. Miyazawa, M.; Tsuji-kawahara, S.; Kanari, Y. Host genetic factors that control immune responses to retrovirus infections. *Vaccine* 2010, *26*, 2981–2996.
54. Kaur, G.; Mehra, N. Genetic determinants of HIV-1 infection and progression to AIDS: Immune response genes. *Tissue Antigens* 2009, *74*, 373–385.
55. Brodie, S. Current concepts in the epizootiology, diagnosis, and economic importance of ovine progressive pneumonia in North America: A review. *Small Rumin. Res.* 1998, *27*, 1–17.
56. Blacklaws, B.A.; Harkiss, G.D. Small ruminant lentiviruses and human immunodeficiency virus: Cousins that take a long view. *Curr. HIV Res.* 2010, *8*, 26–52.
57. Stump, D.S.; VandeWoude, S. Animal models for HIV AIDS: A comparative review. *Comp. Med.* 2007, *57*, 33–43.
58. Angelopoulou, K.; Brellou, G.D.; Vlemmas, I.; Greenland, T. A novel deletion in the LTR region of a Greek small ruminant lentivirus may be associated with low pathogenicity. *Virus Res.* 2006, *118*, 178–184.
59. Oskarsson, T.; Hreggvidsdóttir, H.S.; Agnarsdóttir, G.; Matthíasdóttir, S.; Ogmundsdóttir, M.H.; Jónsson, S.R.; Georgsson, G.; Ingvarsson, S.; Andrésson, O.S.;

Andrésdóttir, V. Duplicated sequence motif in the long terminal repeat of Maedi-Visna Virus extends cell tropism and is associated. *J. Virol.* 2007, *81*, 4052–4057.

60. Leginagoikoa, I.; Minguijón, E.; Juste, R.A.; Barandika, J.; Amorena, B.; de Andrés, D.; Badiola, J.J.; Luján, L.; Berriatua, E.; de Andrés, D. Effects of housing on the incidence of Visna/Maedi virus infection in sheep flocks. *Res. Vet. Sci.* 2010, *88*, 415–421.

61. González, L.; Juste, R.A.; Cuervo, L.A.; Idigoras, I.; Saez de Ocariz, C. Pathological and epidemiological aspects of the coexis- tence of Maedi-Visna and sheep pulmonary adenomatosis. *Res. Vet. Sci.* 1993, *54*, 140–146.

62. Andrésdóttir, V.; Tang, X.; Agnarsdóttir, G.; Andrésson, O.S.; Georgsson, G.; Skraban, R.; Torsteinsdóttir, S.; Rafnar, B.; Benediktsdóttir, E.; Matthíasdóttir, S.; Arnadóttir, S.; *et al.* Biological and genetic differences between lung- and brain-derived isolates of Maedi-Visna Virus. *Virus Genes* 1998, *16*, 281–293.

63. Reina, R.; Grego, E.; Bertolotti, L.; de Meneghi, D.; Rosati, S. Genome analysis of small-ruminant lentivirus genotype E: A caprine lentivirus with natural deletions of the dUTPase subunit, *vpr*-like accessory gene, and 70-base-pair repeat of the U3 region. *J. Virol.* 2009, *83*, 1152–1155.

64. Herrmann-Hoesing, L.M.; White, S.N.; Mousel, M.R.; Lewis, G.S.; Knowles, D.P. Ovine progressive pneumonia provirus levels associate with breed and Ovar-DRB1. *Immunogenetics* 2008, *60*, 749–758.

65. Palsson, P. Maedi and visna in sheep. In *Slow Virus Diseases of Animals and Man*; Kimberlin, R.H., Ed.; North-Holland: Amsterdam, The Netherland, 1976; pp. 17–43.

66. Straub, O.C. Maedi-Visna Virus infection in sheep. History and present knowledge. *Comp. Immunol. Microbiol. Infect. Dis.* 2004, *27*, 1–5.

67. Cutlip, R.C.; Lehmkuhl, H.D.; Brogden, K.A.; Sacks, J.M. Breed susceptibility to ovine progressive pneumonia (Maedi/Visna) virus. *Vet. Microbiol.* 1986, *12*, 283–288.

68. Houwers, D.J.; VIsscher, A.H.; Defise, P.R. Importance of ewe/lamb relationship and breed in the epidemiology of Maedi-Visna VIRUS infections. *Res. Vet. Sci.* 1989, *46*, 5–8.

69. Zink, M.C.; Johnson, L.K. Pathobiology of lentivirus infections of sheep and goats. *Virus Res.* 1994, *32*, 139–154.

70. De la Concha-Bermejillo, A.; Brodie, S.J.; Magnus-Corral, S.; Bowen, R.A.; DeMartini, J.C. Pathologic and serologic responses of isogeneic twin lambs to phenotypically disinct lentiviruses. *J. Acquir. Immune Defic. Syndr. Hum. Retrovirol.* 1995, *8*, 116–123.

71. Gates, N.L.; Winward, L.D.; Gorham, J.R.; Shen, D.T. Serologic survey of prevalence of ovine progressive pneumonia in Idaho range sheep. *J. Am. Vet. Med. Assoc.* 1978, *173*, 1575–1577.

72. Keen, J.E.; Hungerford, L.L.; Wittum, T.E.; Kwang, J.; Littledike, E.T. Risk factors for seroprevalenceof ovine lentivirus in breeding ewe flocks in Nebraska, USA. *Prev. Vet. Med.* 1997, *30*, 81–94.

73. Rowe, J.D.; East, N.E.; Franti, C.E.; Thurmond, M.C.; Pedersen, N.C.; Theilen, G.H. Risk factors associated with the incidence of seroconversion to caprine arthritis-encephalitis virus in goats on California dairies. *Am. J. Vet. Res.* 1992,*53*, 2396–2403.

74. Perk, K. Characteristics of ovine and caprine lentivirus infections. *Leukemia* 1995, *9*, 98–100.

75. Zhang, Z.; Watt, N.J.; Hopkins, J.; Harkiss, G.; Woodall, C.J. Quantitative analysis of Maedi-Visna Virus DNA load in peripheral blood monocytes and alveolar macrophages. *J. Virol. Methods* 2000, *86*, 13–20.

76. Singh, I.; McConnell, I.; Blacklaws, B. Immune response to individual Maedi-Visna Virus gag antigens. *J. Virol.* 2006,*80*, 912–919.

77. Fluri, A.; Nenci, C.; Zahno, M.-L.; Vogt, H.; Charan, S.; Busato, A.; Pancino, G.; Peterhans, E.; Obexer-Ruff, G.; Bertoni, G. The MHC-haplotype influences primary, but not memory, immune responses to an immunodominant peptide containing T- and B-cell epitopes of the caprine arthritis encephalitis virus Gag protein. *Vaccine* 2006, *24*, 597–606.

78. Clements, J.E.; Zink, M.C. Molecular biology and pathogenesis of animal lentivirus infections. *Clin. Microbiol. Rev.*1996, *9*, 100–117.

79. Staskus, K.A.; Couch, L.; Bitterman, P.; Retzel, E.F.; Zupancic, M.; List, J.; Haase, A.T. *In situ* amplification of visna virus DNA in tissue sections reveals a reservoir of latently infected cells. *Microb. Pathog.* 1991, *11*, 67–76.

80. Reina, R.; Glaria, I.; Benavides, J.; de Andrés, X.; Crespo, H.; Solano, C.; Pérez, V.; Luján, L.; Pérez, M.M.; Pérez de la Lastra, J.M.; *et al.* Association of CD80 and CD86 expression levels with disease status of Visna/Maedi virus infected sheep. *Viral Immunol.* 2007, *20*, 609–622.

81. Gudnadóttir, M.; Demosthenous, A.; Hadjisavvas, T. Vaccination delays Maedi-Visna lentivirus infection in a naturally-infected sheep flock. *BMC Vet. Res.* 2013, *9*, e16.

82. Benavides, J.; García-Pariente, C.; Ferreras, M.C.; Fuertes, M.; García-Marín, J.F.; Pérez, V. Diagnosis of clinical cases of the nervous form of Maedi-Visna in 4- and 6-month-old lambs. *Vet. J.* 2007, *174*, 255–258.

83. Brodie, S.J.; Pearson, L.D.; Zink, M.C.; Bickle, H.M.; Anderson, B.C.; Marcom, K.A.; Demartinit, J.C.; DeMartini, J.C. Ovine lentivirus expression and disease. Virus replication, but not entry, is restricted to macrophages of specific tissues. *Am. J. Pathol.* 1995, *146*, 250–263.

84. Agnarsdóttir, G.; Thorsteinsdóttir, H.; Oskarsson, T.; Matthíasdóttir, S.; Haflidadóttir, B.S.; Andrésson, O.S.; Andrésdóttir, V. The long terminal repeat is a determinant of cell tropism of Maedi-Visna Virus. *J. Gen. Virol.* 2000, *81*, 1901–1905.

85. Hötzel, I.; Cheevers, W.P. A maedi-visna virus strain K1514 receptor gene is located in sheep chromosome 3p and the syntenic region of human chromosome 2. *J. Gen. Virol.* 2002, *83*, 1759–1764.

86. Hötzel, I.; Cheevers, W.P. Host range of small-ruminant lentivirus cytopathic variants determined with a selectable caprine arthritis-encephalitis virus pseudotype system. *J. Virol.* 2001, *75*, 7384–7391.

87. Crespo, H.; Jauregui, P.; Glaria, I.; José, I.S.; Polledo, L.; García-Marín, J.F.; Luján, L.; de Andrés, D.; Amorena, B.; Reina, R. Mannose receptor may be involved in small ruminant lentivirus pathogenesis. *Vet. Res.* 2012, *43*, e43.

88. Amills, M.; Ramiya, V.; Norimine, J.; Lewin, H.A. The major histocompatibility complex of ruminants. *Rev. Sci. Tech.*1998, *17*, 108–120.

89. Dukkipati, V.S.R.; Blair, H.T.; Garrick, D.J.; Murray, A. "Ovar-Mhc"—Ovine major histocompatibility complex: Structure and gene polymorphisms. *Genet. Mol. Res.* 2006, *5*, 581–608.

90. Sayers, G.; Sweeney, T. Gastrointestinal nematode infection in sheep—A review of the alternatives to anthelmintics in parasite control. *Anim. Health Res. Rev.* 2005, *6*, 159–172.

91. Lee, W.C.; Bird, P.; McConnell, I.; Watt, N.J.; Blacklaws, B. The phenotype and phagocytic activity of macrophages during Maedi-Visna Virus infection. *Vet. Immunol. Immunopathol.* 1996, *51*, 113–126.

92. Bergsteinsdóttir, K.; Arnadóttir, S.; Torsteinsdóttir, S.; Agnarsdóttir, G.; Andrésdóttir, V.; Péttursson, G.; Georgsson, G. Constitutive and visna virus induced expression of class I and II major histocompatibility complex antigens in the central nervous system of sheep and their role in the pathogenesis of visna lesions. *Neuropathol. Appl. Neurobiol.* 1998,*24*, 224–232.

93. Harkiss, G.D.; Watt, N.J.; King, T.J.; Williams, J.; Hopkins, J. Retroviral arthritis: Phenotypic analysis of cells in the synovial fluid of sheep with inflammatory synovitis associated with visna virus infection. *Clin. Immunol. Immunopathol.* 1991, *60*, 106–117.

94. Anderson, A.A.; Harkiss, G.D.; Watt, N.J. Quantitative analysis of immunohistological changes in the synovial membrane of sheep infected with Maedi-Visna Virus. *Clin. Immunol. Immunopathol.* 1994, *72*, 21–29.

95. Larruskain, A.; Minguijón, E.; García-etxebarria, K.; Moreno, B.; Arostegui, I.; Juste, R.A; Jugo, B.M. MHC class II DRB1 gene polymorphism in the pathogenesis of Maedi-Visna and pulmonary adenocarcinoma viral diseases in sheep. *Immunogenetics* 2010, *62*, 75–83.

96. Larruskain, A.; Minguijón, E.; Arostegui, I.; Moreno, B.; Juste, R.A.; Jugo, B.M. Microsatellites in immune-relevant regions and their associations with Maedi-Visna and ovine pulmonary adenocarcinoma viral diseases. *Vet. Immunol. Immunopathol.* 2012, *145*, 438–446.

97. Ruff, G.; Regli, J.G.; Lazary, S. Occurrence of caprine leucocyte class I and II antigens in Saanen goats affected by caprine arthritis (CAE). *Eur. J. Immunogenet.* 1993, *20*, 285–288.

98. Batalia, M.A.; Collins, E.J.; Carolina, N. Peptide binding by class I and class II MHC molecules. *Biopolymers* 1997, *43*, 281–302.

99. Konnai, S.; Takeshima, S.; Tajima, S.; Yin, S.A.; Okada, K.; Onuma, M.; Aida, Y. The influence of ovine MHC class II DRB1 alleles on immune response in bovine leukemia virus infection. *Microbiol. Immunol.* 2003, *47*, 223–232.

100. De Andrés, D.; Klein, D.; Watt, N.J.; Berriatua, E.; Torsteinsdottir, S.; Blacklaws, B.A.; Harkiss, G.D. Diagnostic tests for small ruminant lentiviruses. *Vet. Microbiol.* 2005, *107*, 49–62.

101. Singh, D.K.; Chebloune, Y.; Mselli-Lakhal, L.; Karr, B.M.; Narayan, O. Ovine lentivirus-infected macrophages mediate productive infection in cell types that are not susceptible to infection with cell-free virus. *J. Gen. Virol.* 1999, *80*, 1437–1444.

102. Torsteinsdóttir, S.; Georgsson, G.; Gísladóttir, E.; Rafnar, B.; Pálsson, P.A.; Pétursson, G. Pathogenesis of central nervous system lesions in visna: Cell-mediated immunity and lymphocyte subsets in blood, brain and cerebrospinal fluid. *J. Neuroimmunol.* 1992, *41*, 149–158.

103. Perry, L.L.; Wilkerson, M.J.; Hullinger, G.A.; Cheevers, W.P. Depressed CD4T lymphocyte proliferative response and enhanced antibody response to viral antigen in chronic lentivirus-induced arthritis. *J. Infect. Dis.* 1995, *171*, 328–334.

104. Trujillo, J.D.; Hotzel, K.J.; Snekvik, K.R.; Cheevers, W.P. Antibody response to the surface envelope of caprine arthritis-encephalitis lentivirus: Disease status is predicted by SU antibody isotype. *Virology* 2004, *325*, 129–136.

105. Bird, P.; Reyburn, H.T.; Blacklaws, B.A.; Allen, D.; Nettleton, P.; Yirrell, D.L.; Watt, N.; Sargan, D.; McConnell, I. The restricted IgG1 antibody response to maedi visna virus is seen following infection but not following immunization with recombinant gag protein. *Clin. Exp. Immunol.* 1995, *102*, 274–280.

106. Watt, N.J.; MacIntyre, N.; Collie, D.; Sargan, D.; McConnell, I. Phenotypic analysis of lymphocyte populations in the lungs and regional lymphoid tissue of sheep naturally infected with Maedi-Visna Virus. *Clin. Exp. Immunol.* 1992, *90*, 204–208.

107. Luján, L.; Begara, I.; Collie, D.D.; Watt, N.J. CD8+ lymphocytes in bronchoalveolar lavage and blood: *In vivo* indicators of lung pathology caused by Maedi-Visna Virus. *Vet. Immunol. Immunopathol.* 1995, *49*, 89–100.

108. Jolly, P.E.; Gangopadhyay, A.; Chen, S.; Reddy, P.G.; Weiss, H.L. Changes in the leukocyte phenotype profile of goats infected with the caprine arthritis encephalitis virus. *Vet. Immunol. Immunopathol.* 1997, *56*, 97–106.

109. Blacklaws, B.A; Bird, P.; Allen, D.; McConnell, I. Circulating cytotoxic T lymphocyte precursors in Maedi-Visna Virus-infected sheep. *J. Gen. Virol.* 1994, *75*, 1589–1596.

110. Lee, W.C.; McConnell, I.; Blacklaws, B.A. Cytotoxic activity against Maedi-Visna Virus-infected macrophages. *J. Virol.*1994, *68*, 8331–8338.

111. Estes, D.M.; Brown, W.C. Type 1 and type 2 responses in regulation of Ig isotype expression in cattle. *Vet. Immunol. Immunopathol.* 2002, *90*, 1–10.

112. Snekvik, K.R.; Beyer, J.C.; Bertoni, G.; von Beust, B.R.; Baszler, T.V; Palmer, G.H.; McElwain, T.F.; Cheevers, W.P. Characterization of caprine interleukin-4. *Vet. Immunol. Immunopathol.* 2001, *78*, 219–229.

113. Lechner, F.; Vogt, H.R.; Seow, H.F.; Bertoni, G.; Cheevers, W.P.; von Bodungen, U.; Zurbriggen, A; Peterhans, E. Expression of cytokine mRNA in lentivirus-induced arthritis. *Am. J. Pathol.* 1997, *151*, 1053–1065.

114. Woodall, C.J.; Maclaren, L.J.; Watt, N.J. Differential levels of mRNAs for cytokines, the interleukin-2 receptor and Class II DR/DQ genes in ovine interstitial pneumonia induced by Maedi visna virus infection. *Vet. Pathol.* 1997, *34*, 204–211.

115. Legastelois, I.; Cottin, V.; Mornex, J.F.; Cordier, G. Alveolar macrophages from sheep naturally infected by Visna-Maedi virus contribute to IL-8 production in the lung. *Vet. Immunol. Immunopathol.* 1997, *59*, 131–139.

116. Zhang, Z.; Harkiss, G.D.; Hopkins, J. Granulocyte macrophage colony stimulating factor is elevated in alveolar macrophages from sheep naturally infected with Maedi-Visna Virus and stimulates Maedi-Visna Virus replication in macrophages *in vitro*. *Clin. Exp. Immunol.* 2002, *129*, 240–246.

117. Legastelois, I.; Cordier, O.; Cozon, G.; Cador, J. Visna-Maedi virus-induced expression of interleukin-8 gene in sheep alveolar cells following experimental *in vitro* and *in vivo* infection. *Res. Virol.* 1996, *147*, 191–197.

118. Ellis, J.A.; DeMartini, J.C. Ovine interleukin-2: Partial purification and assay in normal sheep and sheep with ovine progressive pneumonia. *Vet. Immunol. Immunopathol.* 1985, *8*, 15–25.

119. Legastelois, I.; Levrey, H.; Greenland, T.; Mornex, J.F.; Cordier, G. Visna-Maedi virus induces interleukin-8 in sheep alveolar macrophages through a tyrosine-kinase signaling pathway. *Am. J. Respir. Cell Mol. Biol.* 1998, *18*, 532–537.

120. Larruskain, A.; Bernales, I.; Luján, L.; de Andrés, D.; Amorena, B.; Jugo, B.M. Expression analysis of 13 ovine immune response candidate genes in Visna/Maedi disease progression. *Comp. Immunol. Microbiol. Infect. Dis.* 2013, *36*, 405–413.

121. White, S.N.; Mousel, M.R.; Reynolds, J.O.; Lewis, G.S.; Herrmann-Hoesing, L.M. Common promoter deletion is associated with 3.9-fold differential transcription of ovine CCR5 and reduced proviral level of ovine progressive pneumonia virus. *Anim. Genet.* 2009, *40*, 583–589.

122. Shirakawa, I.; Deichmann, K.A.; Izuhara, I.; Mao, I.; Adra, C.N.; Hopkin, J.M. Atopy and asthma: Genetic variants of IL-4 and IL-13 signalling. *Immunol. Today* 2000, *21*, 60–64.

123. Locati, M.; Otero, K.; Schioppa, T.; Signorelli, P.; Perrier, P.; Baviera, S.; Sozzani, S.; Mantovani, A. The chemokine system: Tuning and shaping by regulation of receptor expression and coupling in polarized responses. *Allergy* 2002,*57*, 972–982.

124. Medzhitov, R. Recognition of microorganisms and activation of the immune response. *Nature* 2007, *449*, 819–826.

125. Werling, D.; Jann, O.; Offord, V.; Glass, E.; Coffey, T. Variation matters: TLR structure and species-specific pathogen recognition. *Trends mmunol.* 2009, *30*, 124–130.

126. Takeda, K.; Kaisho, T.; Akira, S. Toll-like receptors. *Annu. Rev. Immunol.* 2003, *21*, 335–376.

127. Mikula, I.; Bhide, M.; Pastorekova, S. Characterization of ovine TLR7 and TLR8 protein coding regions, detection of mutations and Maedi-Visna Virus infection. *Vet. Immunol. Immunopathol.* 2010, *138*, 51–59.

128. Bell, J.K.; Mullen, G.E.; Leifer, C.A.; Mazzoni, A.; Davies, D.R.; Segal, D.M. Leucine-rich repeats and pathogen recognition in Toll-like receptors. *Trends Immunol.* 2003, *24*, 528–533.

129. Zheng, Y.H.; Peterlin, B.B. Intracellular immunity to HIV-1: Newly defined retroviral battles inside infected cells.*Retrovirology* 2005, *2*, e25.

130. Huthoff, H.; Towers, G.J. Restriction of retroviral replication by APOBEC3G/F and TRIM5alpha. *Trends Microbiol.*2008, *16*, 612–619.

131. Jáuregui, P.; Crespo, H.; Glaria, I.; Luján, L.; Contreras, A.; Rosati, S.; de Andrés, D.; Amorena, B.; Towers, G.J.; Reina, R. Ovine TRIM5 can restrict Visna/Maedi virus. *J. Virol.* 2012, *86*, 9504–9509.

132. Van Manen, D.; Rits, M.A.; Beugeling, C.; van Dort, K.; Schuitemaker, H.; Kootstra, N.A. The effect of Trim5 polymorphisms on the clinical course of HIV-1 infection. *PLoS Pathog.* 2008, *4*, e18.

133. LaRue, R.S.; Jónsson, S.R.; Silverstein, K.A.T.; Lajoie, M.; Bertrand, D.; El-Mabrouk, N.; Hötzel, I.; Andrésdóttir, V.; Smith, T.P.L.; Harris, R.S. The artiodactyl APOBEC3 innate immune repertoire shows evidence for a multi-functional domain organization that existed in the ancestor of placental mammals. *BMC Mol. Biol.* 2008, *9*, 10–1186.

134. LaRue, R.S.; Lengyel, J.; Jonsson, S.R.; Andresdottir, V.; Harris, R.S. Lentiviral Vif degrades the APOBEC3Z3/APOBEC3H protein of its mammalian host and is capable of cross-species activity. *J. Virol.* 2010, *84*, 8193–8201.

135. Jónsson, S.R.; Haché, G.; Stenglein, M.D.; Fahrenkrug, S.C.; Andrésdóttir, V.; Harris, R.S. Evolutionarily conserved and non-conserved retrovirus restriction activities of artiodactyl APOBEC3F proteins. *Nucleic Acids Res.* 2006, *34*, 5683–5694.

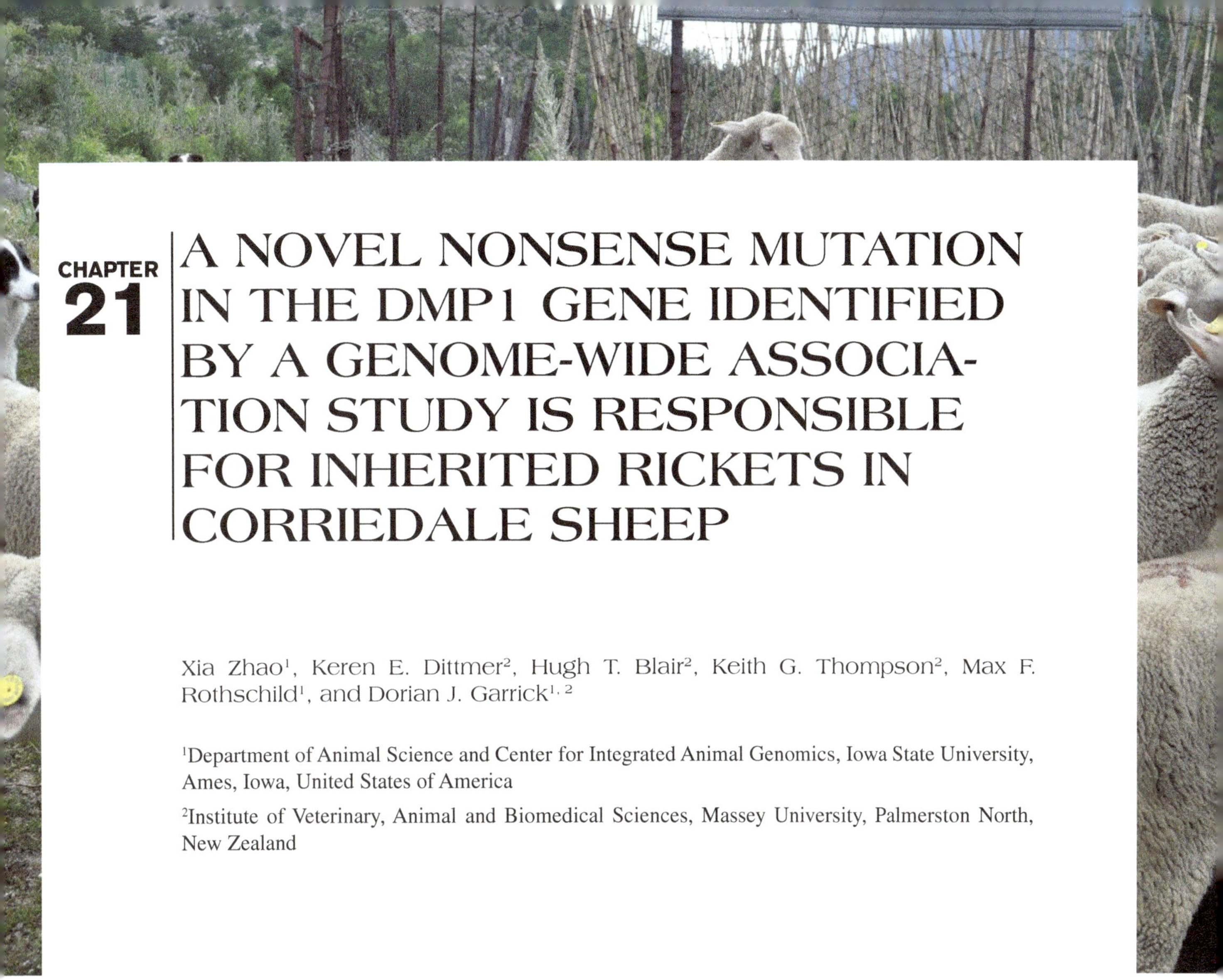

CHAPTER 21 A NOVEL NONSENSE MUTATION IN THE DMP1 GENE IDENTIFIED BY A GENOME-WIDE ASSOCIATION STUDY IS RESPONSIBLE FOR INHERITED RICKETS IN CORRIEDALE SHEEP

Xia Zhao[1], Keren E. Dittmer[2], Hugh T. Blair[2], Keith G. Thompson[2], Max F. Rothschild[1], and Dorian J. Garrick[1, 2]

[1]Department of Animal Science and Center for Integrated Animal Genomics, Iowa State University, Ames, Iowa, United States of America

[2]Institute of Veterinary, Animal and Biomedical Sciences, Massey University, Palmerston North, New Zealand

ABSTRACT

Inherited rickets of Corriedale sheep is characterized by decreased growth rate, thoracic lordosis and angular limb deformities. Previous outcross and backcross studies implicate inheritance as a simple autosomal recessive disorder. A genome wide association study was conducted using the Illumina OvineSNP50 BeadChip on 20 related sheep comprising 17 affected and 3 carriers. A homozygous region of 125 consecutive single-nucleotide polymorphism (SNP) loci was identified in all affected sheep, covering a region of 6 Mb on ovine chromosome 6. Among 35 candidate genes in this region, the dentin matrix protein 1 gene (*DMP1*) was sequenced to reveal a nonsense mutation 250C/T on exon 6. This mutation introduced a stop codon (R145X) and could truncate C-terminal amino acids. Genotyping by PCR-RFLP for this mutation showed all 17 affected sheep were "T T" genotypes; the 3 carriers were "C T"; 24 phenotypically normal related sheep were either "C T" or "C C"; and 46 unrelated normal control sheep from other breeds were all "C C". The other SNPs in *DMP1* were not concordant with the disease and can all be ruled out as candidates. Previous research has shown that mutations in the *DMP1* gene are responsible for autosomal recessive hypophosphatemic rickets in humans. Dmp1_knockout mice exhibit rickets phenotypes. We believe the R145X mutation to be responsible for the inherited rickets found in Corriedale sheep. A simple diagnostic test can be designed to identify carriers with the defective "T" allele. Affected sheep could be used as animal models for this form of human rickets, and for further investigation of the role of DMP1 in phosphate homeostasis.

INTRODUCTION

Rickets is a metabolic bone disease in humans and animals with most cases caused by a nutritional deficiency of either vitamin D or phosphorus. This disease leads to softening and weakening of bone caused by defective mineralization of cartilage at sites of endochondral ossification and potentially causes fractures and limb deformities [1], [2], [3]. Rickets may also result from genetic mutations that disrupt genes whose functions are critical for normal bone metabolism. Five types of rickets have been described in humans with common clinical characteristics of renal phosphate wasting, including X-linked hypophosphatemic rickets (XLH), autosomal dominant hypophosphatemic rickets (ADHR), autosomal

Citation: Xia Zhao, Keren E. Dittmer, Hugh T. Blair, Keith G. Thompson, Max F. Rothschild, Dorian J. Garrick, A Novel Nonsense Mutation in the DMP1 Gene Identified by a Genome-Wide Association Study Is Responsible for Inherited Rickets in Corriedale Sheep, doi: 10.1371/journal.pone.0021739.

recessive hypophosphatemic rickets (ARHR) type 1 and 2, and hereditary hypophosphataemic rickets with hypercalciuria (HHRH). A large number of different mutations comprising single base pair deletions, nonsense and missense mutations have been identified in *PHEX* (phosphate regulation gene with homologies to endopeptidases on the X chromosome) as being responsible for XLH [4], [5], [6]. ADHR is caused by gain of function mutation leading to increased activity of fibroblast growth factor 23 encoded by gene *FGF23* [7], and mutations in the dentin matrix protein 1 gene (*DMP1*) and ecto-nucleotide pyrophosphatase/phosphodiesterase 1 (*ENPP1*) have been identified in autosomal recessive hypophosphataemic rickets type 1 and 2, respectively [8], [9],[10]. The mutation for HHRH occurs in the gene for the NaP_i-IIc protein (or *SLC34A3*, human chromosome 9q34), a renal Na-P co-transporter [11]. Two other recessively inherited forms of rickets in humans are due to the disruptions of either the synthesis or metabolism of vitamin D. Vitamin D-dependent rickets type I (VDDR-I) is caused by mutations in the *CYP27B1* gene, which encodes vitamin D 1-alpha-hydroxylase[12]. Loss of function mutations in the vitamin D receptor gene (VDR) are the genetic basis for vitamin D-dependent rickets type II (VDDR-II), which is also called hereditary vitamin D - resistant rickets (HVDRR)[13], [14].

Inherited forms of rickets have been uncovered frequently in humans but were rare in domestic animals. Recently, an inherited form of rickets has been described in purebred Corriedale sheep from a commercial flock in New Zealand, with an incidence of up to 20 lambs out of 1,600 over a 2-year period. Affected sheep were characterized by decreased growth rate, thoracic lordosis and angular limb deformities (Figure 1) [15], with low serum calcium and phosphate concentrations and normal 25 hydroxyvitamin D and 1,25 dihydroxyvitamin D_3 concentrations [16]. Embryo transfer and backcross breeding trials have determined that this disease is likely a simple autosomal recessive disorder [16].

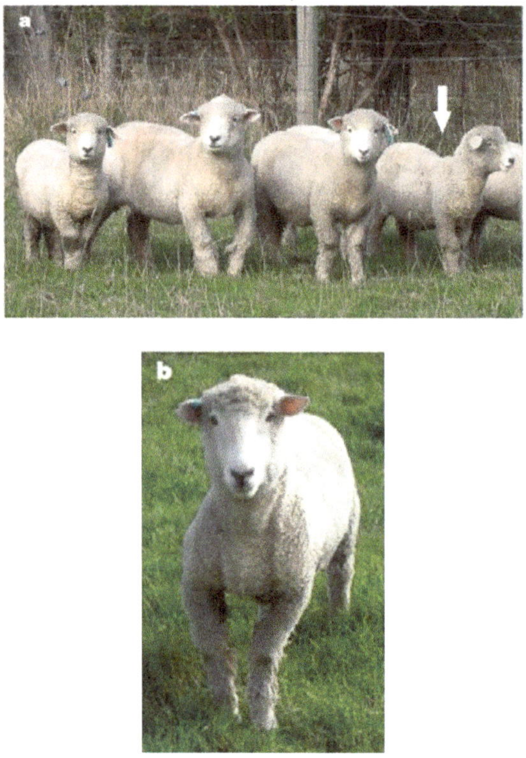

Figure 1: Corriedale sheep with rickets.

Large animal models of human genetic diseases have received extensive clinical attention due to their advantages over rodent models, including greater physiological similarity to human patients, a longer life span and larger body size. Sheep have been used as an animal model for gene therapy (GT) of human diseases, such as post-traumatic osteoarthritis [17] and steroid-induced ocular hypertension [18]. The convenience of performing in utero GT prior to disease onset will help to achieve long-term expression of the exogenous gene without modifying the germ line of the recipient [19]. Based on the hypothesis that inherited rickets-affected Corriedale sheep could be a potential model for human rickets; and a genetic marker could help sheep breeders to avoid at-risk matings, we performed a genome-wide association study by genotyping 54,241 evenly distributed single nucleotide polymorphisms (SNPs) for 17 affected Corriedale sheep and 3 carriers using the Illumina Ovine SNP50 BeadChip. It has been shown that the analysis of genome-wide high-density SNPs is an effective strategy to map and identify causal mutations for recessive diseases [20].

RESULTS

Homozygosity Mapping

The genotyping data using a SNP BeadChip for this study was submitted to the NCBI Gene Expression Omnibus (http://www.ncbi.nlm.nih.gov/geo) under Super Series accession no GSE26310. In our study, exactly 3 homozygous regions of more than 10 consecutive SNPs were identified in all 17 affected sheep whereas the 3 carriers exhibited heterozygosity in those regions.

The largest homozygous segment consisted of 125 consecutive SNP loci, whereas the other two segments had only 19 or 11 consecutive SNPs. The largest 125-SNP region started from SNP OAR6_109334543.1 and extended to SNP s03175.1, covering a region of 5.95 Mb (109,334,543 to 115,285,275 bp) on the long arm of sheep chromosome 6 (OAR 6).

There were 35 genes located in this region based on the bovine reference sequence (Figures 2a, 2b). The size of the second homozygous segment was about 0.70 Mb (OAR6: 118,884,834 to 119,587,883 bp) and had only 3.2 Mb separation from the first homozygous segment on the same chromosome (OAR 6). The third homozygous segment covered a 0.66 Mb region (OAR15: 1,131,166 to 1,654,496 bp) on the short arm of OAR 15. Within the second and third homozygous regions there were 8 and 6 positional candidate genes, respectively.

One gene called *DMP1* in the largest 125-SNP region was considered the most plausible candidate due to its biological functions involved in mineralization and phosphate homeostasis and previous reports of its involvement in human rickets [8], [21]. By comparing with the bovine genomic reference sequence it was found that this gene was at 112.20 Mb on OAR6q, spanned over 16 kb of size and contained 6 exons.

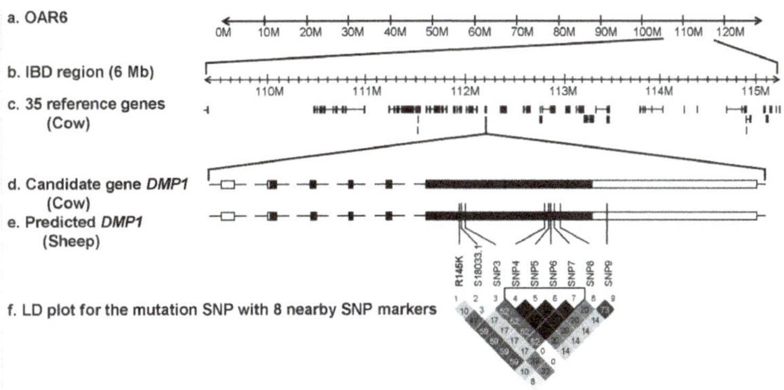

Figure 2: Work flow chart for discovering the mutation locus of inherited rickets in Corriedale sheep.

Candidate Gene Sequencing

Fine mapping was carried out by individual PCR amplification and sequencing of all the exons of the *DMP1*gene to identify the mutation for this disease . After blasting the sheep genomic reference sequence with bovine *DMP1* coding sequence (ENSBTAT00000025468), there were several alignments for exon 6 with high identity rates (91%–96%). As exon 6 is the last and also the largest exon covering 88% of the open reading frame of *DMP1*, it was prioritized for re-sequencing. Direct sequencing from 3 carriers and 1 normal control revealed 1 published SNP (s18093.1, OAR6: 112,213,812 bp) and 8 novel ones in this exon (Figure 2e). The complete genomic sequence of exon 6 for sheep *DMP1* gene was submitted to GenBank (http://www.ncbi.nlm.nih.gov/genbank/) under accession no. HQ600592.

Moreover, we successfully amplified exon 1, exon 3, exon 4 and exon 5 of sheep *DMP1* gene using exon flanked intronic sequences of cow reference for each exon. The amplifications of exon 2 failed after using several pairs of primers. Intronic SNPs (SNP1 and SNP2) and a 1-bp insertion/deletion (indel: A) were identified respectively in intron 1, intron 5 and intron 3 by direct sequencing.

Mutation Analysis

Seventeen base pairs upstream of SNP s18093.1, a SNP (C/T, OAR6:112,213,795 bp) located at +250bp of exon 6 caused a non-synonymous amino acid change in the DMP1 protein. This C -> T transition introduced a stop codon (R145X) that led to a truncated DMP1 protein at the 145th amino acid (Figure 3a, Figure 3b). Genotyping of this mutation by PCR-RFLP (Polymerase Chain Reaction-Restriction Fragment Length Polymorphism) (Figure 3c) and direct sequencing showed all 17 affected animals had the "T T" genotype; the 3 carriers were "C T"; 24 phenotypically normal related sheep were either "C T" or "C C"; and 46 unrelated control sheep of other breeds were only "C C" genotypes (Table 1). This mutation was 100% concordant with the recessive pattern of inheritance in affected, carrier and normal individuals. Moreover, genotyping of the other 8 SNPs in exon 6 which surrounded the R145X mutation in *DMP1*, found incomplete linkage disequilibrium for these markers with either the disease or the mutant SNP (Figure 2f). The 3 genomic variants in introns 1, 3 and 5 identified were not located at either the splicing receptor or acceptor sites. Therefore, those mutations could be ruled out as candidate mutation loci. RT-PCR/RFLP (Figure 3d) was performed for the R145X mutation and showed the same digestion pattern as PCR-RFLP.

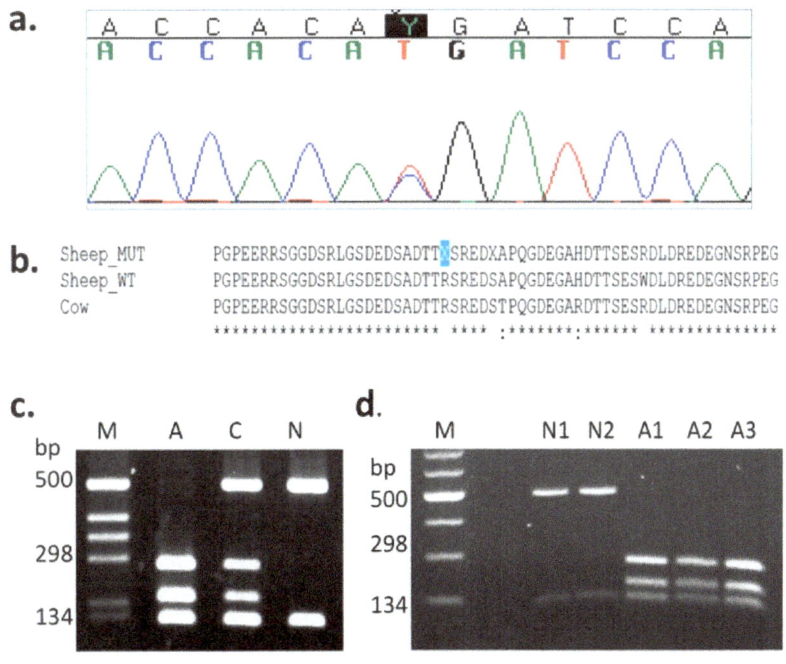

Figure 3: Mutation analyses.

Table 1: The genotyping results of the causative mutation (R145X).

Sheep Breed	Phenotype		Genotype		Rate of Concordance
	Rickets Status	# Sheep	Genotype	# Sheep	
Corriedale	Affected	17	T T	17	100%
	Known Carrier	3	T C	3	100%
	Phenotype Normal[a]	24	T C , C C	24	100%
Texel, Perendale	Normal	46	C C	46	100%

Taken together, our results strongly suggest that the R145X substitution is causative for inherited rickets in Corriedale sheep, disrupting the function of the DMP1 protein, preventing successful bone mineralization and phosphate homeostasis.

DISCUSSION

Homozygosity mapping is a powerful method to map simple recessive traits since the regions immediately flanking the mutation locus will likely be homozygous by descent in closely related offspring. The affected animals in this study resulted from consanguineous mating between pairs of offspring descended from one common male ancestor in the embryo transfer and backcross studies used to characterize the inheritance of the disease [15], [16]. The region containing the mutation should in these circumstances span a large chromosome segment that would be progressively diminished in subsequent meioses when recombination events occur near to the mutation. This mapping strategy has been used successfully for recessive diseases in both animal and human studies [20], [22]. The homozygosity mapping in this study was conducted from knowledge of the SNP genotypes in affected individuals and their genomic location, and used command line UNIX tools including awk, sort and join to identify any regions of at least 10 consecutive homozygous SNPs, equivalent to about 0.5 cM or more. It was presumed that one such region would contain the mutation associated with inherited rickets in Corriedale sheep. In this study, 3 homozygous regions met the criteria of exceeding 10 consecutive homozygous SNP markers. Previously reported rickets genes including *PHEX,FGF23*, *ENPP1*, *SLC34A3*, *CYP27B1* and *VDR* did not show up in any of these homozygous segments based on the ovine genome assembly v1.0, whereas *DMP1* was contained in the largest region. This is not surprising because *PHEX* or *FGF23* related rickets have a distinctive inheritance mode that differs from the autosomal recessive inheritance of the rickets studied here. The severe hypophosphatemia in affected sheep indicates disturbed phosphate balance within the body. Therefore, the *DMP1* gene was considered to be a high priority candidate gene. The nonsense mutation we identified in the *DMP1* gene was 100% concordant with the recessive pattern of inheritance for the disease studied.

DMP1 encodes a serine-rich acidic protein and is a member of Small Integrin-Binding Ligand, N-linked, Glycoprotein family (SIBLING) which mineralizes tissue such as bones and teeth by binding strongly to hydroxyapatite using an Arg-Gly-Asp (RGD) tripeptide [23]. Dual functions of the DMP1 protein have been reported based on the *in vitro* studies. The nonphosphorylated cytoplasmic DMP1 protein translocates to the cell nucleus and initially acts as a transcriptional factor to enhance gene transcription of the osteoblast-specific genes such as alkaline phosphatase and osteocalcin, and then it moves out to the extracellular matrix during the osteoblast to osteocyte transition phase, to promote mineralization and phosphate homeostasis [24], [25]. Loss of function mutations in the human *DMP1* gene have been shown to cause autosomal recessive hypophosphatemic rickets in different ethnic groups including Turkish, consanguineous Spanish, Lebanese and Japanese populations. These variant mutations in *DMP1* include deletions in exon 6, nucleotide substitution in the splice acceptor sequence of intron 2, and missense mutations in exon 2 or exon 3 that introduce the premature termination codon [8], [21], [26]. The *Dmp1*-null mouse model also exhibits hypophosphatemic rickets, which indicates the important role of the *DMP1* gene in the development of normal bone formation [21]. Since the majority of the dentin matrix protein 1 is encoded by the sixth and last exon of *DMP1*, typical for proteins in the SIBLING family [27], the novel nonsense mutation (250C/T, R145X) identified here in ovine *DMP1* gene is a plausible mutation leading to loss of function following nonsense-mediatedmRNA decay shown to occur in human patients. The nonsense-mediated mRNA decay is a post-transcriptional mechanism in eukaryotic species. It likely eliminates the abnormal transcripts produced by prematurely terminated translation [28]. The previous studies strongly support the nonsense mutation we identified in exon 6 as causing loss of function of the DMP1 protein and being responsible for ARHR type 1 in Corriedale sheep.

Despite the wide variety of mutated genes that result in the different forms of hereditary hypophosphatemic rickets, the clinical features are relatively similar (with the exception of HHRH). In XLH, ADHR, ARHR type 1 and 2, the overriding common feature is increased serum concentration and activity of FGF23. FGF23 inhibits a NPT-2a co-transporter (Na-P_i co-transporter) in the kidneys leading to loss of phosphate from renal tubules into the urine (phosphaturia). FGF23 also inhibits the activity of CYP27B1, thereby inhibiting active vitamin D (1,25-dihydroxyvitamin D_3) production [29]. As a result of the increased FGF23 concentrations patients with XLH, ADHR, ARHR type 1 and 2 present with rickets, hypophosphatemia, phosphaturia and inappropriately normal serum 1,25-dihydroxyvitamin D_3 concentrations [9], [30]. Corriedale sheep with the mutation in *DMP1* also developed rickets, were severely hypophosphataemic and had normal serum $1,25(OH)_2D_3$ concentrations [1], [16]. The mechanism by which mutations in *PHEX*, *DMP1* or *ENPP1*result in upregulation of FGF23 is unknown. An unusual feature of ARHR type 2 is that mutations in*ENPP1* are also associated with generalized arterial calcification of infancy, again the mechanism by which a mutation in *ENPP1* can result in a disease characterised by hypomineralization and one characterised by hypermineralization is unknown [9]. In HHRH, CYP27B1 is actually upregulated, resulting in increased $1,25(OH)_2D_3$ concentrations, and perhaps explaining the hypercalciuria [11].

In conclusion, this is the first report of ARHR type 1 caused by a mutation in the *DMP1* gene in a sheep population. In this study, we demonstrate successful use of applying high density SNP arrays for localization of a mutation locus causing a recessive inherited defect. The results can be rapidly applied as a selection marker to identify carriers with the defective "T" allele in order to avoid at-risk matings to improve animal welfare and decrease economic losses. At this stage, the incidence of the mutation in the Corriedale sheep population is unknown, however it is suspected to be widespread and testing of New Zealand Corriedale sheep is planned. More importantly, due to their size and relatively low cost of maintenance, Corriedale sheep with inherited rickets could be used as an animal model for this form of human rickets. Even though the human and sheep mutations are not exactly the same, both disrupt the function of the DMP1 protein. The sheep model can be used for further investigation of the role of DMP1 in phosphate homeostasis and to explore the potential for early medical intervention to reduce the development of the disease in homozygous individuals.

MATERIALS AND METHODS

Ethics Statement

Approvals dealing with DNA or tissue collection from animals were obtained from the Massey University Animal Ethics Committee (APPROVAL NUMBER 05/123) and Iowa State University Animal Care & Use Committee did not require additional approvals.

Animals

In total, 17 affected Corriedale sheep (9 males, 8 females) and 27 phenotypically normal crossbred Corriedale sheep (6 males, 21 females) as well as 46 normal controls (Texel and crossbred Perendale sheep) were examined. The age of examined animals ranged from a fetus of 133 days gestation to a 3 year-old animal. Eight affected sheep were from the original commercial property at Marlborough, New Zealand, and 9 affected sheep were their offspring. The 27 phenotypically normal crossbred Corriedale sheep were progeny from the mating of unrelated Romney ewes with the Corriedale carrier ram (F1 generation from outcross), or progeny of the F1 generation daughters mated back to the carrier ram (F2 generation from backcross). SNP genotypes were obtained for the 17 affected and 3 carrier Corriedale sheep, while fine mapping was conducted on all 44 pure or crossbred Corriedale sheep. The 46 normal control sheep used for validation of the mutation were from unrelated populations without evidence of rickets.

SNP Genotyping

DNA was extracted from blood using a Roche MagNA Pure automated analyser. DNA samples were randomized on genotyping plates according to disease status. The genotyping was performed using the Ovine SNP50 BeadChip containing 54,241 SNPs (Illumina, San Diego, CA, USA) with standard procedures at GeneSeek Inc. Lincoln, NE, USA. The SNPs retained had to get a call rate >80% and a minimum GenTrain score of 0.25. All genotypes with satisfactory call rate and GenTrain score were used regardless of minor allele frequency (MAF).

SNP Chip Data Analyses

The IBD program used awk, join and sort UNIX commands to scan the whole genome of the genotyped affected cases, to produce a list of all the strings of consensus homozygous markers with a length of more than 10 SNPs. The same process was repeated in the carriers to ensure the regions identified in the affected individuals were not homozygous in the carriers. The homozygosity mapping algorithm involved the following: first, SNPs in the Illumina ovine 50K map file were sorted by chromosome and position, and numerically coded in contiguous order. Second, the names of the "A/B" genotypes (provided by GeneSeek Inc.) for each individual were joined with the renumbered map file to identify the genotypes by their locations. The joined file was separated into three groups according to the disease status of affected, carrier and normal. Third, the number of occurrences of genotypes ("AA", "AB", "BB" and no call "—") for each SNP was counted in the affected and carrier groups. Fourth, the genotype frequencies were calculated for each SNP. In the frequency calculation, the numerator was the count of genotypes being either "AA", "AB" or "BB", and the denominator was the total count excluding the category of no call. Finally, if the highest genotype frequency for a SNP was equal to 1 and the two alleles of this genotype were the same, such as "AA" or "BB", this SNP was considered a homozygous locus. The span of contiguous homozygous loci were accumulated and reported if the region included more than 10 loci. Genes in these IBD regions were examined for potential involvement using comparative maps between the ovine and bovine genomes through the Ovine Genome Assembly v1.0 (http://www.livestockgenomics.csiro.au/perl/gbrowse.cgi/oar1.0/#search).

DMP1 Gene Sequencing

Primers were designed to amplify all 6 exons for sheep *DMP1*. Cow *DMP1* genomic sequence was used as a template for primer designing in order to amplify the first 5 exons of sheep *DMP1* gene. PCR was performed using a 10 µl system with GoTaq DNA polymerase (Promega, Madison, WI). The annealing temperatures were 58°C or 60°C. PCR products were purified with ExoSAP-IT® (USB, Cleveland, OH), before pooling from 3 carriers and sequencing commercially using a 3730xl DNA Analyzer.

Mutation Analyses

Sheep EST sequence (DY509762) encompassing exon 1 to exon 5 of sheep *DMP1* along with re-sequencing results were used to predict the DMP1 protein sequence by applying the ExPASy translate tool (http://ca.expasy.org/tools/dna.html). The predicted sheep DMP1 protein was compared to the wild type (normal) of sheep and cow (AAI49017) using the CLUSTALW alignment tool (http://align.genome.jp/). Each SNP variant was analyzed to check whether it could induce a missense or nonsense mutation. The identified SNPs were genotyped on all 44 related Corriedale sheep and/or 46 normal controls by restriction enzyme digestion (PCR-RFLP) or direct sequencing. The genotyping results from all 9 SNPs distributed in exon 6 of the *DMP1* gene were formatted and put into Haploview software (http://www.broadinstitute.org/haploview/haploview). The linkage disequilibrium (LD) between pairs of SNPs in exon 6 was analyzed by Haploview software. Under the LD tabs, r^2, the correlation coefficient, was saved to show the LD between each pair of SNPs. The related LD color scheme was produced accordingly.

RNA Extraction and Reverse Transcriptase-Polymerase Chain Reaction (RT-PCR)

RNA was extracted from fibroblast cells cultured *in vitro* from skin biopsies of affected and control sheep to confirm the mutation existed at the transcript level. The fibroblast cell culture is as previously described [16]. Total RNA was extracted using Tri Reagent as per the manufacturer›s instructions (Sigma-Aldrich Co., USA). RT-PCR was performed using the Superscript® one-step RT-PCR system with Platinum® Taq polymerase (Invitrogen Corp., USA). The RT-PCR conditions were: 55°C for 30 min, 94°C for 2 min, 40 cycles of 30 s at 94°C, 30 s at 58° and 30 s at 72°C, and finally a 5 min elongation step at 72°C.

Restriction Enzyme Digestion

The nonsense mutation (C -> T) created a new recognition site for the restriction enzyme NlaIII (New England Biolabs Inc., USA). DNA fragments from the PCR and RT-PCR reactions were subjected to restriction enzyme digestion with NlaIII. The reaction mix was incubated at 37°C overnight, and the products were analyzed on a 2.5% (w/v) ultra-pure agarose gel.

REFERENCES

1. Dittmer KE, Thompson KG, Blair HT. Pathology of inherited rickets in Corriedale sheep. J Comp Pathol.2009;141:147–155.
2. Fitch LWN. Rickets in hoggets, with a note on the aetiology and definition of the disease. Australian Vet J.1943;19:2.
3. Ozkan B. Nutritional rickets. J Clin Res Pediatr Endocrinol. 2010;2:137–143.
4. HYP Consortium. A gene (HYP) with homologies to endopeptidases is mutated in patients with X-linked hypophosphatemic rickets. Nature Genet. 1995;11:130–136.
5. Sabbagh Y, Jones AO, Tenenhouse HS. PHEXdb, a locus-specific database for mutations causing X-linked hypophosphatemia. Hum. Mutat. 2000;16:1–6.
6. Ichikawa S, Traxler EA, Estwick SA, Curry LR, Johnson ML, et al. Mutational survey of the PHEX gene in patients with X-linked hypophosphatemic rickets. Bone. 2008;43:663–666.
7. ADHR Consortium. Autosomal dominant hypophosphataemic rickets is associated with mutations in FGF23. Nat Genet. 2000;26:345–348.
8. Lorenz-Depiereux B, Bastepe M, Benet-Pages A, Amyere M, Wagenstaller J, et al. DMP1 mutations in autosomal recessive hypophosphatemia implicate a bone matrix protein in the regulation of phosphate homeostasis. Nat Genet. 2006;38:1248–1250.
9. Lorenz-Depiereux B, Schnabel D, Tiosano D, Hausler G, Strom TM. Loss-of-function ENPP1 mutations cause both generalised arterial calcification of infancy and autosomal-recessive hypophosphatemic rickets.Am J Hum Genet. 2010;86:267–272.
10. Levy-Litan V, Hershkovitz E, Avizov L, Leventhal N, Bercovich D, et al. Autosomal-recessive hypophosphatemic rickets is associated with an inactivation mutation in the ENPP1 gene. Am J Hum Genet.2010;86:273–278.
11. Bergwitz C, Roslin NM, Tieder M, Loredo-Osti JC, Bastepe M, et al. SLC34A3 mutations in patients with hereditary hypophosphatemic rickets with hypercalciuria predict a key role for the sodium-phosphate cotransporter NaPi-IIc in maintaining phosphate homeostasis. Am J Hum Genet. 2006;78:179–192.
12. Alzahrani AS, Zou M, Baitei EY, Alshaikh OM, Al-Rijjal RA, et al. A novel G102E mutation of CYP27B1 in a large family with vitamin D-dependent rickets type 1. Clin Endocrinol Metab. 2010;95:4176–4183.
13. Malloy PJ, Pike JW, Feldman D. The vitamin D receptor and the syndrome of hereditary 1,25-dihydroxyvitamin D-resistant rickets. Endo Rev. 1999;20:156–188.
14. Malloy PJ, Xu R, Peng L, Peleg S, Al-Ashwal A, et al. Hereditary 1,25-dihydroxyvitamin D resistant rickets due to a mutation causing multiple defects in vitamin D receptor function. Endocrine. 2004;145:5106–511.
15. Thompson KG, Dittmer KE, Blair HT, Fairley RA, Sim DF. An outbreak of rickets in Corriedale sheep: evidence for a genetic aetiology. N Z Vet J. 2007;55:137–142.
16. Dittmer KE, Howe L, Thompson KG, Stowell KM, Blair HT, et al. Res Vet Sci [Epub ahead of print]; 2010. Normal vitamin D receptor function with increased expression of 25-hydroxyvitamin D(3)-24-hydroxylase in Corriedale sheep with inherited rickets.
17. Hurtig M, Frederic D, Darilyn F, Betina L, Antonio C, et al. BMP-7 Gene Therapy for Mitigation of Post-traumatic Osteoarthritis in Sheep. Eur Cell Mater. 2008;16:52.
18. Gerometta R, Spiga MG, Borras T, Candia OA. Treatment of sheep steroid-induced ocular hypertension with a glucocorticoid-inducible MMP1 gene therapy virus. Invest Ophthalmol Vis Sci. 2010;51:3042–3048.
19. Porada CD, Tran N, Eglitis M, Moen RC, Troutman L, et al. In utero gene therapy: transfer and long-term expression of the bacterial neo(r) gene in sheep after direct injection of retroviral vectors into preimmune fetuses. Hum Gene Ther. 1998;9:1571–1585.
20. Charlier C, Coppieters W, Rollin F, Desmecht D, Agerholm JS, et al. Highly effective SNP-based association mapping and management of recessive defects in livestock. Nat Genet. 2008;40:449–454.
21. Feng JQ, Ward LM, Liu S, Lu Y, Xie Y, et al. Loss of DMP1 causes rickets and osteomalacia and identifies a role for osteocytes in mineral metabolism. Nat Genet. 2006;38:1310–1315.
22. Lander ES, Botstein D. Homozygosity mapping: a way to map human recessive traits with the DNA of inbred children. Science. 1987;236:1567–1570.
23. Fisher LW, Fedarko NS. Six genes expressed in bones and teeth encode the current members of the SIBLING family of proteins. Connect Tissue Res. 2003;44(Suppl 1):33–40.
24. Narayanan K, Ramachandran A, Hao J, He G, Park KW, et al. Dual functional roles of dentin matrix protein 1. Implications in biomineralization and gene transcription

by activation of intracellular Ca2+ store. J Biol Chem. 2003;278:17500–17508.

25. Schiavi SC. Bone talk. Nat Genet. 2006;38:1230–1231.

26. Koshida R, Yamaguchi H, Yamasaki K, Tsuchimochi W, Yonekawa T, et al. A novel nonsense mutation in the DMP1 gene in a Japanese family with autosomal recessive hypophosphatemic rickets. J Bone Miner Metab. 2010;28:585–590.

27. Fisher LW, Torchia DA, Fohr B, Young MF, Fedarko NS. Flexible structures of SIBLING proteins, bone sialoprotein, and osteopontin. Biochem Biophys Res Commun. 2001;280:460–465.

28. Maquat LE. Nonsense-mediated mRNA decay: splicing, translation and mRNP dynamics. Nat Rev Mol Cell Biol. 2004;5:89–99.

29. Bergwitz C, Jüppner H. Regulation of Phosphate Homeostasis by PTH, Vitamin D, and FGF23. Annu Rev Med. 2010;61:91–104.

30. Dittmer KE, Thompson KG. Vitamin D metabolism and rickets in domestic animals: a review. Vet Pathol. 2011;48:389–407.

CHAPTER 22

PRP GENE POLYMORPHISM IN MEDIEVAL REMAINS OF SICILIAN SHEEP

Stefano Reale[1], Mario Cosenza[1], Luca Sìneo[2], Letizia Arcoleo[2], Gabriele Zaffora[1], Daniele Macrì[1], Fabrizio Vitale[1]

[1]Molecular Biology Department, Istituto Zooprofilattico Sperimentale della Sicilia "A. Mirri", Palermo, Italy

[2]Laboratory of Anthropology, STEBICEF Department, University of Palermo, Palermo, Italy

ABSTRACT

Encephalopathy in sheep was at first described in Ireland in 1732 and was called scrapie. Ancient DNA in archaeogenetics represents an effective method to evaluate the ancestral pedigree of living animals and track evolutionary changes occurred between the past and the present day. Since several point mutations are today widely described in modern scrapie, no data about both sequence and frequency are still available for the prion protein (PrP) gene in ancient breeds. In order to evaluate whether the haplotypes distribution in ancient sheep differed from those of the modern population we evaluated polymorphism at four well know codons of the Prp Open Reading Frame. In the present work, we collected 37 medieval sheep bone remains found at the Calathamet (n = 11), Palazzo Bonagia (n = 12) and Palazzo Steri (n = 14) Sicilians archeological sites and dated back between 9th - 15th century. Single nucleotide polymorphisms (SNPs) at codons 136, 141, 154 and 171 of the prion protein (PrP) were investigated using cycle sequencing. Sequenom Mass ARRAYiPLEX platform confirmed the results for 5 individuals out of 37. Cycle sequencing showed at all samples the $AA_{136}LL_{141}RR_{154}QQ_{171}$(hereafter ALRQ/ALRQ) genotype except at 2 individuals showing the very susceptible genotype VLRQ/VLRQ (n = 1) and the resistant (ALRR/ ALRR) (n = 1) respectively. Supported by a high incidence of susceptible genotype to prion infection we concluded that presumably scrapie was already widespread enough in the medieval Sicily. Moreover, we described conceivable scenarios that could have underlain evolutionary changes in the medieval sheep population.

INTRODUCTION

Scrapie or prion disease belongs to the transmissible spongiform encephalopathies (TSEs) together with bovine spongiform encephalopathy (BSE) in cattle and chronic wasting disease (CWD) in deer. Scrapie is a fatal neurodegenerative disorder that affects genetically susceptible sheep and goat and it is characterized by the deposition of the aberrant isoform of the natural prion glycoprotein. It is revealed that the PrP abnormal prion protein form, consist of an approximately 40% of beta sheet folding that makes it protease resistant and infectious [1] . Scrapie disease is also the oldest form of TSEs and various data indicate that it was already present in Europe in eighteenth century or earlier. The first description of scrapie case came back to the year 1750 by Leopoldt [2] who reported

Citation: Reale, S. , Cosenza, M. , Sìneo, L. , Arcoleo, L. , Zaffora, G. , Macrì, D. and Vitale, F. (2015) PrP Gene Polymorphism in Medieval Remains of Sicilian Sheep. Open Journal of Animal Sciences, 5, 486-494. doi: 10.4236/ojas.2015.54050.

the infectious nature. Since that time several studies were conducted to describe the early history of the TSEs [3] and only two centuries later it was reported the first signal of scrapie in Italy, in the Biellese breed (Piedmonte), described by Cravero et al., 1976 [4] . PrP polymorphisms are highly debated and to date their involvement in scrapie is not completely clear. Specific point mutations in the coding region are widely linked to susceptibility in sheep to develop prion disease [5] . Several SNPs are currently reported [6] and four well- known codons show crucial importance in modulate genetic susceptibility to classical scrapie. Amino acid polymorphism at codon 136 (Alanine/Valine; A/V), codon 141 (Leucine/Phenylalanine; L/F), codon 154 (Arginine/ Histidine; R/H) and codon 171 (Arginine/Glutamine/Histidine; R/Q/H) are extensively described in literature [7] -[9] . The ARR/ARR is associated with a high resistant genotype to natural scrapie [7] [9] [10] , while AHQ haplotype is associated only in some breeds with the resistance to disease [11] . In contrast, the VRQ confers high susceptibility both homozygosis and heterozygosis [12] [13] . The ARQ represents the most common haplotype [14] and exhibits high to moderate susceptibility to disease while the ARH allele seems to be neutral [15] . Based on the above evidence, several PrP genotypes subsist within the population and each of them is related with a different degree of proneness to develop scrapie (R1 - R5, respectively from very low risk to high susceptibility). When DNA are well preserved, direct sequencing represents definitely the most reliable and powerful tools to decode ancient genes and to track genetic variability along the time-scale. In line with this premises, we thought the PrP gene as a target of possible evolutionary pressure reflecting the characteristics of living animals.

To date, Italian data on the amino acid frequencies at PrP gene are available and show the prevalence of the ARQ both homozygosis and heterozygosis with the ARR [16] . In the Sicilian sheep the haplotypes distributions follow the same trend as the rest of the Italian population [17] despite the genetic isolation that characterizes the native sheep breeds. Since there are no data available on the ancestral genotype distribution for the Sicilian sheep, through a retrospective study we evaluated PrP allelic profile using aDNA analysis directly from archaeological samples. To this aim we searched for amino acid variations in order to assess whether the ancestral sheep already had at that time a certain level of susceptibility to prion infection. We estimated the ancestral genotype and compared them with those of the contemporary sheep by employing direct sequencing and mass spectrometry MALDI-TOF.

MATERIALS AND METHODS

A specimen of 37 ovine bones (Ovis aries) from medieval periods was examined. Samples came from three different ancient sites of the town of Palermo in Italy: Palazzo Bonagia (12 specimens), Palazzo Steri (14 specimens) and Calathamet (11 specimens) [18] [19] in the north-west of Sicily. Scans and analysis of the artifacts discovered in the proximity of the specimens revealed that the relics of Palazzo Bonagia can be dated back to a period between the end of the 9th century and the beginning of the 11th century A.D.; the specimens of Calathamet can be dated back to 11th - 14th century A.D. [18] whereas the specimens of Palazzo Steri can be dated back to 11th - 15th century A.D. For the site of Calathamet only the samples attributed to 13th century A.D. were analyzed and, analogously for Palazzo Steri, only the relics of the "Chiaramonte" period (14th - 15th century A.D.) were considered. Since some skeletal remains were badly preserved and damaged, various bone elements were sampled in order to form the highest Minimum Number of Individuals (MNI). Samples were selected by choosing the same anatomical part and the same side, in order to be sure not to collect and analyze twice the same individual. Young-to-adults individuals with an age of death included in a range of 18 to 36 months represented the specimen. We managed directly aDNA from the sheep skeletal remains according to the strict practices provided by Cooper and Poinar, 2000 [20] . To assure sterility, all the work surfaces were treated with 1% sodium hypochlorite solution and equipment and pipettors exposed to UV rays. Latex gloves, mask and body suit were used by researchers during handling of the bones. A fragment for each animal was collected under sterile conditions in a pre-PCR area exclusively dedicated and soaked in 10% bleach. A 80 - 100 mg were powdered mechanically in a homogenizer. Ancient DNA was extracted according to Yang's et al. protocol, 1998 [21] in a dedicate extractions area within the laboratory and in a laminar flow hood (HEPA-filtered) in order to avoid cross-contamination with modern DNA. Bone powder was decalcified with EDTA 0.5 M pH 8 at room temperature for 48 h and then incubated in a thermo mixer at 55°C overnight with 20 mg/ml proteinase K and 0.5% SDS. The solution was centrifuged at 2000 × g for 5 minutes and the supernatant was transferred into a sterile microtube to perform DNA purification with the QIAquick PCR Purification Kit (Qiagen, Sweden) following the manufacturer's instructions. New reagents for aDNA extraction, PCR amplification and multiple downstream applications were used. Non-template control and reagent blanks were employed to check exogenous contamination throughout working procedure. Direct sequencing was initially performed on a 225 bp fragment using a couple of primer provided by Acutis et al. (2010) [22] including all codons investigated in one amplicon. At this condition PCR amplification did not showed any amplicon because of the too high dimension of the fragment to be amplified related to the degree of degradation of the aDNA. In light of this we amplified each codon independently, except at codons 136 and 141 because of their closeness. For this purpose, new mini primer for the selective amplification of the codons 136/141, 154 and 171 were suitably in-house designed, as illustrates Table 1. The oligos hybridize on the PrP open reading frame at positions 386 - 407 and 506 - 485 for the codon 136 - 141 (respectively forward and reverse); 429 - 447 and 558 - 539 for the codon 154; 504 - 523 and 619 - 599 for the codon 171 [GenBank:AJ000739]. The couple of primers for each codon annealed at strategic positions so that SNPs were identified close to the reverse primer. The amplification was performed in a final reaction volume of 50 μl using AmpliTaq Gold 360 DNA Polymerase (Applied Biosystems, Foster City, California, USA). The amplification was performed in a GeneAmp PCR system 9700 (Applied Biosystems, Foster City, California) with an initial hold of 8 min at 95°C followed by 40 cycle of 45 sec at 95°C, 50 sec at 56°C and 30 sec at 72°C; a final extension period of 10 min at 72°C was employed. Products were ran on the automated capillary electrophoresis device QIAxcel (Qiagen, Milano, Italy) to avoid handling of samples, cleaned up and started toward the cycle sequencing using BigDye Terminator v3.1chemistry(Applied Biosystems, Foster City, California, USA). The amplicon was newly cleaned up with BigDye X-Terminator purification kit and running on a ABI Prism 3130 Genetic Analyzer (Applied Biosystems, Foster City, California, USA). Each sequence was submitted to the BLAST alignment tool to be sure not to have contamination and aligned using SeqScape Software v2.7 (Applied Biosystems, Foster City, California, USA) to check PrP polymorphisms. Each sample was also amplified using a specific iPLEX Genotyping kit named MyriapodScrapie (DiatechPharmacogenetics, Jesi, Italy) exclusively designed for the detection at the same time of the polymorphism at codons 136, 141, 154 and 171. A first PCR amplification was performed using AMP-Mix prepared according to the manufacturer's instructions. Briefly three microliters were dispensed in each tube and 2 µl of DNA (1 - 100 ng/µl) were used. The plate was sealed using a SQ foil and amplified on a Labcycler (SensoQuest, GmbH) using the following protocol: initial hold of 95°C for 2 min followed by 45 cycle of 30 sec at 95°C, 30 sec at 56°C and 1 min at 72°C. Two additional sequential hold of 72°C and 4°C each for 5 min were also performed. After the first amplification, a SAP treatment is required to cleans up left over primers and dNTPs using 2 µl of a specific SAP-Mix in 5 µl of PCR product; the following thermal profile was applied: 37°C for 40 min, 85°C for 5 min and 4°C for 5 min. Afterwards a primer single-base extension was performed preparing a specific EXT-Mix following the manufacturer's instructions. Two microliter of the mix were added to previous tube reaching a final volume of 9 µl. A specific iPLEX PCR protocol was applied: 94°C for 30 sec followed by 40 cycle of 94°C for 5 sec and annealing and extension repeated 5 times for each cycle, respectively of 52°C and 80°C for 5 sec. A further hold of 72°C for 3 min and 4°C for 5 min was also applied. Extension products were nanodispensed to a SpectroCHIParray and transferred to the MassARRAY for the analysis of the fragments of allele-specific mass. The mass difference allows the software to discriminate between different SNP alleles at each codon using the Sequenom MassARRAY Analyzer 4 (Diatech Pharmacogenetics, Jesi, Italy). For the same reasons mentioned above, the allele-mass peak was not always detected because of the amplicon length (~400 bp).

Table 1: Mini primer for the selective amplification of the codons 136/141, 154 and 171; Ta, annealing temperature

Primer Name	Primer 5' - 3'	Size (bp)	Ta (°C)
MC136/141-F	CAGTAAGCCAAAAACCAACATG	121	56
MC136/141-R	GCCAAAATGTATAAGAGGCCTG		
MC154-F	GCAGCTGGAGCAGTGGTAG	130	
MC154-R	GGTTGGGGTAACGGTACATG		
MC171-F	GGCAATGACTATGAGGACCG	116	
MC171-R	ACACAGTCATGCACAAAGTTG		

RESULTS

Despite some badly preservation and dating of the bones, ancient DNA resulted in a positive amplification for all codons investigated (Figure 1). Sheep skeletal remains were analyzed in double, confirming the results without any incongruence and therefore considering it as authentic. Sequencing analysis showed for all sample a 94.6% of ALRQ/ALRQ genotype; the remaining was VLRQ/VLRQ and ALRR/ALRR (2.7% each). We have not found nucleotide mutation leading to amino acid change or synonymous substitution so that we excluded artifacts in a DNA amplification induced by e.g. deamination of cytosine [23] . We have detected triplets GCC (Ala/Ala) and GTC (Val/Val) at codon 136, CTT at codon 141 (Leu/Leu), CGT at codon 154 (Arg/Arg), CGG (Arg/Arg) and CAG (Gln/Gln) at codon 171. Sequencing positive control was heterozygote at codon 171 (ARR/ARQ). Mass spectrum results confirmed cycle sequencing data for four ARQ homozygotes and one susceptible VRQ both belonging to the Calathamet site, showing a better DNA preservation of these samples (Figure 2(a) and Figure 2(b)). The remaining samples did not revealed any signal on mass array.

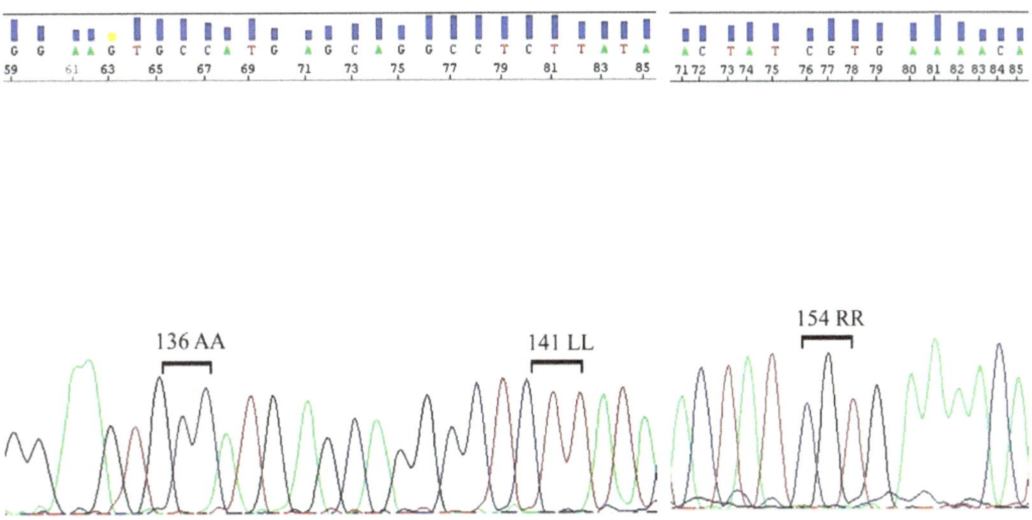

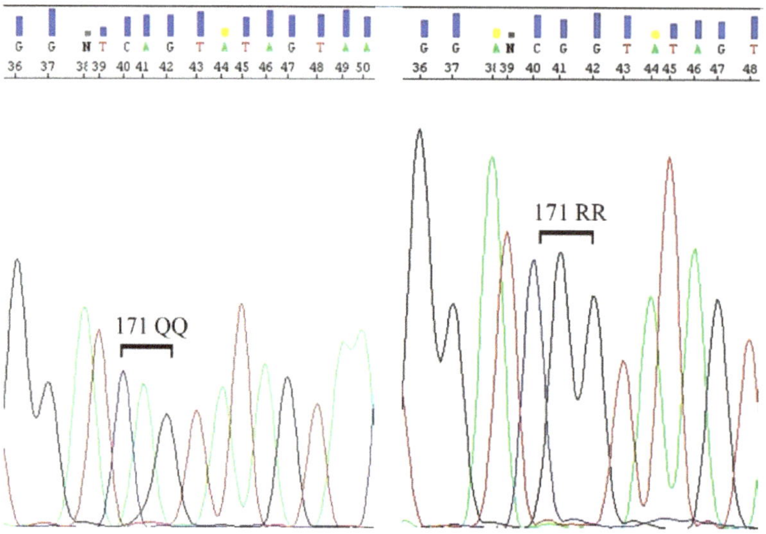

Figure 1: Cycle sequencing of the codons 136 - 141, 154 and 171.

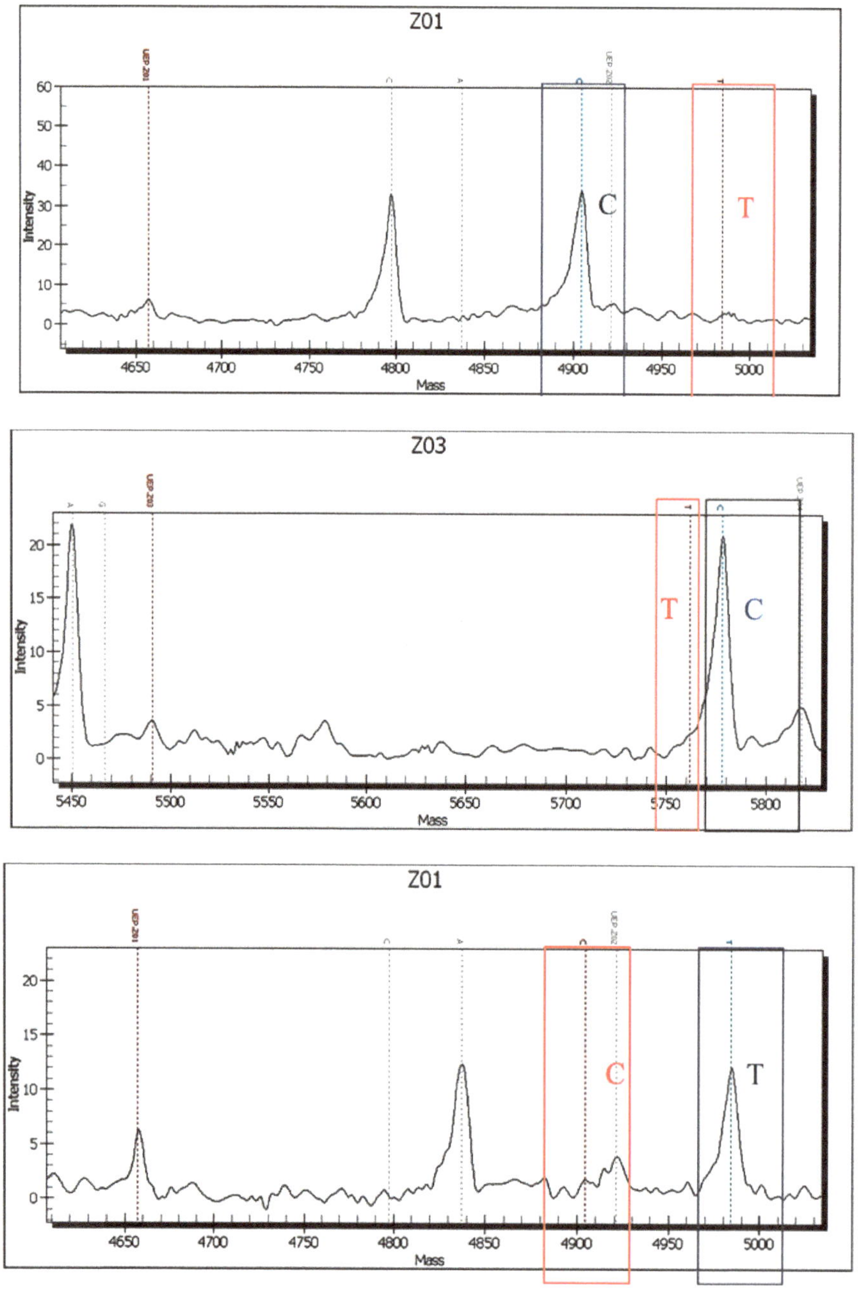

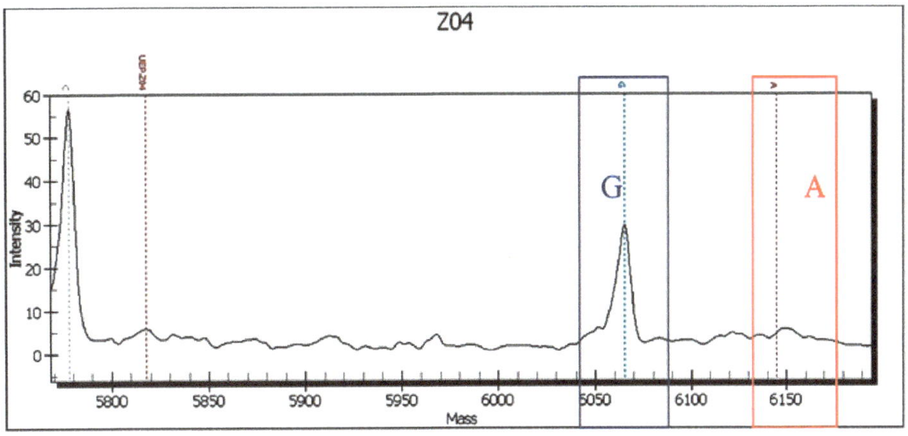
Z04
Intensity
Mass
G
A
60
50
40
30
20
10
0
5800
5850
5900
5950
6000
6050
6100
6150

(a)

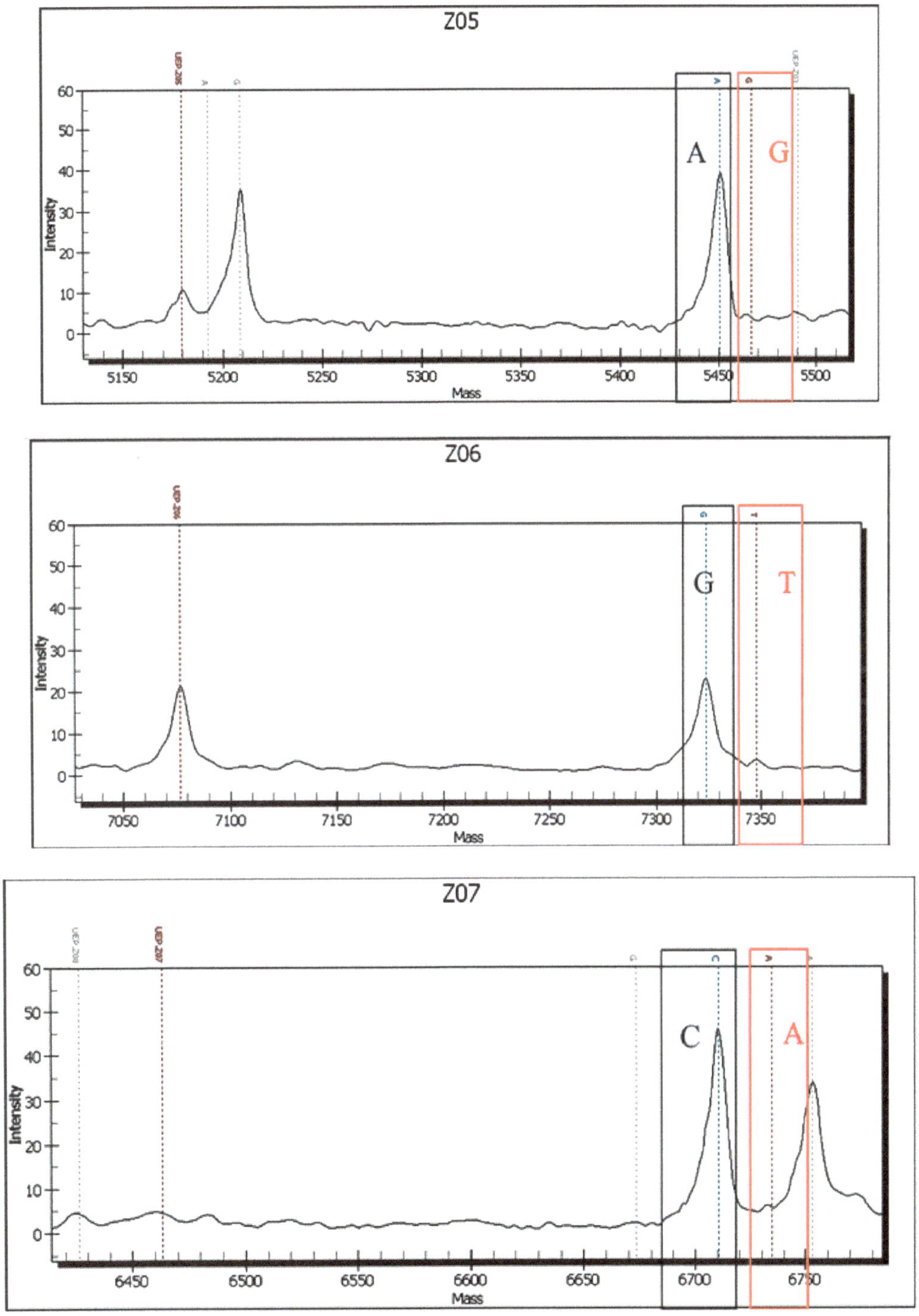
Z05
Intensity
Mass
A
G
5150
5200
5250
5300
5350
5400
5450
5500
Z06
Intensity
Mass
G
T
7050
7100
7150
7200
7250
7300
7350
Z07
Intensity
Mass
C
A
6450
6500
6550
6600
6650
6700
6750

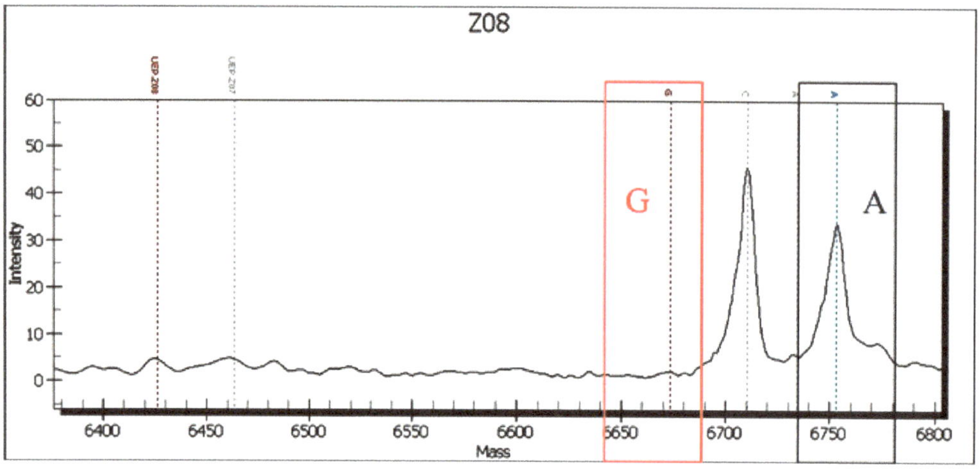

(b)

Figure 2: (a) Mass spectrum chromatogram. Panels Z1 to Z4 represent a definite nucleotide assay at one specific codon. Z1 A136V (GCC - GTC); Z3 L141F (CTT - TTT); Z4 R154H (CGT - CAT). (b) Mass Array spectrum for the codon 171. Panels Z5 to Z8 represent a definite nucleotide assay at codon 171. Z5 Q171R (CAG - CGG); Z6 Q171H (CAG - CAT); Z7 Q171K (CAG - AAG); Z8 work as control of Z5 analysis (A → G) using a different primer.

DISCUSSION AND CONCLUSIONS

Scrapie disease is a lethal disorder affecting genetically susceptible sheep. The aim of this study was to assess the allelic pattern at codons 136, 141, 154 and 171 in order to estimate whether scrapie was already infectious in medieval era. Moreover, we presumed genetic forces driving evolutionary changes occurred in the ancestral sheep population. The predominant ALRQ haplotypes found in this study are in line with the modern allelic distribution in Sicily [17] . According to the Van Kaam study, currently the ARQ haplotype mean frequency in Sicilians sheep is much higher (56.2%) compared to the resistant ARR (34.8%). Despite this, the heterozygotes ARR/ARQ are today the most representative genotypes of the Sicilian ovine population (mean 39.9%) and only secondly the homozygotes ARQ/ARQ (mean 31.4%). The ARR/ARR genotype is poorly represented within the population (mean 12.1%) tending to its increase using selective mating strategies under EU member states plan. In our study, the ancestral ALRQ/ALRQ appears to be the predominant genotype for the Sicilian sheep. Only one sample showed the Valine (V) allele at codon 136 whereas another sample displayed the Arginine (R) allele at codon 171. No heterozygotes were detected showing slightly differences among ancient and contemporary sheep breeds. In light of this, we wondered why the prion protein gene already had in the middle age a scrapie- susceptible form. Lacking or poorness of scrapie resistant genotype in European sheep [24] -[26] could be due to anthropic and selective pressures that have acted in past affecting genetics of the present days. It's clear today that domestication took place about in 4000 B.C. by Neolithic settlers as shown by findings of skeletal remains. During that time, the most common use of medieval sheep was to provide milk, wool and meat and as results of anthropic pressure probably they were selected for their somatic characteristics (e.g. long or short wools, white-faced, polled or horned). Unfortunately, to our knowledge no study was conducted nor results are reported linking phenotype with polymorphisms of susceptibility. On the other hand, evolutionary changes may have took place over the last centuries in the Sicilian Island involving sheep population. As shown in this work, a small proportion of resistant alleles were already present and only secondly lost or strongly reduced perhaps due to accidental crossing with breeds carrying the susceptible alleles. Alternatively, it might be also possible that migrations of incoming sheep population could have interacted genetically with the autochthonous with a significative changing in the haplotype frequencies. Unfortunately these happenings may be difficult to investigate. Moreover Sicilians sheep might have been progressively selected for different alleles due to stochastic effects such as genetic drift and bottlenecks. In line with this assumptions, founder effect could have supported the selection process by forming a new population starting from a few number of sheep survived and carrying e.g. the Q_{171} allele. These occurrences most likely have led to the differentiation of the sheep breeds as we know them today and to the fragmentation of their genetic variability. It would be reasonable to consider a driving force favoring the protective form (e.g. RR_{171}) rather than those susceptible. This might suggest more simply that selective pressure acting on the PrP alleles could be also the answer to an evolutionary adaptation to date unknown. From a contemporary point of view, artificial selection could be responsible for the large Q_{171} increase within the modern Sicilian sheep population due to a wrong in-house breeding program. This issue is strengthened by the disproportion between male and female that form today the Italians sheep flock. In such breeding program, Sicilian sires carrying glutamine allele at codon 171 are unknowingly used as reproducers, spreading the susceptible haplotype. This led to consolidate and disseminate the current frequencies. For reasons to date unclear, the genotype obtained from the medieval sheep bones differs if compared to the modern sheep. In our study, the ancient haplotypes seem to be lacking at codon 171 of the resistant triplet leading to the amino acid Arginine or could be simply infrequent variants within the ancient sheep and therefore hard to detect [27] . On the other hand, the high ALRQ proportion could be overestimated precluding the possibility to find coding mutations. Despite the limited number of bones analyzed, we assumed however that sampling derived from the different ancient sites was considered representative of the historical period. We concluded that scrapie mutation was observed in any of the samples analyzed. On the basis of objective observations, we could confirm that in the period 9th - 15th century scrapie was widespread as demonstrated by the high incidence of susceptible genotype found. Our data represent only a piece of a larger scenario that need of insights but that may contribute to shed some light on the geneflow phenomena occurred between present and past as well in tracking selection events.

REFERENCES

1. 1. Prusiner, S.B. (1991) Molecular Biology of Prion Diseases. Science, 252, 1515-1522.http://dx.doi.org/10.1126/science.1675487
2. 2. Leopoldt, J.G. (1750) Nutzliche und auf die Erfahrung gegrundete Einleitung zu der Land-Wirthschafft, 5, Johann Gottlieb Rothen, Sorau.
3. 3. Schneider, K., Fangerau, H., Michaelsen, B. and Raab, W.H.M. (2008) The Early History of the Transmissible Spongiform Encephalopathies Exemplified by Scrapie. Brain ResearchBulletin, 77, 343-355. http://dx.doi.org/10.1016/j.brainresbull.2008.09.012
4. 4. Cravero, G., Guarda, F., Dotta, U. and Guglielmino, R. (1976) La scrapie in pecore di razza biellese. Prima segnalazione in Italia. La Clinica Veterinaria, 100, 1-14.
5. 5. Bossers, A., Belt, P.B.G.M., Raymond, G.J., Caughey, B., de Vries, R. and Smits, M.A. (1997) Scrapie Susceptibility- Linked Polymorphismsmodulate the in Vitro Conversion of Sheep Prion Protein to Protease Resistantforms. Proceedings of the National Academy of Sciences, USA, 94, 4931-4936. http://dx.doi.org/10.1073/pnas.94.10.4931
6. 6. Heaton, M.P., Leymaster, K.A., Freking, B.A, Hawk, D.A., Smith, T.P., Keele, J.W., Senlling, W.M., Fox, J.M., Chitko-McKown, C.G. and Laegreid, W.W. (2003) Prion Gene Sequence Variation within Diverse Groups of U.S. Sheep, Beef Cattle, and Deer. Mammalian Genome, 14, 765-777. http://dx.doi.org/10.1007/s00335-003-2283-y
7. 7. Goldmann, W., Hunter, N., Smith, G., Foster, J. and Hope, J. (1994) PrP Genotype and Agent Effects in Scrapie: change in Allelic Interaction with Different Isolates of Agent in Sheep, a Natural Host of Scrapie. Journal of General Virology, 75, 989-995.http://dx.doi.org/10.1099/0022-1317-75-5-989
8. 8. Clouscard, C., Beaudry, P., Elsen, J.M., Milan, D., Dussaucy M., Bounneau C., Schelcher, F., Chatelain, J., Launay, J. M. and Laplanche, J.L. (1995) Different Allelic Effects of the Codons 136 and 171 of the Prion Protein Gene in Sheep with Natural Scrapie. Journal of General Virology, 76, 2097-2101. http://dx.doi.org/10.1099/0022-1317-76-8-2097
9. 9. Hunter, N., Goldmann, W., Smith, G. and Hope, J. (1994) The Association of a Codon 136 PrP Gene Variant with the Occurrence of Natural Scrapie. Archives of Virology, 137, 171-177. http://dx.doi.org/10.1007/BF01311184
10. 10. Baylis, M., Goldmann, W., Houston, F., Cairns, D., Chong, A., Ross, A., Smith, A., Hunter, N. and McLean, A.R. (2002) Scrapie Epidemic in a Fully PrP-Genotyped Sheep Flock. Journal of General Virology, 83, 2907-2914. http://dx.doi.org/10.1099/0022-1317-83-11-2907
11. 11. Thorgeirsdottir, S., Sigurdarson, S., Thorisson, H.M., Georgsson, G. and Palsdottir, A. (1999) PrP Gene Polymorphism and Natural Scrapie in Icelandic Sheep. Journal of General Virology, 80, 2527-2534. http://dx.doi.org/10.1099/0022-1317-80-9-2527
12. 12. Belt, P.B., Muileman, I.H., Schreuder, B.E., Bos-de Ruijter, J., Gielkens, A.L. and Smits, M.A. (1995) Identification of Five Allelic Variants of the Sheep PrP Gene and Their Association with Natural Scrapie. Journal of General Virology, 76, 509-517.http://dx.doi.org/10.1099/0022-1317-76-3-509
13. 13. Hunter, N., Foster, J.D., Goldmann, W., Stear, M.J., Hope, J. and Bostock, C. (1996) Natural Scrapie in a Closed Flock of Cheviot Sheep Occurs Only in Specific PrP Genotypes. Archives of Virology, 141, 809-824. http://dx.doi.org/10.1007/BF01718157
14. 14. Baylis, M. and Goldmann, W. (2004) The Genetics of Scrapie in Sheep and Goats. Current Molecular Medicine, 4, 385-396. http://dx.doi.org/10.2174/1566524043360672
15. 15. Dawson, M., Hoinville, L.J., Hosie, B.D. and Hunter, N. (1998) Guidance on the Use of PrP Genotyping as an Aid to the Control of Clinical Scrapie. Veterinary Record, 142, 623-625.
16. 16. Pongolini, S., Bergamini, F., Iori A., Migliore, S., Corradi, A. and Bassi, S. (2009) Prion Protein Genotypes of Italian Sheep Breeds with Lysine-171 and Phenylalanine-141 Detection. Veterinary Microbiology, 137, 18-23.http://dx.doi.org/10.1016/j.vetmic.2008.12.012
17. 17. Van Kaam, J.B.C.H.M., Finocchiaro, R., Vitale, M., Pinelli, F., Scimonelli, M., Vitale, F., Portolano, B., Oltenacu, P.A. and Caracappa, S., (2008) Prion Protein Gene Frequencies in Three Sicilian Dairy Sheep Populations. Italian Journal of Animal Science, 7, 87-94. http://dx.doi.org/10.4081/ijas.2008.87
18. 18. Di Patti, C., Di Salvo, R., Di Trapani, F. and Schimmenti, V. (2013) Les restesfauniques du déportoir. In: Lesnes, é. and Poisson, J.M., Eds., Calathamet. Archéologie et histoire d'un chateau normand en Sicile, école francaise de Rome, Rome, 283-298.
19. 19. Sarà, M. (2013) Les restes fauniques du déportoir. In: Lesnes, é. and Poisson, J.M., Eds., Calathamet. Archéologie et histoire d'un chateau normand en Sicile, école francaise de Rome, Rome, 299-304.
20. 20. Cooper, A. and Poinar, H.N. (2000) Ancient DNA: Do It Right or Not at All. Science, 289, 1139. http://dx.doi.org/10.1126/science.289.5482.1139b
21. 21. Yang, D.Y., Eng, B., Waye, J.S., Dudar, J.C. and Saunders, S.R. (1998) Technical Note: Improved DNA Extraction from Ancient Bones Using Silica-Based Spin Columns. American Journal of Physical Anthropology, 105, 539-543.http://dx.doi.org/10.1002/(SICI)1096-8644(199804)105:4<539::AID-AJPA10>3.0.CO;2-1

22. 22. Acutis, P.L., Colussi, S., Riina, M.V., Giovannini, T., Trisorio, S., Maniaci, M.G., Zuccon, F. and Peletto, S. (2010) Absence of the Alleles AT137RQ e ARQK176 Protective to Scrapie in Ovine Piedmontese Breeds. Proceedings of 19th SIPAOC Conference, Rimini, 16, 53.

23. 23. Hofreiter, M., Jaenicke, V., Serre, D., Haeseler, A.V. and Paabo, S. (2001) DNA Sequences from Multiple Amplifications Reveal Artefacts Induced by Cytosine Deamination in Ancient DNA. Nucleic Acids Research, 29, 4793-4799.http://dx.doi.org/10.1093/nar/29.23.4793

24. 24. Acín, C., Martìn-Burriel, I., Goldmann, W., Lyahyai, J., Monzòn, M., Bolea, R., Smith, A., Rodellar, C., Badiola, J.J. and Zaragoza, P. (2004) Prion Protein Gene Polymorphisms in Healthy and Scrapie-Affected Spanish Sheep. Journal of General Virology, 85, 2103-2110.http://dx.doi.org/10.1099/vir.0.80047-0

25. 25. Hunter, N., Goldmann W., Foster J.D., Cairns, D. and Smith, G. (1997) Natural Scrapie and PrP Genotype: Case-Control Studies in British Sheep. Veterinary Record, 141, 137-140. http://dx.doi.org/10.1136/vr.141.6.137

26. 26. Sipos, W., Kraus, M., Schmool, F., Achmann, R. and Baumgartner, W. (2002) PrP Genotyping of Austrian Sheep Breeds. Journal of Veterinary Medicine Series A, 49, 415-418. http://dx.doi.org/10.1046/j.1439-0442.2002.00472.x

27. 27. Reale, S., Sìneo, L., Macrì, D., Bivona, M., Arcoleo, L., Risi, M., Cosenza, M. and Vitale, F. (2014) Ancient DNA Polymorphisms Analysis to Investigate Scrapie Susceptibility in Sicilian Sheep Remains from Medieval Archaeological Sites. Proceedings of PRION 2014 Conference, 8, 67.

CHAPTER 23

MOLECULAR CHARACTERIZATION OF ORF VIRUS FROM SHEEP AND GOATS IN ETHIOPIA, 2008–2013

Esayas Gelaye[1,2,3], Jenna Elizabeth Achenbach[1], Shiferaw Jenberie[3], Gelagay Ayelet[3], Alebachew Belay[3], Martha Yami[3], Angelika Loitsch[4], Reingard Grabherr[5], Adama Diallo[1] and Charles Euloge Lamien[1]

[1]Animal Production and Health Laboratory, Joint FAO/IAEA Division of Nuclear Techniques in Food and Agriculture, Department of Nuclear Sciences and Applications, International Atomic Energy Agency, Wagramer Strasse 5, Vienna, Austria

[2]Institute of Applied Genetics and Cell Biology, University of Natural Resources and Life Sciences, Muthgasse 18, A-1190 Vienna, Austria

[3]Research and Diagnostic Laboratories, National Veterinary Institute, Debre Zeit, Ethiopia

[4]Institute for Veterinary Disease Control, Austrian Agency for Health and Food Safety, Robert Koch-Gasse 17, A-2340 Mödling, Austria

[5]Institute of Applied Microbiology, University of Natural Resources and Life Sciences, Muthgasse 11, 1190 Vienna, Austria

ABSTRACT

Background

Orf is a contagious disease of sheep, goats and wild ungulates caused by orf virus (ORFV) a member of the genus Parapoxvirus, Poxviridae family. Although orf is endemic in Ethiopia, little attention has been given so far as it is not a notifiable disease by the World Organization for Animal Health. In this work, we have investigated orf outbreaks representing five different geographical locations of Ethiopia, in Amba Giorgis, Gondar zuria, Adet, Debre zeit and Adami Tulu, between 2008 and 2013.

Results

The viral isolation and the sequence analysis of the A32L and the B2L genes of eighteen representative isolates confirmed that sampled animals were infected by ORFVs. The phylogenetic study and the comparative analysis of the deduced amino acid profile suggests that there were two main clusters of ORFV isolates which were responsible for the investigated outbreaks. Additionally the analysis of these two genes showed limited variability to ORFVs encountered elsewhere. This is the first report on the genetic characterization of the ORFV isolates from sheep and goats in Ethiopia.

Conclusion

The molecular characterization of Ethiopian ORFV isolates highlighted the circulation of two main clusters causing orf disease in sheep and goats. The use of laboratory based methods and a constant monitoring of Ethiopian ORFV isolates is needed to better understand the dynamic of ORFV circulating in the country and facilitate the implementation of control measures.

Citation: Esayas Gelaye, Jenna Elizabeth Achenbach, Shiferaw Jenberie, Gelagay Ayelet, Alebachew Belay, Martha Yami, Angelika Loitsch, Reingard Grabherr, Adama Diallo and Charles Euloge Lamien, Molecular characterization of orf virus from sheep and goats in Ethiopia, 2008–2013, DOI 10.1186/s12985-016-0489-3.

BACKGROUND

Orf is an acute, contagious, debilitating and economically important zoonotic viral skin disease of sheep, goats and wild ruminants caused by orf virus (ORFV). ORFV, a prototype of *Parapoxvirus* genus of *Chordopoxvirinae*subfamily within the *Poxviridae* family, has a size of approximately 260 nm length and 160 nm width comprised of a linear double-stranded DNA genome (134–139 kbp) with high GC content (63–64 %) in comparison with other poxviruses [1, 2, 3, 4, 5]. The genus *Parapoxvirus* also includes pseudocowpox virus (PCPV), bovine papular stomatitis virus (BPSV) and parapoxvirus of red deer in New Zealand [3, 4, 5].

ORFV infection in sheep and goats is generally known as orf, contagious ecthyma, infectious labial dermatitis, scabby mouth, contagious pustular dermatitis, or sore mouth. Lesions of orf progress from erythema, vesicle formation, pustules and then scabs [3, 4, 5, 6]. The disease not only has an economic impact on farmers worldwide but also has a considerable negative effect on animal welfare. Infected animals are sickly, fail to thrive, and are more susceptible to bacterial infections. Characteristic of the disease are proliferative and often self-limiting lesions (3–4 weeks) on the skin of the lips, on the oral mucosa and around the nostrils. Lesions can also be found occasionally on the teats of nursing animals but rarely on other organs [3, 4, 5, 6]. Depending on the location of the lesions, animals may be unwilling to nurse, eat, or walk. The mortality rate related to orf is usually low, but it may be very high when bacterial or fungal secondary infections occur.

The disease also has zoonotic potential, although it is more of occupational hazard to people working with animals (farmers, animal caretakers, veterinarians), characterized by nodular and papillomatous lesions mainly on the hands, face, and mouth [3, 5, 6, 7].

A number of natural outbreaks of suspected infections of ORFV are frequently observed in sheep and goats reared under different production systems in Ethiopia. Until now only the observation of clinical signs formed the basis of orf diagnosis in the country. Owing to the existence of several diseases which can potentially present similar lesions on the mouth and related symptoms such as sheep pox, goat pox, peste des petits ruminants, dermatophylosis and foot and mouth disease, laboratory diagnostic of orf is urgently needed in the country to confirm any suspected orf outbreaks. Even though outbreaks of ORFV infections are endemic and develop severe ecthyma lesions in sheep and goats in most of the agro-climatic regions of Ethiopia, no attempt has been made until now to isolate, identify and molecularly characterize the circulating virus isolates. Orf disease is neglected by the veterinary service, however, owing to its zoonotic potential and impact on animal production, more attention needs to be given to the disease.

Two genes are widely used to molecularly characterize ORFV and reveal the genetic variation of parapoxviruses: the A32L gene homologue of vaccinia virus, encoding the viral ATPase protein which plays a role in viral DNA packaging [1, 4, 8, 9, 10, 11], and the B2L gene encoding the major virus envelope protein [1,4, 8, 9, 10, 11]. Five functional predicted motifs (motif I-V), which have synergistic activities on the virus-host cell interaction through enzymatic processes, characterize the ATPase protein sequence [2, 4, 12, 13, 14, 15]. The C-terminal of the ATPase gene displays high heterogeneity, which makes it suitable for viral strain differentiation [2, 12].

In the present study, we have investigated suspected orf outbreaks occurred at different geographical locations of Ethiopia between 2008 and 2013, and have confirmed the disease and characterized the isolates. The analysis of the isolates, their comparison among each other and to foreign isolates and the implications are discussed to allow a better understanding of ORFV dynamics in the country.

METHODS

Outbreak Areas

From 2008 to 2013, pox crusted samples were collected from sick sheep and goats presenting pox-like lesions and suspected to have pox disease. The samples were collected from the five following geographical locations of Ethiopia: Northern Ethiopia (Amba Giorgis [12°46□05.52□ N, 37°37□46.76□ E], Gondar zuria [12°3559.54□ N, 37°28□00.36□ E], and Adet [11°15□51.36□ N, 37°29□31.72□ E]), central Ethiopia (Debre zeit [8°45□32.12□ N, 39°01□19.87□ E]), and southern Ethiopia (Adami Tulu [7°51□33.20□ N, 38°42□24.72□ E]) (Fig. 1). Adet and Adami Tulu are agriculture research centers where animals were kept in a controlled environment while the remaining three outbreaks occurred in herds where animals are reared by individual owners and graze on communal grazing land. All six outbreaks were attended by veterinary professionals.

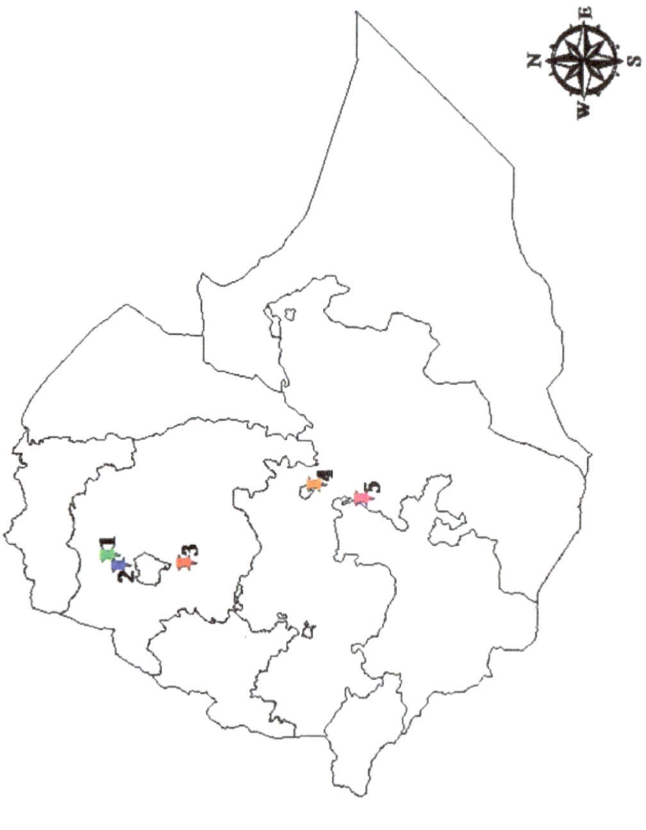

Figure 1: Study area. Representative scabby lesion samples have been collected during orf suspected outbreaks from clinically sick sheep and goats in: 1. Amba Giorgis, 2. Gondar zuria, 3. Adet, 4. Debre zeit, and 5. Adami Tulu. The map was sketched using ArcGIS 9 software (ArcMap™ version 9.3, California, USA).

Sample and Outbreak Data Collection

Representative tissue samples of scab lesion scrapings were collected from a total of 24 sheep and goats showing suspected clinical signs of poxvirus infection. About 2 g of tissue samples were collected from each animal and placed in a labeled sterile universal tube containing phosphate buffered saline (PBS), pH 7.2 supplemented with antibiotics and antifungal. Samples were immediately transferred into a cold box and transported to the National Veterinary Institute using the cold-chain system. The samples were then stored at −20 °C until laboratory analysis. All the clinical parameters were recorded during collection of samples.

For all outbreak areas, a physical inspection of the diseased sheep and goats was undertaken by veterinary professionals to record the clinical observations. Additional data were collected through an interview of the farmers and animal keepers using a questionnaire. These data included: vaccination history, mortality and morbidity rates, and date of appearance of the disease in the farm or herd, as well as the appearance of lesions on humans in close contact with the diseased animals.

Ethics Statement

Samples were collected on diseased animal during outbreak for disease confirmation. No animal experiment was conducted. Sample collection and their use were approved by the joint animal ethical committee of the National Veterinary Institute and the College of Veterinary Medicine and Agriculture, Addis Ababa University. All efforts were made to minimize animal suffering during the course of sample collection in orf suspected outbreak areas. Consent was obtained from the animal owners for the collection of tissue samples by a veterinarian.

Virus Isolation

Samples were washed three times with sterile PBS containing antibiotics and antifungal. Tissue homogenates (10 % w/v) were prepared using sterile PBS and centrifuged at high speed using a refrigerated centrifuge. 0.5 mL of the supernatant was inoculated onto a confluent layer of Vero cells grown in a 25 cm^2 tissue culture flask containing10mL Glasgow Minimum Essential Medium (Sigma-Aldrich) supplemented with 10 % fetal calf serum (Gibco). The inoculated cultures were incubated at 37 °C, 5 % CO_2 and observed daily for the appearance of virus-induced cytopathic effects (CPE). Samples were considered negative when no CPE was observed following three blind passages.

Virus DNA Extraction and Preliminary Screening by PCR

The pathological tissue homogenates (10 % w/v in PBS) were centrifuged at 10,000 g for 10 min at +4 °C. The supernatant was used for virus DNA extraction using the DNeasy Blood and Tissue kit (Qiagen) following the manufacturer's instruction. The eluted DNA was labeled and stored at −20 °C until further testing. All samples were first screened by ORFV specific PCR [16], using a C1000 Touch thermal cycler (Bio-Rad, Foster City, CA, USA).

Amplification, Cloning and Sequencing of Fragments Containing the Full A32L and B2L Genes

Primers (Table 1) were designed for the amplification of fragments containing the full B2L and A32L genes using Allele ID version 6 software package (Premier Biosoft International, Palo Alto, CA, USA), using ORFV strain OV-SA00 as template (Accession number: NC005336); The primers binding sites in the genome for B2L gene were ORFV-B2Lf-For =10838-10857 and ORFV-B2Lf-Rev =12030-12047; and for A32L gene ORFV-A32f-For =110603-110622, and ORFV-A32f-Rev=111681-111700). Internal primers were also designed for sequencing (Table 1). Primers were synthesized by VBC Biotech, Austria.

Table 1: Primers used in this study. Primers orf1 and orf2 [16] were used for the preliminary screening of the clinical samples. The remaining primers were used for the amplification and sequencing of the full-length A32L (825 nt) and B2L (1137 nt) genes of ORFV. The estimated PCR product sizes are presented

S I No	Primer name	Sequences (5'– 3')	Application	PCR product size (base pair)
1	Orf1	CGCAGACGTGGCTGAGTACGT	PCR	140
2	Orf2	TGAGCTGGTTGGCGCTGTCCT		
3	ORFV-A32f-For	CTCCATTTAGAGGCCGTGAG	PCR/Sequencing	1098
4	ORFV-A32f-Rev	CGTGTTATGTGCCATCTTGC		
5	ORFV-A32i-For	GGTCGAGACAGCGCTTGA	Sequencing	-
6	ORFV-A32i-Rev	CGTCTACAACGCCGCCTAC		
7	ORFV-B2Lf-For	GACCTTCCGCGCTTTAATTT	PCR/Sequencing	1210
8	ORFV-B2Lf-Rev	CCCGCCTGCTAAAAGACT		
9	ORFV-B2Li-For	GTCCGCGTTCTTCCACTC	Sequencing	-
10	ORFV-B2Li-Rev	GCGGGCGTCAACTACTACA		
11	SP6	ATTTAGGTGACACTATAG	Sequencing	-
12	T7	TAATACGACTCACTATAGGG		

For the molecular characterization, DNA extracts from tissue homogenates were used. Fragments containing the full B2L and A32L genes were amplified by PCR in a reaction volume of 25 μL containing 500 nM forward primer, 500 nM reverse primer, 2 mM dNTPs, 1x PCR Buffer (Qiagen), 2.5 U Taq Polymerase (Qiagen) and 5 μL template DNA. The cycling conditions for the full A32L gene were: initial denaturation at 95 °C for 5 min, followed by 35 cycles at 95 °C for 50 s, 55 °C for 60 s and 72 °C for 90 s, and final extension at 72 °C for 7 min. The same protocol was used for the B2L gene except that the annealing was at 52 °C instead of 55 °C. For each PCR run, a negative control consisting of 5 μL of water instead of the template DNA was included. Aliquots of the PCR products were checked using electrophoresis on a 1.5 % agarose gel stained with ethidium bromide for 1 h at 100 V.

The amplified products of A32L and B2L genes were purified using Wizard SV Gel and PCR clean-up system kit (Promega), ligated into the pGEM-T vector (Promega) and transformed into SURE® 2 Supercompetent cells (Stratagene). Positive clones were selected and plasmids were purified using PureYield™ Plasmid Midiprep System (Promega). Sequencing of the plasmids was achieved using six primers indicated in Table 1. The plasmids were sequenced by LGC Genomics (Germany).

Sequence and Phylogenetic Analysis

The sequences were assembled and edited using Vector NTI Advance™ 11.5 software (Invitrogen, Carlsbad, CA, USA). The full-length A32L and B2L gene sequences of the Ethiopian ORFV isolates (Table 2) together with those of homologue genes of parapoxviruses retrieved from GenBank (Table 3) were aligned using BioEdit software. All sequences were deposited in GenBank under accession numbers KT438513 to KT438530 for the B2L gene and KT438531 to KT438548 for the A32L gene.

Table 2: Ethiopian orf virus field isolates (*n*= 18) characterized in this study. The isolate's names, area of collection, animal species and GenBank accession number for the A32L (ORF011) and B2L (ORF108) genes are provided

Sl No	Strain name	Area of collection	Animal species/Host	GenBank accession number	
				A32 gene	**B2L gene**
1	Adet/O01/2012	Adet	Sheep	KT438531	KT438513
2	Adet/O02/2012	Adet	Sheep	KT438532	KT438514
3	Adet/O03/2012	Adet	Sheep	KT438533	KT438515
4	Adet/O04/2012	Adet	Sheep	KT438534	KT438516
5	Adet/O05/2012	Adet	Sheep	KT438535	KT438517
6	Amba G/O01/2012	Amba Giorgis	Sheep	KT438537	KT438519
7	Amba G/C02/2012	Amba Giorgis	Goat	KT438536	KT438518
8	Amba G/O03/2012	Amba Giorgis	Sheep	KT438538	KT438520
9	ATARC/O01/2008	Adami Tulu	Sheep	KT438539	KT438521
10	ATARC/O02/2008	Adami Tulu	Sheep	KT438541	KT438523
11	ATARC/O01/2010	Adami Tulu	Sheep	KT438540	KT438522
12	ATARC/O02/2010	Adami Tulu	Sheep	KT438542	KT438524
13	Debre zeit/O01/2012	Debre zeit	Sheep	KT438543	KT438525
14	Debre zeit/O02/2012	Debre zeit	Sheep	KT438544	KT438526
15	Gondar z/C01/2013	Gondar zuria	Goat	KT438545	KT438527
16	Gondar z/C02/2013	Gondar zuria	Goat	KT438546	KT438528
17	Gondar z/C03/2013	Gondar zuria	Goat	KT438547	KT438529
18	Gondar z/O04/2013	Gondar zuria	Sheep	KT438548	KT438530

ATARC Adami Tulu Agriculture Research Center, *C* Caprine, *O* Ovine

Table 3: List of representative Parapoxvirus A32L (*n*= 12) and B2L (*n*= 13) genes nucleotide sequences retrieved from the GenBank for comparative sequence analysis and phylogenetic tree construction

Sl No	Strain	Gene name	Animal species	Country	GenBank accession no	Reference
1	ORFV-Nantou	A32L	Goat	Taiwan	EU327509	[17]
2	ORFV-NZ2	A32L	Sheep	New Zealand	DQ184476	[8]
3	ORFV-OV-IA82	A32L	Sheep	USA	AY386263	[1]

4	ORFV-OV-SA00	A32L	Goat	USA	AY386264	[1]
5	ORFV-67/04	A32L	Sheep	India	JN183066	[9]
6	ORFV-TN/2008	A32L	Sheep	India	JN183076	[9]
7	ORFV-Mys/2010	A32L	Sheep	India	JN183075	[9]
8	ORFV-Meg/2003	A32L	Goat	India	JN183073	[9]
9	ORFV-59/05	A32L	Goat	India	JN183074	[9]
10	ORFV-Ass/2010	A32L	Goat	India	JN183069	[9]
11	PCPV-VR634	A32L	Bovine	New Zealand	GQ329670	[18]
12	BPSV-BV-AR02	A32L	Bovine	USA	AY386265	[1]
13	ORFV/2009	B2L	Goat	Korea	GQ328006	[19]
14	ORFV/2003	B2L	Goat	USA	AY278208	[20]
15	ORFV/2004	B2L	Sheep	USA	AY424970	[21]
16	ORFV-India 82/04	B2L	Goat	India	DQ263303	[22]
17	ORFV-India 67/04	B2L	Sheep	India	DQ263305	[22]
18	ORFV-India 79/04	B2L	Sheep	India	DQ263306	[22]
19	ORFV/GanSu/2009	B2L	Sheep	China	HQ694772	Unpublished
20	ORFV-Assam/09	B2L	Goat	India	JN846834	[23]
21	ORF-Vaccine strain	B2L	NA	USA	AY278209	[20]
22	ORFV-D	B2L	Sheep	Brazil	JN088052	Unpublished
23	ORFV-NE2	B2L	Goat	Brazil	JN088051	Unpublished
24	PCPV	B2L	Sheep	USA	AY424972	[21]
25	BPSV	B2L	Sheep	USA	AY424973	[21]

For phylogenetic reconstructions of the A32L and the B2L gene trees, sequences were aligned with Muscle using the aligned codon option of MEGA 6 [24]. The file with aligned sequences was exported into MrBayes compatible Nexus file using Mesquite 2.74. For both A32L and B2L genes, the Tamura 3-parameter model of nucleotide substitution with gamma-distributed rate variation across sites was selected as best-fit model with MEGA 6. MrBayes3.2.2 was then used to produce a tree.

The MCMC method was run for 10,000,000 generations, with a sampling frequency of 1,000, until model convergence was reached. Four independent chains were run with the chain heating temperature set to 0.2. At the convergence, 25 % of the initial trees were discarded for all analyses. A 50 % majority rule consensus tree was built from the resulting trees. The tree was visualized using Figtree 1.4.2 program. Bovine popular stomatitis virus and pseudocowpox virus were used as outgroups.

Additionally, the amino acid sequences of the ATPase were aligned, using BioEdit 7.2.3, to analyze the presence of five predicted functional motifs and its C-terminal heterogeneity. For a more comprehensive analysis of the C-terminal heterogeneity, all publicly available aa sequences of ORFV ATPase protein were included.

RESULTS

Outbreaks Description, Preliminary Screening and Viral Isolation

The first orf outbreak investigated in this study occurred in November 2008, in sheep reared at the Adami tulu agriculture research center (ATARC) causing specific lesions (Fig. 2a) in 10 % of the animals. The outbreak occurred 4 months after vaccination of the animals with a capripox vaccine, strain KS1-O180, leading the researchers of this center to suspect capripoxvirus infections. In 2010, the same center experienced a second outbreak of pox disease in sheep with a morbidity rate of about 3 %. The third outbreak occurred in June 2012 at the Adet sheep research center where the diseased sheep presented with pox lesions at different sites of the body (Fig. 2b) with a morbidity rate of 22 % (25/112). During the same month, on 26 June 2012, the fourth outbreak occurred in Debre Zeit, where an animal owner presented two diseased sheep to the veterinary clinic with lesions around the muzzle and nostrils (Fig. 2c and d).

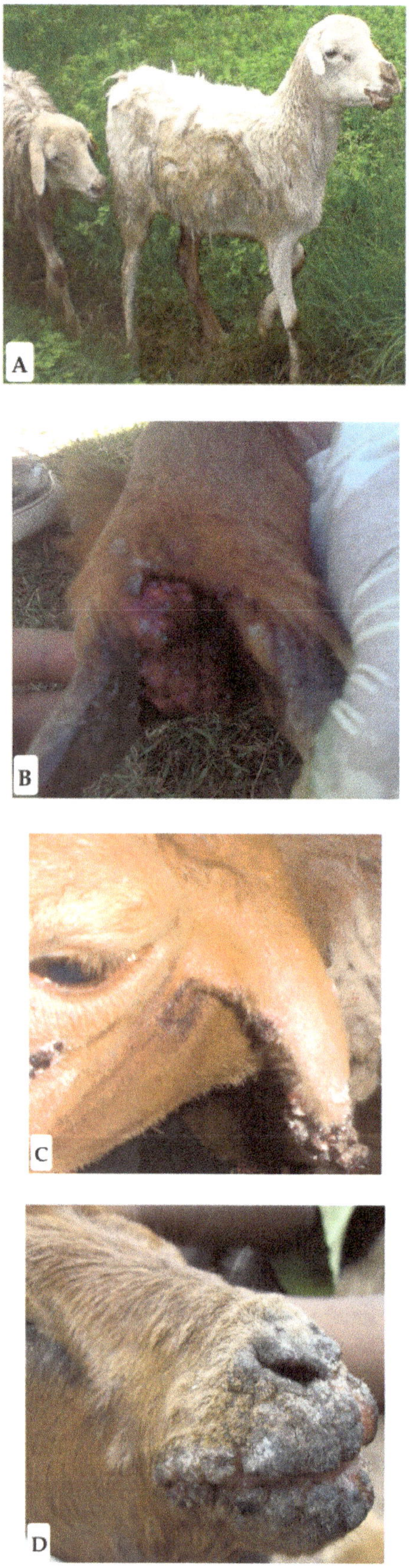

Figure 2: Representative clinical sign of orf virus infection observed during outbreaks investigation. a Scabby and ulcerated ecthyma lesions around oral commissures, muzzle, lower jaw and knee region in sheep. b Severe bloody tissue growth lesion in the interdigital space in sheep. c Growth of tumor-like lesions on the ear skin in sheep. d Severely crusted wart-like multiple lesions on the oral commissures, lips and nostril area in goat.

The fifth and the sixth outbreaks were in the Amba Giorgis on 21 November 2012 and, in Gondar zuria on 20 January 2013 in sheep and goats reared by individual farmers sharing common grazing land and pasture. Animals presented with lesions on the muzzle, nostril and interdigital spaces and the morbidity rates were estimated to be around 4 % and 3 %, respectively.

In general, for all outbreaks areas, there was no recorded mortality associated with ORFV infections and no human infections were reported. Animals which had developed severe lesions around the mouth and interdigital spaces were unable to walk and graze freely which resulted in a reduction in body weight and production loss. The dry crusted skin lesions led to secondary complications and worsened the health of the animal. Severe lesions were observed in young lambs and kids which had close contact with diseased parents. Eighteen out of 24 samples collected during these outbreaks tested positive using ORFV specific PCR primers orf 1 and orf 2 which produced the expected fragment size of 140 bp (Table 1). The distribution of the positive samples was as follows: ATARC, 2008 (2/4), ATARC, 2010 (2/2); Adet 2012 (5/6); Debre zeit 2012 (2/2); Amba Giorgis 2012 (3/4); Gondar zuria 2013 (4/7). For each positive sample, the complete B2L and A32L genes were amplified, sequenced and used for comparative analysis.

>Infected Vero cell cultures developed characteristic poxvirus-induced cytopathic effects (CPE), with rounded cell detaching from monolayer, after 3–5 days in culture for either the first or second blind passage (data not shown). This result, taken together with the results from PCR screening, confirmed the presence of infectious ORFV in all attended herds.

Sequence Analysis and Phylogenetic Tree Construction

Comparative sequence analysis of the Ethiopian ORFV isolates based on A32L and B2L genes was carried out including homologous genes from a selection of parapoxviruses (Table 3) using MEGA.6. The arithmetic means of nucleotide and amino acid substitutions per site between the Ethiopian isolates only (within group mean distance) and between the Ethiopian isolates and foreign isolates (between groups mean distance) were estimated using MEGA. The within group mean distance was 0.01 at both the nucleotide and aa levels for the Ethiopian isolates based on their A32L gene nucleotide sequences and the deduced aa sequences. The mean distance between Ethiopian isolates and foreign isolates was 0.020 at both the nucleotide and aa levels. Likewise, for the B2L gene, the within group mean distance for the Ethiopian isolates was 0.010 at both the nucleotide and aa levels. The mean distance between Ethiopian isolates and foreign isolates was 0.020 at both the nucleotide and aa levels. This shows that the Ethiopian ORFV isolates are more similar to each other than to foreign isolates.

In the phylogenetic tree reconstructions, based on the nucleotide sequences of the B2L gene, the Ethiopian ORFV isolates grouped into two major clusters. Cluster I included fourteen local ORFV isolates (Adet, Amba Giorgis, Gondar zuria and Debre zeit) and eight foreign ORFV strains from India, Taiwan and USA; whereas the four ATARC ORFV isolates and three strains from New Zealand, Taiwan and USA were grouped within cluster II (Fig. 3).

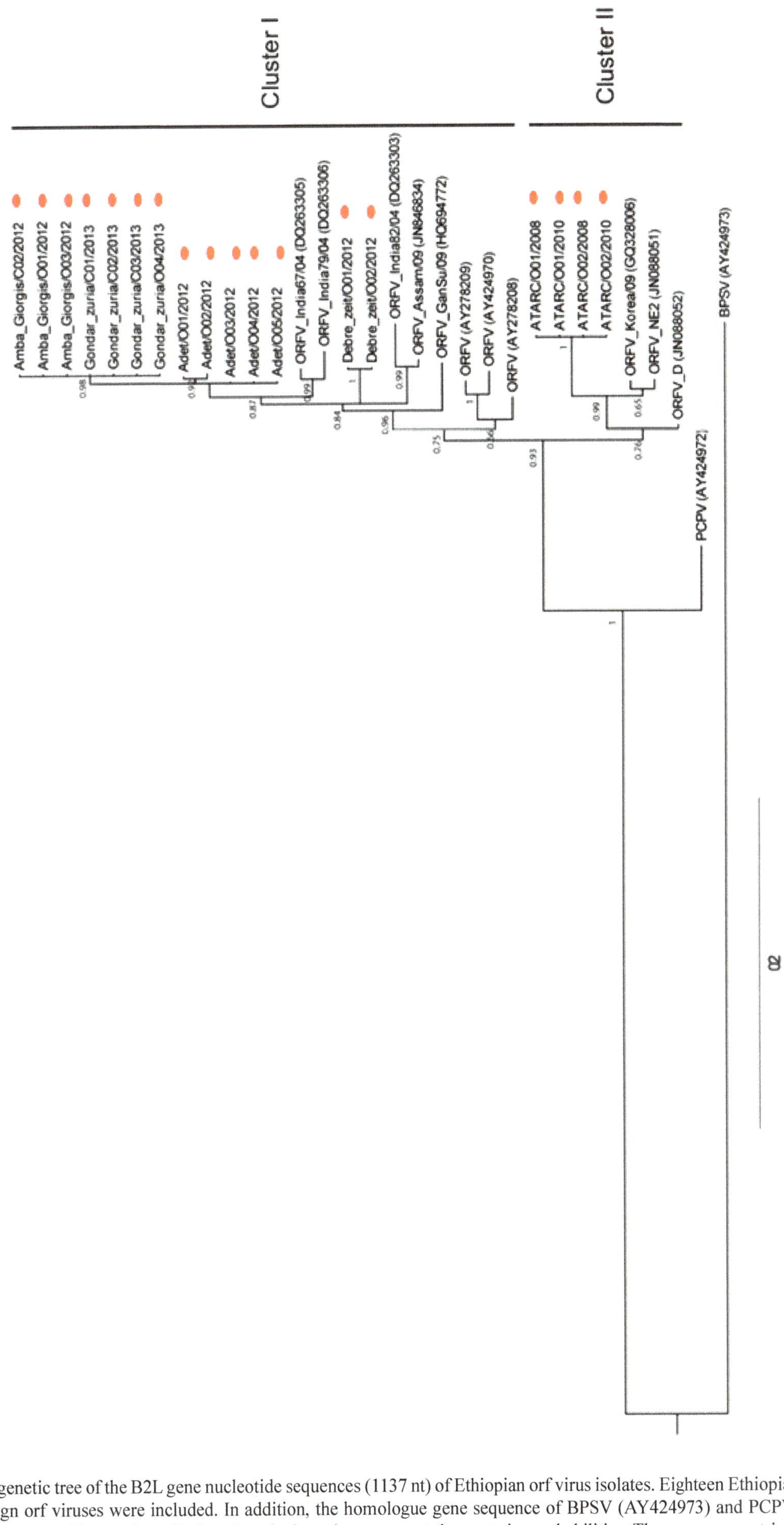

Figure 3: Phylogenetic tree of the B2L gene nucleotide sequences (1137 nt) of Ethiopian orf virus isolates. Eighteen Ethiopian orf virus isolates and eleven foreign orf viruses were included. In addition, the homologue gene sequence of BPSV (AY424973) and PCPV (AY424972) and were used as out-groups. The numbers displayed on the branches represent the posterior probabilities. The sequences retrieved from GenBank are indicated with accession number under bracket and those of this study were highlighted with red bubbles.

In the A32L gene tree, two major clusters were observed, with all Ethiopia isolates falling within cluster I. However, the four ATARC isolates formed a separate sub-cluster as compared to the other Ethiopian and foreign ORFV isolates of this cluster I (Fig. 4).

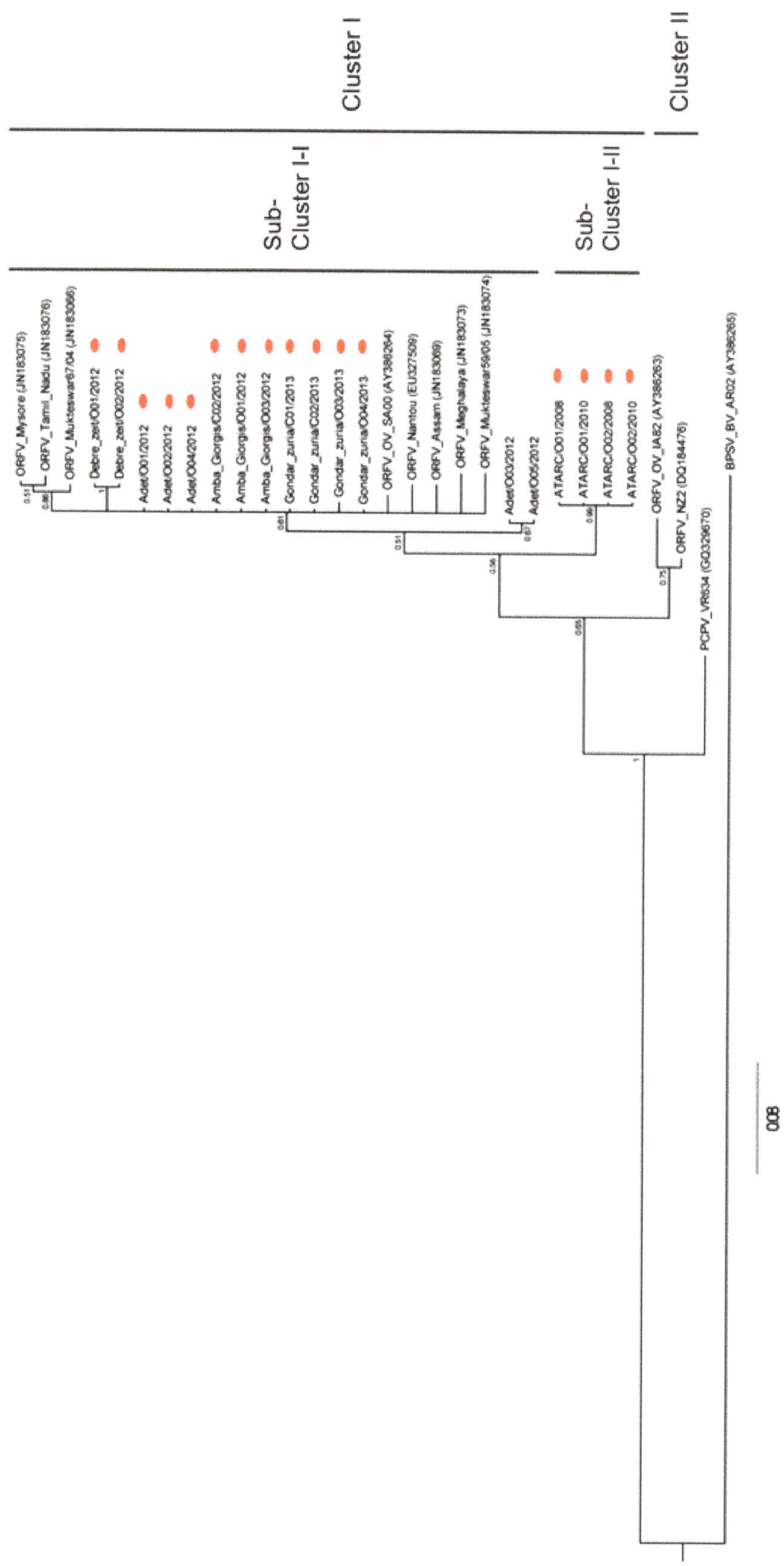

Figure 4: Phylogenetic tree of the A32L gene nucleotide sequence (825 nt) of Ethiopian isolates orf virus isolates. Eighteen Ethiopian orf virus isolates and ten foreign orf viruses were compared. Additionally, the homologue gene sequence of BPSV (AY386265) and PCPV (GQ329670) were used as out-groups. The numbers displayed on the branches represent the posterior probabilities. The sequences retrieved from GenBank are indicated with accession number under bracket and those of this study were highlighted with red bubbles.

C-Terminal Heterogeneity of Ethiopian ORFVs ATPase

The analysis of the aa sequences of Ethiopian ORFV isolates confirmed the high level of conservation of the N-terminal region of the ATPase encoded by the A32L gene. No aa change was observed until residue position 249. All predicted five functional motifs of the ATPase protein were found in all Ethiopian ORFV isolates sequences.

In contrast to the N-terminal, the C-terminal displayed a high variability among the Ethiopian isolates and also when compared to foreign isolates.

Six different profiles were observed at the C-terminal of the ATPase protein of the Ethiopian ORFV isolates (Fig. 5). Two isolates, Adet/O02/2012 and Adet/O04/2012, contained repeats of three KGD sequences (position 247 – 255), a KGD at position 270–272, and their protein sequences ended with an ADSND. The ATPase protein of isolate Adet/O01/2012 had two repeats of KGD sequences (position 247 – 252), a KGD at position 270–272 and ended with an ADSND. The ATPase protein sequence of isolate Adet/O01/2012 was completely similar to that of the ORFV isolate Orissa 14/06 from India.

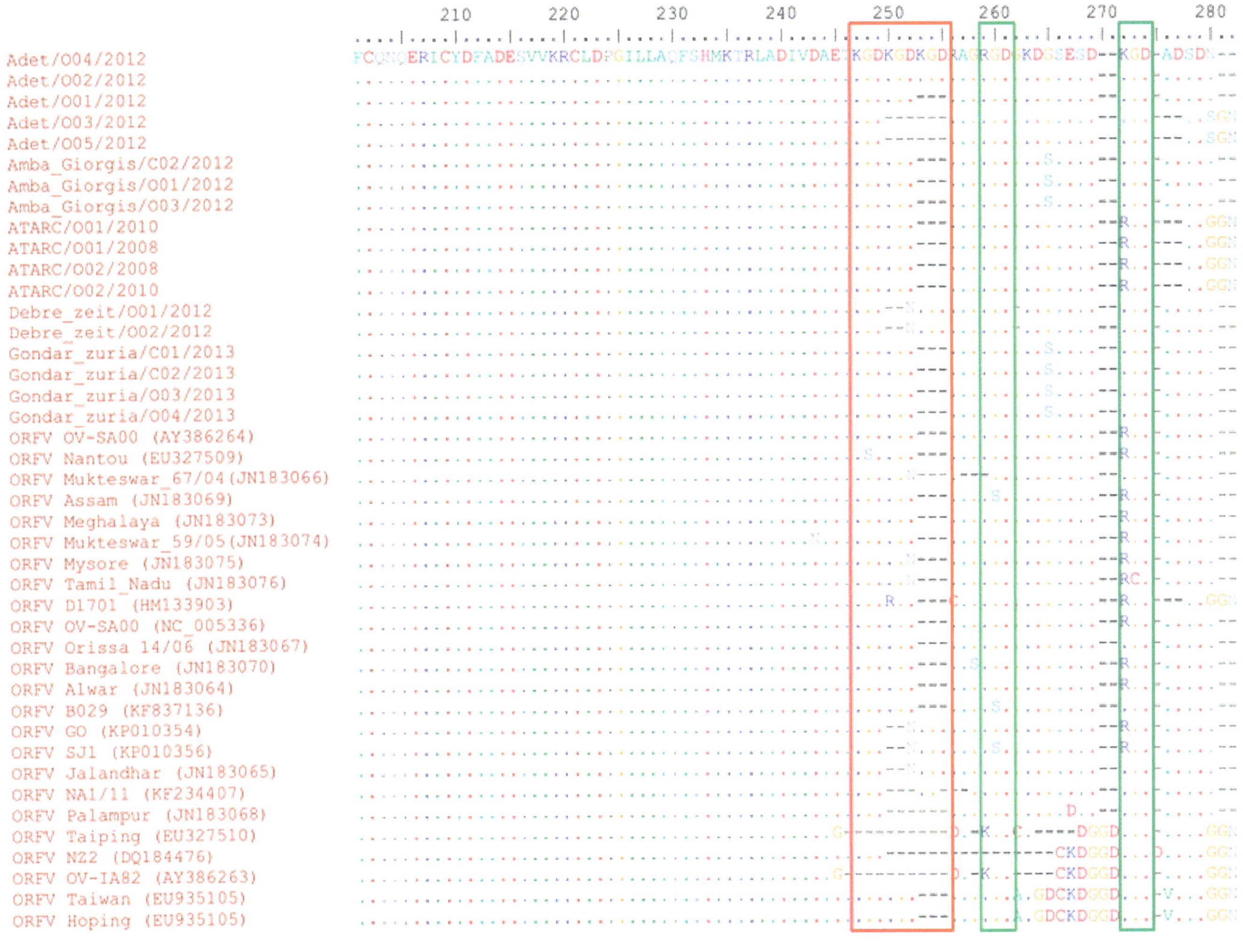

Figure 5: Multiple sequence alignment of the deduced amino acid sequence of the A32L gene of the Ethiopian orf virus isolates. The deduced amino acid sequence of the A32L gene of twenty four foreign orf virus strains retrieved from GenBank were added of comparison. The analysis revealed a high divergence in the carboxyl terminal region of ATPase protein sequence unlike the N-terminal region. The three repeats of KGD amino acid residues are highlighted with red color box. The two green color boxes indicate the presence of RGD sequences at two sites.

All three ORFV isolates from Amba Giorgis, and four from Gondar zuria had two repeats of KGD sequences (position 247 – 252), a KGD at position 270–272, and ended with an ADSND. Additionally, these isolates presented a G265S aa substitution when compared to other Ethiopian ORFVs and all publicly available ORFV ATPase protein sequences.

The four isolates from ATARC also presented two repeats of KGD sequences (position 247 – 252) at the C-terminal of the ATPase protein, but a RGD was present at position 270–272 instead of a KDG, and ended with a SDGGN.

The isolates Adet/03/2012 and Adet/05/2012 had only one KGD at position 247–249, a KGD at position 270–272 and their ATPase protein sequence ended with a SGSGN.

The two isolates from Debre zeit presented two KGDs, at position 247–249 and 253–255 interrupted by a two aa deletion at position 250–251 and an N at position 252, and their sequence ended with an ADSND. Additionally they presented a deletion of a G at position 262.

An additional copy of RGD sequence was present at position 259–261 of all sequenced isolates, but was not specific to the Ethiopian isolates.

DISCUSSION

ORFV infection of sheep and goats is generally neglected worldwide due to the low morbidity rates. In Ethiopia, despite the increased frequency of orf disease outbreaks, there hasn't been any attempt to further investigate the disease.

This study describes for the first time, the molecular characterization of ORFV isolates collected from sheep and goats during six suspected orf disease outbreaks in Ethiopia.

Our phylogenetic analyses suggest two main clusters of ORFV infecting sheep and goats in Ethiopia. All isolates collected from both sheep and goats in Amba Giorgis, Gondar zuria, Adet and Debre zeit grouped in cluster I of the B2L tree, while those from ATARC were located separately in cluster II.

In addition to the clear separation of the Ethiopian ORFV isolates into 2 clusters on the B2L tree, two isolates from Debre zeit further diverged from other isolates of cluster I, forming their own sub-cluster.

The analysis of the C-terminal domain of their A32 protein revealed six different amino acid profiles among the Ethiopian ORFV isolates, of which the G265S was unique to the Ethiopian ORFV isolates of Amba Giorgis, Gondar zuria, and the SGSGN ending of the protein was present only in isolates Adet/03/2012 and Adet/05/2012 of Ethiopia. Additionally, two ORFV isolates from Debre zeit also showed a unique deletion of a G at position 265.

Overall the Ethiopian ORFV isolates showed high similarity to previously sequenced foreign ORFV isolates on either the B2L or the A32L gene. Nevertheless, they carried specific mutations that differentiated them from previously sequenced isolates [1, 4, 8, 9, 10, 11].

Interestingly, there was a good agreement between the phylogenetic analysis and the profile of the C-terminal of the Ethiopian isolates. All ATARC isolates of the cluster II presented two RGD attachment sequences in the C-terminal of the ATPase gene at position 259–261 and 270–272, whereas other Ethiopian isolates belonging to cluster I contained only one RGD at position 259–261. The RGD at position 270–272 was replaced by a KGD for the Ethiopian ORFV isolates of cluster I.

We have also noticed the presence of variant KGD repeat motifs of one to three copies in all Ethiopian ORFV isolates. Although, these KGD motifs were found in previously sequenced ORFV isolates [1, 4, 8, 9, 10, 11], the presence of a repeat with 3 consecutive KGD units was a unique feature of two Ethiopian isolates (Adet/O02/2012 and Adet/O04/2012) collected in Adet research centre. Interestingly, other isolates collected from the same outbreak, presented with either 2 KGD repeats (isolate Adet/O01/2012) or only 1 KGD (Adet/03/2012 and Adet/05/2012).

The presence of all three KGD repeat variants within the same farm highlights the possibility of a rapid mutation of the A32L gene, probably during chronicity, or during adaptation to new tissues or to improve virus shedding and increase its spreading potential.

It is interesting to note that the Adet research centre, where all 3 variants of KGD motifs were recorded, also presented the highest morbidity rate as compared to other outbreak areas indicating a high infectivity rate. However, the fact that the animals of the Adet research centre are reared in a confined environment could also increase the chance of ORFV transmission from infected animals to those susceptible.

In addition to the major clinical signs of orf disease in sheep and goats, as described elsewhere [25, 26, 27], we have also documented the appearance of less specific skin lesions in areas other than the nose and mouth which could be easily confused with sheep pox, goat pox, peste des petits ruminants, FMD and dermathophilosis lesions [3]. This could explain why the ATARC researchers suspected capripox disease during the first outbreak that occurred on their farm, four months after vaccination against sheep pox. This highlights the need to perform laboratory confirmation of ORFV suspected infection using molecular tools.

Since ORFV infections may induce lesions that are similar to other economically important diseases, it is urgent to adopt multiparamatric pathogen detection methods for screening samples from animals presenting pox-like lesions. The screening for eventual asymptomatic carriers as well as wildlife is also needed to identify potential reservoirs.

An important reason for investigating orf disease remains it zoonotic potential [3]. Although no human infections were reported in this study, it is not possible to completely rule out the presence of zoonotic ORFV infections in Ethiopia, as human infections may be self-limiting, and occur without the presence of severe disease [28].

CONCLUSION

This paper reports the first characterization of ORFVs circulating in Ethiopia. It shows that two main clusters of ORFVs were involved in the investigated outbreaks in Ethiopia.

The endemicity of orf in the country calls for the urgent adoption of appropriate diagnostic tools and a better monitoring of the isolates circulating within the country.

The use of appropriate personal protective equipment such as gloves and proper hygiene while handling diseased animals and carcasses of dead animals is also recommended to reduce the risk of zoonotic infections.

ACKNOWLEDGEMENTS

The authors would like to thank Prof. Lukas Mach for helpful discussions. We also like to thank field veterinarians and researchers from Amba Giorgis, Gondar zuria, Adet, Debre zeit and Adami Tulu for facilitating the samples collection.

AUTHORS' CONTRIBUTIONS

Conceived and designed the experiments: CEL, EG. Performed the experiments: EG, SJ, AB. Analyzed the data: EG, CEL. Contributed reagents/materials/analysis tools: MY, AL, SJ, GA. Wrote the paper: EG, CEL, AD, MY, RG, JEA. Supervised the study: AD, CEL. Edited the final manuscript: AD, RG, AL, JEA, GA. All authors read and approved the final manuscript.

REFERENCES

1. Delhon G, Tulman ER, Afonso CL, Lu Z, de la Concha-Bermejillo A, Lehmkuhl HD, et al. Genomes of the parapoxviruses ORF virus and bovine papular stomatitis virus. J Virol. 2004;78:168–77.

2. Chan KW, Yang CH, Lin JW, Wang HC, Lin FY, Kuo ST, et al. Phylogenetic analysis of parapoxviruses and the C-terminal heterogeneity of viral ATPase proteins. Gene. 2009;432:44–53.
3. Hosamani M, Scagliarini A, Bhanuprakash V, McInnes CJ, Singh RK. Orf: an update on current research and future perspectives. Expert Rev Anti Infect Ther. 2009;7:879–93.
4. Li W, Ning Z, Hao W, Song D, Gao F, Zhao K, et al. Isolation and phylogenetic analysis of orf virus from the sheep herd outbreak in northeast China. BMC Vet Res. 2012;8:229.
5. Nandi S, De UK, Chowdhury S. Current status of contagious ecthyma or orf disease in goat and sheepGÇöA global perspective. Small Ruminant Research. 2011;96:73–82.
6. MacLachlan NJ, Dubovi EJ. Poxviridae. In: Fenner's Veterinary Virology. 4th ed. London: Academic; 2011. p. 151–65.
7. Zhang K, Liu Y, Kong H, Shang Y, Liu X. Human infection with ORF virus from goats in China, 2012. Vector Borne Zoonotic Dis. 2014;14:365–7.
8. Mercer AA, Ueda N, Friederichs SM, Hofmann K, Fraser KM, Bateman T, et al. Comparative analysis of genome sequences of three isolates of Orf virus reveals unexpected sequence variation. Virus Res. 2006;116:146–58.
9. Yogisharadhya R, Bhanuprakash V, Venkatesan G, Balamurugan V, Pandey AB, Shivachandra SB. Comparative sequence analysis of poxvirus A32 gene encoded ATPase protein and carboxyl terminal heterogeneity of Indian orf viruses. Vet Microbiol. 2012;156:72–80.
10. Billinis C, Mavrogianni VS, Spyrou V, Fthenakis GC. Phylogenetic analysis of strains of Orf virus isolated from two outbreaks of the disease in sheep in Greece. Virol J. 2012;9:24.
11. Zhang K, Liu Y, Kong H, Shang Y, Liu X. Comparison and phylogenetic analysis based on the B2L gene of orf virus from goats and sheep in China during 2009–2011. Arch Virol. 2014;159:1475–9.
12. Koonin EV, Senkevich TG, Chernos VI. Gene A32 product of vaccinia virus may be an ATPase involved in viral DNA packaging as indicated by sequence comparisons with other putative viral ATPases. Virus Genes. 1993;7:89–94.
13. Ogura T, Wilkinson AJ. AAA+ superfamily ATPases: common structure--diverse function. Genes Cells. 2001;6:575–97.
14. Burroughs AM, Iyer LM, Aravind L. Comparative genomics and evolutionary trajectories of viral ATP dependent DNA-packaging systems. Genome Dyn. 2007;3:48–65.
15. Lin FY, Chan KW, Wang CY, Wong ML, Hsu WL. Purification and functional motifs of the recombinant ATPase of orf virus. Protein Expr Purif. 2011;79:210–6.
16. Torfason EG, Gunadottir S. Polymerase chain reaction for laboratory diagnosis of orf virus infections. J Clin Virol. 2002;24:79–84.
17. Chan KW, Yang CH, Lin JW, Wang HC, Lin FY, Kuo ST, et al. Phylogenetic analysis of parapoxviruses and the C-terminal heterogeneity of viral ATPase proteins. Gene. 2009;432:44–53.
18. Hautaniemi M, Ueda N, Tuimala J, Mercer AA, Lahdenperä J, McInnes CJ. The genome of pseudocowpoxvirus: comparison of a reindeer isolate and a reference strain. J Gen Virol. 2010; 91:1560–76.
19. Oem JK, Roh IS, Lee KH, Lee KK, Kim HR, Jean YH, et al. Phylogenetic analysis and characterization of Korean orf virus from dairy goats: case report. Virol J. 2009;6:167.
20. Guo J, Zhang Z, Edwards JF, Ermel RW, Taylor C Jr, de la Concha-Bermejillo A. Characterization of a North American orf virus isolated from a goat with persistent, proliferative dermatitis. Virus Res. 2003;93:169–79.
21. Guo J, Rasmussen J, Wünschmann A, de La Concha-Bermejillo A. Genetic characterization of orf viruses isolated from various ruminant species of a zoo. Vet Microbiol. 2004;99:81–92.
22. Hosamani M, Bhanuprakash V, Scagliarini A, Singh RK. Comparative sequence analysis of major envelope protein gene (B2L) of Indian orf viruses isolated from sheep and goats. Vet Microbiol. 2006;116:317–24.
23. Bora DP, Barman NN, Das SK, Bhanuprakash V, Yogisharadhya R, Venkatesan G, et al. Identification and phylogenetic analysis of orf viruses isolated from outbreaks in goats of Assam, a northeastern state of India. Virus Genes. 2012;45:98–104.
24. Tamura K, Peterson D, Peterson N, Stecher G, Nei M, Kumar S. MEGA5: molecular evolutionary genetics analysis using maximum likelihood, evolutionary distance, and maximum parsimony methods. Mol Biol Evol. 2011;28:2731–9.
25. Zhang K, Shang Y, Jin Y, Wang G, Zheng H, He J, et al. Diagnosis and phylogenetic analysis of Orf virus from goats in China: a case report. Virol J. 2010;7:78.
26. Lojkic I, Cac Z, Beck A, Bedekovic T, Cvetnic Z, Sostaric B. Phylogenetic analysis of Croatian orf viruses isolated from sheep and goats. Virol J. 2010;7:314.
27. Oem JK, Chung JY, Kim YJ, Lee KK, Kim SH, Jung BY, et al. Isolation and characterization of orf viruses from Korean black goats. J Vet Sci. 2013;14:227–30.
28. Roess AA, Galan A, Kitces E, Li Y, Zhao H, Paddock CD, et al. Novel deer-associated parapoxvirus infection in deer hunters. N Engl J Med. 2010;363:2621–7.

CHAPTER 24

A CASE PRESENTATION OF SPIDER LAMB SYNDROME IN A KERMANIAN BREED LAMB

Mohammad Naser Nazem[1], Bahador Shojaei[1], Akbar Asadi[2], and Mohammad Hasanzadeh[1]

[1]Department of Basic Sciences, Faculty of Veterinary Medicine, Shahid Bahonar University of Kerman, Kerman, Iran

[2]Department of Basic Sciences, Faculty of Veterinary Medicine, Islamic Azad University, Shahre Babak Branch, Kerman, Iran

ABSTRACT

Skeletal abnormalities are most often used to describe defects in the arms or legs that are associated with genes or chromosomes, or that occur due to an event that happens during pregnancy. Spider lamb syndrome (SLS) is a congenital disorder in sheep breeding that is recognized by some deformities in skeletal system especially in the limbs. A dead day-old cross-breed white lamb with deformed limbs was referred to the anatomy hall of the Veterinary Faculty of Shahid Bahonar University of Kerman. In the external examination, the lamb was very skinny and in the facial region, superior brachygnathia with a slight Roman nose were observed. Metacarpal and metatarsal regions were more elongated than that expected. Also Metacarpal and metatarsal bones were as long as the antebrachial and crural regions, respectively. This paper, the first report of this syndrome in Iran, described the anatomic and radiographic features of the skeletal deformities in a day-old dead Kermanian breed lamb.

INTRODUCTION

Skeletal limb abnormalities are most often used to describe defects in the arms or legs that are associated with genes or chromosomes, or that occur due to an event that happens during pregnancy. The abnormalities are often present at birth.[1] One of these disorders in sheep is spider lamb syndrome (SLS),[2] also known more formally as hereditary chondrodysplasia.[2,3] It is a congenital osteopathy first described in young lambs during the early 1970s.[3] Several skeletal abnormalities are associated with the syndrome, including disproportionately long, spider like legs, curvature of the spine, deformed ribs and sterna, facial deformities, lack of body fat and muscular atrophy.[3,4] The most noticeable condition is an outward bending of the forelimbs from the carpal joints, with many lambs also having a crooked spine (mentioned before) in the thoracic area and a marked Roman nose. In addition, these lambs show extreme height, fineness of bone, poor muscling and failure to thrive.[2] Embryonic development at the ends of the long bones is impaired and lambs end up on the ground with their legs splayed like a spider.[5]

This syndrome was primarily observed in United State black – faced Suffolk and Hampshire sheep.2[4,6,]7According to some researches the presence of SLS was originally confined to sheep derived from Suffolk breeding stock, suggesting the mutation most likely arose within this breed.[8] As mentioned before, it is speculated that the mutation probably occurred in

Citation: Mohammad Naser Nazem, Bahador Shojaei, Akbar Asadi, Mohammad Hasanzadeh, A case presentation of spider lamb syndrome in a Kermanian breed lamb, Vet Res Forum. 2015 Autumn; 6(4): 343–347.

the late 1960s and was disseminated through the use of a popular genetic for its production and show – ring performance. Within the last two decades, the syndrome has been reported in several sheep breeds, presumably due to crossbreeding.[4,9] Reduction in the number of viable lambs born per ewe can have a major economic impact on lamb production systems.[4,10] Thus, the presence of a congenital disorder such as SLS can have a significant effect on production efficiency. The elimination of SLS from affected sheep population by identifying individuals that are carriers of the mutation would be of benefit to the sheep industry.[4] The aim of this article was is to describe the anatomical features of a lamb affected with the spider lamb syndrome.

CASE DESCRIPTION

A dead one day-old cross-breed white lamb with deformed limbs was referred to the anatomy hall of the Veterinary faculty of Shahid Bahonar University of Kerman on March 2014. In the physical examinations, the lamb was very skinny and there wasn't a notable fat layer under the skin. In the facial region, superior brachygnathia with a slight Roman nose was observed. Also there was an ankylosis in the tarsal joint.

Metacarpal and metatarsal regions were more elongated than that should be expected. Also metacarpal and metatarsal bones were as long as the antebrachial and crural regions, respectively (Fig. 1). The dorsoventral and latero-medial radiographic images were acquired using 60 kVp and 5 mAs with FFD of 80 cm (Xvision EX; Toshiba, Nasu, Japan). Finally in order to reveal the abnormal structures the lamb was dissected carefully.

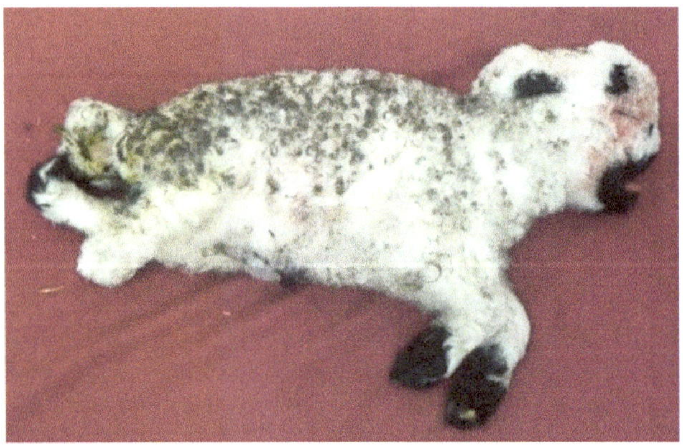

Figure 1: Cross-breed white Kermanian lamb. Superior brachygnathia with a slight Roman nose is observed in the skull. Deformed limbs and mild kyphosis in the thoracic region are also seen.

Dissection of the forelimb revealed that extensor muscles of the digits were originated normally from the lateral surface of the radius, but their tendons were run at the lateral border of the radius to the carpal joint and finally deviated to the caudolateral aspect of the carpal joint to reach to the metacarpal bone. At the metacarpal region according to the outward bending of the forelimb distal to the carpal joint, extensor tendons run slightly to the cranial surface. It had resulted in the change of dorsopalmar axis of metacarpal to the lateromedial one. According to this change, extensor digital tendons in the metacarpal region were observed on the lateral surface of the metacarpal bone but their divisions were normal proximal to the fetlock. Due to these events, normal lateromedial arrangement of the extensor tendons of the metacarpal region had been changed to the caudocranial position (Fig. 1). The cranial tendon, extensor digitrum communis, was divided into the two lateral and medial branches proximal to the fetlock. Medial branch was continued to the medial digit while lateral one divided to two lateral and medial branches which were run to the lateral and medial digits, respectively. The tendon of caudal muscle, extensor digitrum lateralis, was continued to the lateral digit similar to normal arrangement.

The flexor muscles of the digits were originated from the caudoproximal part of the radius except superficial digital flexor muscle which originated normally from the medial epicondyle of the humerus. According to the radius deviation, flexor tendons were passed to the medial side. At the carpal region, they were seen on the caudomedial surface. Also superficial digital flexor tendon was situated medially in compared to the deep digital flexor tendon.

According to our examinations, the axis of carpus was dorsolateral to mediopalmar instead of dorsopalmar. This position caused the carpal canal to displace to the mediopalmar of the forelimb. This malposition had led to move the accessory carpal bone to displace to the mediopalmar surface.

In the distal joint, the lateral phalanges were deviated to lateral while medial ones turned to the medial surface. Phalanges at the proximal and middle joints were normal.

Dissection of the hind limb showed a medial rotation in the tarsus which caused replacement of the calcaneus and associated tendons to the lateral side (Fig. 2). Superficial digital flexor tendon was passed from the medioplantar of the tarsal joint and positioned at the plantar surface of the metatars.

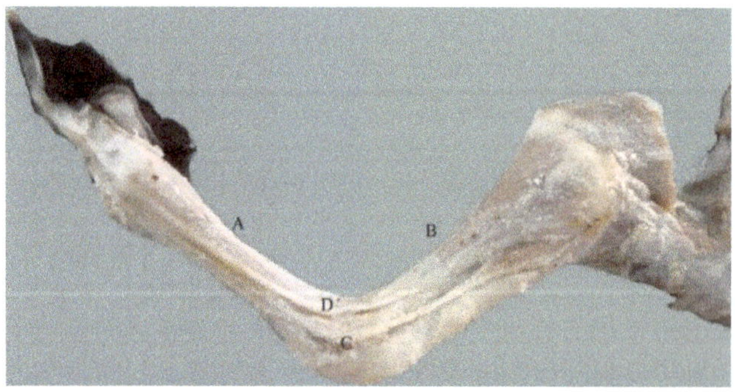

Figure 2: Antebrachial and metacarpal regions. Metacarpal bone (A) is as long as the antebrachial (B). Extensor digitrum communis tendon (C) and extensor digitrum lateralis (D) are shown. Rotation of carpal joint is changed the dorsopalmar axis of this joint.

Deep digital flexor tendon was seen under the superficial one which passed distally to the medioplantar surface of the metatarsal bone. All of the components of the common calcaneal tendon were seen, however with a distolateral direction. It meant that an inward rotation of the hind limbs was taken place.

The fetlock joint in the hindlimb showed inward rotation as well (Fig. 3). According to the medial rotation, tendon of extensor digitrum lateralis muscle was displace to the dorsal surface of the tars and lateral to the extensor digitrum commonis tendon. These tendons were positioned normally proximal to the fetlock. Radiographic examination of the vertebral column in dorsoventral view showed scoliosis in the thoracic region (Fig. 4).

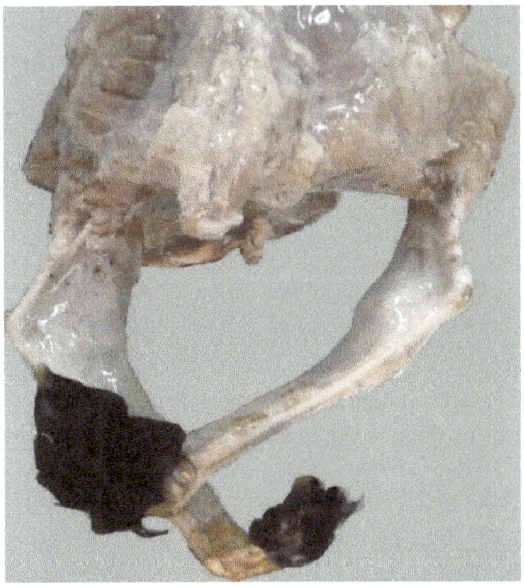

Figure 3: Medial rotation in the tarsal joint that caused replacement of the calcaneus to the lateral side.

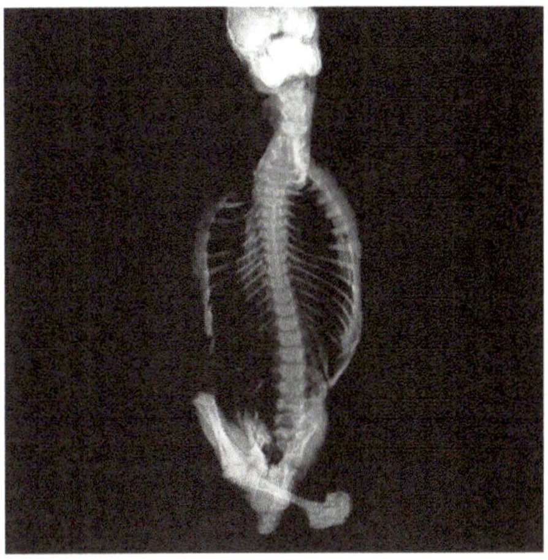

Figure 4: Dorsoventral radiograph shows a scoliosis in the thoracic vertebrae region that continued to the lumbar region.

Lateral radiographs of the skull confirmed superior brachygnathia (Fig. 5).

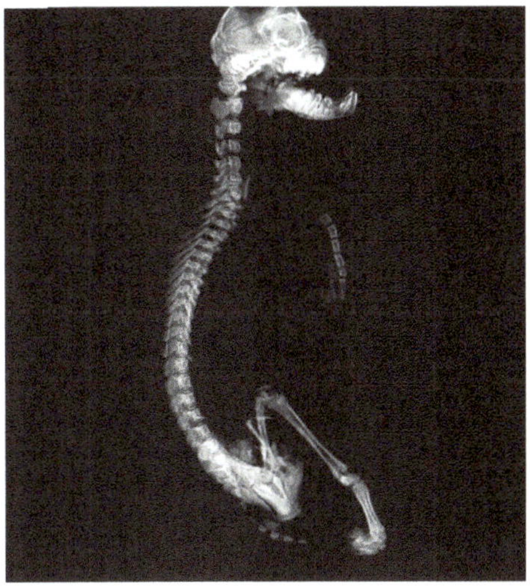

Figure 5: Lateromedial radiograph shows superior brachygnathia, thoracic vertebra spinous process with more caudally oriented with no anticlinal vertebrae and a mild kyphosis.

In the lateromedial view of the thoracic vertebrae, spinous processes of thoracic vertebra were observed more caudally oriented (Fig. 5). Also spines in all thoracic vertebrae were inclined caudally. Anticlinal vertebra wasn't seen (Fig. 5). Radiography of the trunk showed a mild kyphosis in the thoracic region and a concavity in the sternum in this view (Fig. 5).

The assessment of the total length of the scapula, distal extremity of the humerus, distal extremity of the radius, total length of the ulna, proximal end of the metacarp, proximal extremity of the femur, total length of the tibia and metatars did not show any growth plate (Fig. 5). Radiographs of the tarsal joint showed the fusion of the calcaneus, talus and central tarsal bones. This fusion was also occurred in the distal row of tarsal bones (Fig. 6).

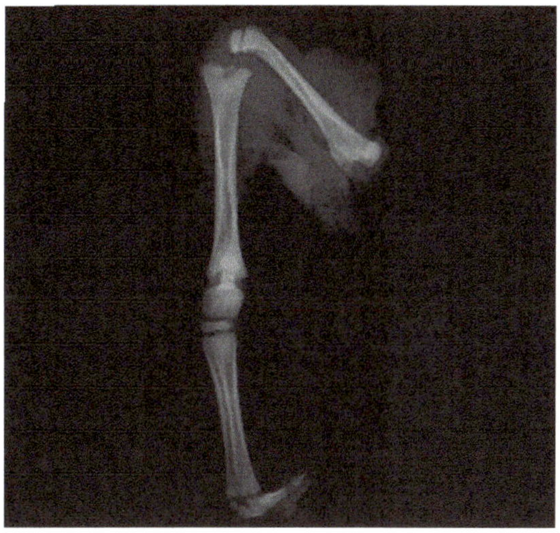

Figure 6: Hind limb radiograph. Absence of growth plate in all bones is seen. The fusion of the calcaneus, talus and central tarsal bones are visible.

DISCUSSION

Spider lamb syndrome is characterized by generalized chondrodysplasia and is apparently a semi lethal auto-somal recessive trait. Variable expressivity of the trait may occur in the homozygous animals.[2] Within the last two decades, the syndrome has been reported in several sheep breeds, presumably due to crossbreeding. Included breeds are North American Suffolks and Hampshires,[6,9] and more recently U.S. Southdowns, Shropshires, and Oxfords. In addition, there are reported cases of SLS in Australia and New Zealand following exportation of several U.S. Suffolk sheep to Australia in 1987.[4,11] The syndrome has not been reported in Iran. Arachnomelia (arachno = spider and melia = limb) is other name of SLS. Inherited arachnomelia or inherited chondrodysplasia reported by batavani *et al.*, in Iran, previously.[12] Also, non-carrier identification of spider lamb syndrome in Iranian Baluchi and Karakul sheep has been reported by Nassiry *et al.*[13] The lamb of this study was a cross breed of Kermanian.

The lamb in this report was dead at the birth and had some deformities which some of them have been mentioned in references. According to Rook *et al.*,[14] clinical presentation of the spider lamb syndrome is highly variable, while some lambs were severely affected at birth. The condition develops in the others at 3 to 4 or 3 to 8 weeks of age.[4,13] It is characterized by overall appendicular and axial deformities, including kyphosis, scoliosis, concavity of the sternum, lateroventral deviation of the maxilla (crooked nose and Roman nose), and angular deformities.[2] According to our findings, this lamb had long bent bones in its limbs especially in the zeugo and autopodium. Because of abnormal asymmetrical growth, the positions of the tendons in these regions, the lamb was showed varus/ valgus abnormality. It means that a non-symmetrical growth has been taken place in affected bones.

One method to recognize the spider lamb syndrome is the evaluation of the radiographic changes. Radiological evaluation of the shoulders, elbows, and sternum from affected lambs reveals multiple irregular islands of ossification and the sternebrae appear irregularly in sized and symmetry.[2,8,14] The most constant radiographic sign is in the olecranon, which exhibits multiple islands of ossification instead of the uniform, nonmineralized cartilage surrounded by dense bone in a normal lamb.[2] In the radiographic assessments, there were not growth plates in some appendicular bones which is the first report on this syndrome. Also we could not observed islands of ossification in the fore and hind limb in radiographs. It is in agreement with Smith that stillborn lambs or those that died in the first week of life did not exhibit radiographic abnormalities in growth plates associated with spider syndrome.[2]

Some abnormalities of the skeletal system of the current case such as scoliosis, mild kyphosis, concavity of the sternum, long bent limbs and angular deformities have been reported by other researchers[2-4] while some of our observations such as deformities in spinous process of vertebrae, brachygnathia superior absence of the anticlinal vertebra, lack of growth plate in some appendicular bones and ankylosis of tarsal bones have not been recorded previously. In the skull the dorsal surface of the nose was dome shaped denoted as Roman nose.[2]

Sheep have 54 chromosomes, with 26 pairs of auto-somes and two sex chromosomes.[3] Many researchers have mapped the spider lamb syndrome locus to the distal end of ovine chromosome.[3,7] Comparative analysis of genome maps between sheep, cattle and humans, combined with the results of knockout studies in mice, has identified fibroblast growth factor receptor 3 (FGFR3) as a positional candidate for the disorder.[3]Lambs homozygous for the SLS allele (FGFR3 SLS/SLS) have bone deformities. In contrast, heterozygous lambs (FGFR3SLS/+) appear normal, though perhaps through relaxed inhibition of chondrocyte proliferation at the growth plate, are physically larger than normal lambs.[15,16] Smith *et al.* and Beever *et al.* proposed that FGFR3SLS/+ sheep will exhibit enhanced long bone growth and greater frame sizes at all ages, which translates to greater BW and a larger LM area.[16,17]

The FGFR3 loss-of-function mutations (i.e, SLS) cause skeletal overgrowth.[17] It can be an appropriate response to increase the height of the appendicular bones such as this case.

In order to control this SLS, all the carrier breeders must be actively omitted from the flocks. Traditional breeding methods such as progeny testing of potential breeding rams would reduce the frequency; however, they are time consuming and unaffordable strategies. Thus, the identification of a genetic marker for SLS would be of benefit for monitoring or eliminating it from affected sheep populations. Additionally, the chromosomal localization of the SLS locus is the first step toward positional cloning of the gene responsible for the syndrome.[2]

REFERENCES

1. Knobloch J, Shaughnessy JD, Ruther U. Thalidomide induces limb deformities by perturbing the Bmp/Dkk1/ Wnt signaling pathway. FASEB J. 2007;21(7):1410–1421.
2. Smith BP. Large animal medicine. 4th ed. St. Louis, USA: Mosby; 2009. pp. 1197–1199.
3. Cockett NE. Genomics of Sheep. Ag Biotech Net. 1999;1:1–4.
4. Cockett NE, Shay TL, Beever JE, et al. Localization of the locus causing spider lamb syndrome to the distal end of ovine chromosome 6. Mamm Genome. 1999;10:35–38.
5. Blood DC, Studdert VP, Gay CC. Saunders comprehensive veterinary dictionary. Amsterdam, The Netherlands: WB Saunders; 2006. p. 305.
6. Drogemuller C, Wohlke A, Distl O. Spider lamb syndrome (SLS) mutation frequency in German Suffolk sheep. Anim Genet. 2005;36(6):511–542.
7. Cockett NE, Shay TL, Beever JE. Screening for the molecular defect causing spider lamb syndrome in sheep. United State Patent. 2001;6:306.
8. Vanek JA, Alstad AD, Berg IE, et al. spider syndrome in lambs: A clinical and postmortem analysis. Vet Med. 1986;81:663–668.
9. Vanek JA, Walter PA, Alstad AD. Comparing spider syndrome in Hampshire and Suffolk sheep. Food Anim Prac. 1987;82:430–437.
10. Wang CT, Dickerson GE. Simulated effects of reproductive performance on life-cycle efficiency of lamb and wool production at three lambing intervals. J Anim Sci. 1991;69:4338–4347.
11. Phillips PH, Bunn CM, Anderson CE. Ovine hereditary chondrodysplasia (spider syndrome) in Suffolk lambs. Aust Vet J. 1993;70:73–74.
12. Batavani RA, Aligholi R, Ghafari R. proceedings: 4th convention of Iranian veterinary clinicians. Urmia, Iran: 2005. Arachnomellia in lambs of sheeps; p. 33.
13. Nassiry MR, Eftekhari Shahroudi F, Rezaee AR, et al. Non-carrier identification of spider lamb syndrome in Iranian Baluchi and Karakul sheep by PCR-RFLP. Biotechnology. 2008;7(3):586–588.
14. Rook JS, Kopcha M, Spaulding K, et al. Diagnosis of hereditary chondrodysplasia (spider lamb syndrome) in sheep. J Am Vet Med Assoc. 1989;193(6):713–718.
15. Troyer DL, Thomas DL, Stein LE. A morphologic and biochemical evaluation of the spider syndrome in Suffolk sheep. Anat Histol Embryol. 1988;17:289–300.
16. Smith LB, Dally MR, Sainz RD, et al. Enhanced skeletal growth of sheep heterozygous for an inactivated fibroblast growth factor receptor 3. J Anim Sci. 2006;84:2942–2949.
17. Beever JE, Smit MA, Meyers SN, et al. A single – base change in the tyrosine kinase II domain of ovine FGFR3 causes hereditary chondrodysplasia in sheep. Anim Genet. 2006;37(1):66–71.

INDEX